THE EMERGING ROLE OF COUNSELING PSYCHOLOGY IN HEALTH CARE

THE EMERGING ROLE OF COUNSELING PSYCHOLOGY IN HEALTH CARE

Sari Roth-Roemer, Ph.D.
Sharon E. Robinson Kurpius, Ph.D.
Cheryl Carmin, Ph.D.
Editors

W.W. Norton & Company
New York • London

Copyright © 1998 by
Sari Roth-Roemer, Sharon E. Robinson Kurpius, and Cheryl Carmin

All rights reserved
Printed in the United States of America
First Edition

For information about permission to reproduce selections
from this book, write to
Permissions, W. W. Norton & Company, Inc., 500 Fifth Avenue,
New York, NY 10110.

The text of the book is composed in Times Roman
with the display set in Futura Condensed
Book design and composition by Paradigm Graphics
Manufacturing by Royal Book

Library of Congress Cataloging-in-Publication Data

The Emerging role of counseling psychology in health care / Sari Roth-Roemer,
Sharon E. Robinson Kurpius, Cheryl Carmin, editors.
p. cm.
"A Norton professional book."
Includes bibliographical references and index.
ISBN 0-393-70268-5
1. Health counseling.   2. Health counseling—Vocational guidance.
I. Roth-Roemer, Sari. II. Kurpius, Sharon E. Robinson. III. Carmin, Cheryl Nina.
R727.4.E47   1998
362. 1'04256—dc21   98-7625 CIP

W.W. Norton & Company, Inc., 500 Fifth Avenue, New York, N.Y. 10110
http://www.wwnorton.com
W.W. Norton & Company Ltd., 10 Coptic Street, London WC1A 1PU

1   2   3   4   5   6   7   8   9   0

For my dearest Douglas and my sweet baby Adin
(SRR)

To the three women who have helped
me become who I am:
My mother, Nora Ekern
My daughter, Erin (Emmy) Robinson
My dear friend, Judith Hasting Hamilton
(SRK)

To Henry Borow, who taught me how to be a counseling
psychologist, and to my parents, Malvin and Dolores Carmin,
who supported me through that process
(CNC)

CONTENTS

ACKNOWLEDGMENTS

I would like to especially thank my valued colleagues, Karen Syrjala, Janet Abrams, and the whole Biobehavioral Science team for their continued support and patience throughout the writing of this book. I also wish to thank my father, Sanford Roth, for all of his hard work and effort—our book is next. And a special acknowledgment to my mother, Marcia Roth, for her inspiring climb back to health. (SRR)

I would like to thank the ongoing support of my colleagues on the Counseling and Counseling Psychology faculties at Arizona State University. They make work a pleasure and were very supportive of the extra time I needed to bring this book to fruition. (SRK)

No endeavor of this sort comes to fruition without the help of any number of people. The Resource Center staff and my secretary at UIC assisted in innumerable ways. The physicians with whom I have worked have also made an indelible contribution to my education and understanding of issues, both academic and political, and have taken the time to provide that information. If not more importantly, I want to thank all of the patients with whom I have worked for what they have taught me.

The year over which this book was written was also one which provided new insights into the workings of the medical system due to chronic illness, and in the case of my father, his death. These experiences, as emotional as they have been, have also provided firsthand experience as to what it is like to be a family member of someone who is chronically and critically ill or what it is like to be waiting on an intensive care unit to speak with a physician. It is much easier to be the professional than the family member, no matter how familiar one is with the workings of hospitals or critical care units. I wish to thank the physicians, nurses, and other staff who could appreciate my persistence when it came to insisting that both patient and family be involved in the health care process. (CNC)

CONTRIBUTORS

John D. Alcorn, Ph.D.
Professor, Department of Psychology
University of Southern Mississippi
Hattiesburg, Mississippi

Elizabeth M. Altmaier, Ph.D.
Professor, Counseling Psychology
College of Education
University of Iowa
Iowa City, Iowa

Cheryl Carmin, Ph.D.
Associate Professor, Department of
    Psychiatry
Director, Cognitive Behavior Therapy
    Program and Stress and Anxiety
    Disorders Clinic
University of Illinois at Chicago
Chicago, Illinois

Kathleen Chwalisz, Ph.D.
Associate Professor, Department of
    Psychology
Southern Illinois University
Carbondale, Illinois

Jesse R. Fann, M.D., M.P.H.
Acting Assistant Professor
Department of Psychiatry and
    Behavioral Sciences
University of Washington
Seattle, Washington

Katherine Vaughn Fielder, M.C.
Doctoral Student, Counseling Psychology
Arizona State University
Tempe, Arizona

Mary Jean Formati, M.A.
Doctoral Student, Department of
    Counseling
University of North Dakota
Grand Forks, North Dakota

Jennifer Hoffman Goldberg, B.A.
Doctoral Student, School of Education
Stanford University
Stanford, California

Sue C. Jacobs, Ph.D.
Associate Professor, Department of
    Counseling
University of North Dakota
Grand Forks, North Dakota

Brian D. Johnson, Ph.D.
Assistant Professor
University of Northern Colorado
Loveland, Colorado

Cynthia R. Kalodner, Ph.D.
Associate Professor
Department of Counseling, Rehabilitation
    Counseling, and Counseling Psychology
West Virginia University
Morgantown, West Virginia

Sharon E. Robinson Kurpius, Ph.D.
Professor of Counseling Psychology
Arizona State University
Tempe, Arizona

Susan E. Maresh, Ph.D.
Psychology Intern
McKennan Hospital
Sioux Falls, South Dakota

Bonnie J. McIntosh, B.S.
Doctoral Candidate, Department of
    Counseling Psychology
State University of New York at Albany
Albany, New York

Cynthia McRae, Ph.D.
Associate Professor, Counseling
    Psychology
College of Education
University of Denver
Denver, Colorado

Thomas V. Merluzzi, Ph.D.
Associate Professor
University of Notre Dame
Notre Dame, Indiana

Sloan L. Norman, Ph.D.
Psychological Assistant, Department
    of Psychiatry
Kaiser Permanente Medical Center
San Francisco, California

Jeffrey L. Okey, Ph.D.
Director
Northwest Center for Integrative
    Medicine
Tacoma, Washington

Raymond L. Ownby, M.D., Ph.D., ABPP
Associate Professor, Department of
    Psychiatry and Behavioral Sciences
University of Miami School of Medicine
Miami, Florida

Jane S. Paulsen, Ph.D.
Associate Professor, Departments of
    Psychiatry and Neurology
University of Iowa
Iowa City, Iowa

Sari Roth-Roemer, Ph.D.
Staff Scientist
Fred Hutchinson Cancer Research Center
Seattle, Washington

Ester Ruiz Rodriguez, R.N., Ph.D.
Assistant Professor, College of Nursing
Arizona State University
Tempe, Arizona

Mary Ann Martinez Sanchez, Ph.D.
Pima Community College
Tucson, Arizona

Charlie H. Smith, M.A.
Doctoral Psychology Intern
College of Education
University of Denver
Denver, Colorado

Marilyn Stern, Ph.D.
Associate Professor, Department of
    Counseling Psychology
State University of New York at Albany
Albany, New York

Carl E. Thoresen, Ph.D.
Professor of Education, Psychology, and
    Psychiatry
School of Education
Stanford University
Stanford, California

THE EMERGING ROLE OF COUNSELING PSYCHOLOGY IN HEALTH CARE

Counseling Psychology in Health Care: An Introduction

Sari Roth-Roemer
Sharon E. Robinson Kurpius
Cheryl Carmin

There is little dispute that health care throughout the world is rapidly chang-ing. As a result, the role of counseling psychology has been adapting and expanding to meet these evolving needs. Counseling psychologists are now emerging from the primary contexts of schools of education and counseling centers, and transformations are even occurring within these settings. As roles and functions change, an opportunity for redefinition arises. This book outlines and discusses the trajectory of these changes as they apply to health care settings.

Although individuals within counseling psychology have been sensitive to both needs and opportunities in the field of health care for close to two decades, the profession of counseling psychology has been slow to claim health care as a domain of practice. While the Veterans Administration, as opposed to other medical institutions, has a long history of employing and training counseling psychologists, it was not until the 1980s that our profes-sional literature began discussing the health concerns of our clients and the roles that counseling psychologists could play in assisting them. In the mid 1980s, *The Counseling Psychologist* focused for the first time on issues of health psychology (Thoresen & Eagleston, 1985), and the *Handbook of Counseling Psychology* included a discussion of health psychology as a main area of practice and research (Brown & Lent, 1984). A parallel movement was occurring in counselor education. The first national conference for the Association of Counselor Education and Supervision in 1988 highlighted three roles for counselors; one of these was health counseling (Robinson & Roth, 1991). Now, over a decade later, counselors, counseling psychologists, and other mental health professionals are entering the field of health psychology in rapidly growing numbers.

In addition to the increasing employment and research opportunities in counseling health psychology, many of our colleagues are choosing to work in health care because of their belief in a holistic approach to wellness. The biopsychosocial model of health and well-being has provided a natural entryway for those interested in linking psychology and medicine. Simply put, the biopsychosocial model emphasizes the nonlinear interaction among biological, psychological, and social factors that influence health. Since all three aspects need to be taken into account in fostering wellness, this has led naturally to the development of interdisciplinary collaboration.

Counseling psychologists have a myriad of roles to play in health care. Health psychology, behavioral medicine, and/or consultation liaison psychiatry services have all been developed either as specialty or interdisciplinary services to address the needs of medical patients who are experiencing some form of emotional distress (Bieliauskas, 1995), who need assistance coping with the losses brought on by physical illness, and who need help with symptom management. Research opportunities for interdisciplinary programs are expanding from federal (e.g., National Institutes of Health, National Institutes of Mental Health), national (e.g., American Heart Association, American Cancer Society, Arthritis Foundation), and local (universities and private foundations) sources.

To help counselors, counseling psychologists, and other health care professionals to be better prepared to meet these growing needs, *The Emerging Role of Counseling Psychology in Health Care* introduces the numerous aspects of practice in health care settings. The goal of the book is to provide an extensive overview for those who want to know more about working in the health care arena; it is not intended to be a "how to" book. The authors were selected for their notable contributions in wedding counseling psychology with health psychology. Each is a recognized expert in the area he or she addresses.

The first section of the book covers the important professional issues that must be considered by anyone entering the health care arena. The lead chapter points out that counseling psychologists do not forsake their professional identity when they apply their expertise to health problems and settings. The authors elaborate on the "goodness of fit" between counseling psychology and health care. The training and experience required for functioning effectively as a counseling health psychologist is elaborated on in the second chapter. The section closes with an overview of the ethical considerations unique to working in the field of health care.

The chapters in the second section of the book are devoted to specific areas of practice. Setting the stage for these chapters, Carmin and Roth-Roemer orient the reader to the diagnostic, practice, and professional issues related to working in medical settings. The following chapters focus on coronary heart disease, chronic disease, life-threatening illness, pain management, rehabilitation medicine, neuropsychology, and eating disorders. Each author presents an overview of a specific health practice area and its psychosocial concomitants. Diagnosis and assessment issues, as well as research-based interventions, are discussed. Current controversies in each of the areas are highlighted. Finally, each author suggests resources for further reading.

The four chapters that comprise the third section of this book highlight issues relevant to working with special populations. Specific populations addressed include children and adolescents, older adults, women, and diverse racial and ethnic populations. Each author addresses the unique health concerns of a select population, as well as outlining relevant practice, assessment, diagnostic, and treatment issues.

The last section, Special Issues, provides additional perspectives on the role of counseling psychology in health care. First, it is a forum for a psychiatrist to offer his views and experiences in collaborating with psychologists in medical practice and research. Second, the spiritual aspects of health and wellness are discussed. Finally, the book closes with a look to the future of this expanding field.

The reader may note an inconsistency among authors regarding terminology. For example, while we prefer the use of "counseling health psychology," other authors refer to "behavioral medicine" or "health psychology." In addition, the frequently used term "mental health professional" includes, and is used interchangeably with, counseling psychologists, counselors, and other mental health providers, such as social workers and marriage and family therapists. While counseling psychologists are most often trained to discuss the people they serve as "clients," in the medical arena the more appropriate term is "patient."

The authors in this book are enthusiastic about the roles and functions that counseling psychologists can play in health care. Their excitement is due, at least in part, to the rapid growth of the health and human services field in addition to the opportunities for clinical research and academic careers. As Klippel and DeJoy (1985) stated, the only limiting factor to our ability to work in health care is "counseling psychology's willingness and ability to respond to the challenges associated with studying the relationship of behavior to health" (p. 219).

References

Bieliauskas, L. A. (1995). Critical issues in consultation and liaison: Adults. In J. J. Sweet, R. H. Rozensky, & S. M. Tovian (Eds.), *Handbook of clinical psychology in medical settings* (pp. 187–199). New York: Plenum.

Brown, S. D., & Lent, R. W. (1984). *The handbook of counseling psychology.* New York: Wiley.

Klippel, J. A., & DeJoy, D. M. (1985). Counseling psychology in behavioral medicine and health psychology. *Journal of Counseling Psychology, 31,* 219–227.

Robinson, S. E., & Roth, S. L. (1991). Health needs facing our nation: A life-span perspective. In H. Hackney (Ed.), *Changing contexts for counselor preparation in the 1990s* (pp. 37–54). Alexandria, VA: AACD.

Thoresen, C. E., & Eagleston, J. R. (1985). Counseling for health. *The Counseling Psychologist, 13,* 15–87.

I
PROFESSIONAL ISSUES

1

Issues in Professional Identity

Elizabeth M. Altmaier
Brian D. Johnson
Jane S. Paulsen

This chapter introduces the reader to issues related to professional identity. It may seem strange to have this material come early in the book, before we have considered which areas of practice in health care are key ones for counseling psychologists. The point in considering professional identity first is to emphasize that we do not cease to be counseling psychologists and become other professionals when we work in health care settings with problems of chronic pain, neuropsychology, geriatrics, and the like. We believe success in applying counseling psychology to health problems and in health care settings lies in our adherence to the identity of counseling psychology as a distinct specialty in psychology. Grounding in our specialty's strengths allows us freedom to enter areas of practice different from those we have traditionally targeted and to join in work with other professionals in collaborative ways. One focus of this chapter, then, is that not only do counseling psychologists not have to "lose their identity" as counseling psychologists in health care applications, but they will also gain immeasurably in the quality of their research, conceptualization, and practice as they remain counseling psychologists—and the specialty will be correspondingly enriched.

A second focus of this chapter is the excitement that we, and other counseling psychologists we know, have found in bringing counseling psychology to health care problems and settings. Many of the authors in this book were early converts to this area of application. (As a later section of this chapter will describe, counseling psychologists' involvement in health care has a short history.) However, we believe this area of application, for both research and interventions, holds great promise for counseling psychology. We hope to convey a sense of this promise and know that the authors who follow will be working toward that same goal.

Our emphasis, then, is on identity, that is, how we maintain counseling psychology's traditional strengths and emphases when applying them to problems of health care. We should begin with the definition of counseling psychology. The Division of Counseling Psychology (1994) defines our specialty as follows:

> Counseling psychology as a psychological specialty facilitates personal and interpersonal functioning across the life span with a focus on emotional, social, vocational, education, health–related, developmental, and organizational concerns. Through the integration of theory, research, and practice, and with a sensitivity to multicultural issues, this specialty encompasses a broad range of practices that help people improve their well-being, alleviate distress and maladjustment, resolve crises, and increase their ability to live more highly functioning lives. Counseling psychology is unique in its attention both to normal developmental issues and to problems associated with physical, emotional, and mental disorders.
>
> Populations served by Counseling Psychologists include persons of all ages and cultural backgrounds. Examples of those populations would include late adolescents or adults with career/educational concerns and children or adults facing severe personal difficulties. Counseling Psychologists also consult with organizations seeking to enhance their effectiveness or the well-being of their members.
>
> Counseling Psychologists adhere to the standards and ethics established by the American Psychological Association.

What are the distinctive aspects of counseling psychology that we have found have value in their application to problems of health?

1. Emphasis on mobilization of strengths. Conceptualizing a patient's problem, a health care team's issue, or a family's response to a critically ill family member from the perspective of identifying strengths and coping resources to be mobilized is tremendously helpful. It gives all involved parties a sense of efficacy in coping and provides dignity in situations where it is lacking.
2. Involvement in problem solving and, more broadly, in psychoeduca-

tional approaches. Today's health care environment demands interventions that are focused and efficient and, more importantly, build in accountability. When patients work collaboratively with counseling psychologists to design interventions, identify life components to be changed, and assist in the measurement of such change, traditional medical health care is powerfully enhanced.

3. Systematic approach to assessment. Counseling psychologists understand the roles of family, the health care environment, other health care professionals, and so on in the genesis of problems and in their remediation. Thus, our integrative understanding of problems and solutions serves us well.

In this chapter, we will:

1. review briefly the evolution of psychology in health care, highlighting the increasing role of counseling psychologists in this change;
2. consider the "roles" of counseling psychology in health care; and
3. provide some needed cautions so that applications can be made carefully, ethically, and with sensitivity.

Our goal is to define a balance: It is possible to be a counseling psychologist, whose values and emphases are clearly recognizable as such, while working in settings that are uncharacteristic, with clients who are not typical, with interventions that are adapted from their traditional format, and with collaborative teams. As an example, it is possible to work side by side with neurologists and with neuropsychologists but remain a counseling psychologist. How is this done? In this chapter, we describe not only how but also why this goal is so critical.

The Evolution of Psychology in Health Care

Health psychology has become an important and influential area in the field of psychology. Its influence is particularly impressive given that it has been formally recognized as a specialty area for fewer than two decades. Most writers credit the beginning of health psychology to William Schofield's 1969 article in the *American Psychologist*. In this article, Schofield cogently argued that psychology is a "health science" and psychologists are health professionals. He noted that, while psychologists' primary research and service endeavors involve mental health issues, critical new directions for psychological research and service include applications related to physical health. His arguments were so persuasive that, in 1973, he was asked to chair a task force established by the American Psychological Association (APA) on health-related research.

In 1976, the Division of Psychologists in Public Service (Division 18) established a section on health research, which was the precursor of the current division on health psychology. That division (Division 38) was formally recognized as an independent division of the APA in 1978. At that time, it had over 700 charter members. Joseph Matarazzo served as its first president. Shortly thereafter, the Division's newsletter, *The Health Psychologist,* began publication. In 1979, the first textbook to have the words "health psychology" in its title was published (Stone, Cohen, & Adler, 1979). The inaugural issue of Division 38's journal, *Health Psychology,* was published in 1982. This journal continues to be influential in the fields of health psychology and behavioral medicine.

At this same time, the field of medicine was beginning to recognize, in a formal way, the important role of psychological variables in physical health. John Knowles (1977) wrote that "over 99% of us are born healthy and made sick as a result of personal misbehavior and environmental conditions" (p. 58). George Engel (1977) concluded that, while the biomedical model of disease had produced many important cures (e.g., polio, smallpox), the model appeared to have limited applicability for the current diseases that result in the highest mortality rates, such as heart disease, stroke, and cancer. Engel articulated the argument and model that are prevalent today: The biomedical model's approach to isolating a single cause is too simplistic and a broader approach to treating and curing these diseases is needed. His proposed biopsychosocial model for contemporary medicine underlies much of the increased contribution of psychologists to health care. First, there is an increasing recognition that many illnesses have their genesis in behavioral factors, for example, the risk that unhealthy eating habits pose for coronary heart disease or the risk that people take on when they fail to engage in preventive health behaviors such as regular seat belt use or breast self-examination. Second, there is also an increasing recognition that health is more than the absence of illness. The growing use of health quality of life as an endpoint in clinical trials reflects the medical profession's acceptance of psychosocial variables as key in defining health.

Although there was increasing acceptance of the importance of applying a broad model to disease and health care, there was a period of time where definitions of the scope and content of health psychology were debated (Matarazzo, 1980, 1982; Millon, 1982; Singer & Krantz, 1982). Partly at issue was the question of which health problems were relevant: those with clearly identified psychological components, such as the risk for heart disease posed by lifestyle, or those with less obvious components, such as the role of psychology in alleviating the stress of cancer. Also partly at issue were the most important contributions of psychologists: in assessment of psychological variables, in applying traditional psychological treatments, or in research.

Millon (1982) proposed a widely accepted definition for clinical health psychology:

> The application of knowledge and methods from all substantive fields of psychology to the promotion and maintenance of mental and physical health of the individual and the prevention, assessment and treatment of all forms of mental and physical disorder in which psychological influences either contribute to or can be used to relieve an individual's distress or dysfunction. (p. 9)

This "broad brush" definition did not provide clear limits, however, and the debate continued. A related area for discussion was the limit of application. Were certain psychological interventions to be applied to health care problems prior to their careful evaluation in those contexts? Researchers continued to evaluate the effectiveness of treatments, while practitioners, responding to the demands of patients, were incorporating them into practice before their efficacy could be demonstrated.

The first doctoral training program in health psychology was established in 1977 at the University of California at San Francisco. Today, over 50 institutions offer predoctoral or postdoctoral training in health psychology. While there is not currently a standardized training model for health psychologists, and emphases in programs vary from research to practice, some have suggested that a model for training counseling psychologists, as opposed to clinical psychologists, should be adopted in health psychology training programs (Wallston, 1993). With the recent expansion of the scope of accreditation by the APA to programs in "emerging specialties," it is likely that health psychology programs with a practice focus will apply for accreditation. It is unclear what effect that change will have on the present qualifications of health psychologists, who typically have their doctoral degrees in clinical psychology or counseling psychology. Chapter 2 will address training issues in more detail.

The first time that health care applications were directly addressed relative to counseling psychology appears to be in the 1979 *Annual Review* chapter on counseling psychology (Krumboltz, Becker-Haven, & Burnett, 1979). In that review, the authors discussed psychological treatments for insomnia, pain control, weight control, and smoking cessation in a four-page section entitled "Health Related Outcomes." In 1984, at the American Psychological Association convention, the first symposium to consider counseling psychology in its relationship to health psychology was held (Howard, 1984).

In 1984, Thoresen and Eagleston wrote a chapter on health psychology in the first edition of the *Handbook of Counseling Psychology*. This was the last chapter in the book and was located in a section entitled "Special Issues and Emerging Areas." In that chapter, Thoresen and Eagleston discussed the limitations of the biomedical model, with a particular focus on the importance of psychological interventions in the treatment of Type A behaviors and heart disease. By the time a second edition of the handbook was published in 1992, the health chapter was located in the section on "Development, Prevention, and Advocacy." In that chapter, Altmaier and Johnson (1992) attempted to move beyond the "tried and true" areas of health practice, such as Type A behavior modification and heart disease prevention, to broaden the scope of areas where counseling psychologists could define health-related applications. The chapter discussed how psychologists have influenced our understanding of the patient-physician relationship and considered psychological treatments for childhood leukemia, chronic back pain, and caregiving of patients with dementia. These are areas where counseling psychologists have made important contributions, although there are many others.

In 1997, at the writing of this chapter, there are 3,146 members of Division 17 (Counseling Psychology). Of those, 189 also hold membership in Division 38 (Health Psychology), which has 3,011 members. More importantly for counseling psychologists interested in health issues, the second section formally recognized by Division 17 was the section related to health applications. This section currently sends its monthly newsletter to over 200 individuals. Clearly, issues related to health and illness will remain important areas of research and practice for counseling psychologists well into the next century.

Roles for Counseling Psychologists

The table of contents of this book lists a variety of ways in which the chapter authors believe counseling psychologists have made or can make important contributions. In many of these areas, counseling psychologists function as researchers, identifying key psychosocial or systemic variables whose alteration can affect the course of illness. Counseling psychologists also function as practitioners, working in multidisciplinary teams to treat patients or families. It is also important to note that counseling psychologists can influence the selection and training of health care professionals.

To give readers a sense of possible roles for counseling psychologists, three counseling psychologists have agreed to describe their work lives. In each of these descriptions, the reader will note the strong emphasis on mobilizing patient strengths, working collaboratively with other health care providers, and educating patients, families, other providers, and the public on the role of psychology in health care. While assessment and treatment are prime responsibilities, they rest within a larger context of attention to environmental and systemic issues. The reader will also note a great variety in settings: from hospital to private practice to an alternative educational setting. It is important to keep in mind that the setting does not have to impose limits on the applicability of counseling psychology to health problems, or on the maintenance of our core values.

A Day in the Life of Katherine Morris

Katherine Morris is a staff psychologist at the Salem Regional Rehabilitation Hospital, Salem, Oregon.

"Often during my daily commute through the Oregon countryside, I introspect on the day to come and the experiences waiting for me at the Physical Rehabilitation Hospital. I switch on the parallel processing circuit that interfaces my frontal and temporal lobes with my limbic system. My attention is diverted from the sunrise to the clients I will see, the meetings I can expect, and the members of the multiple disciplines I will need to contact to coordinate patients' treatment.

"I see myself as a parallel processor, as I am not only a therapist for the client, but also a consultant either to the team of health professionals also treating the patient or to the referring physician. I must sequence data the patient has given me with that from the medical records or other treating professionals and simultaneously understand the patient's life context and the context offered for treatment within the hospital. My aim is to benefit the patient; at times, I also target the education of the treating professionals as to how they may alter their relationship with the patient and be more effective.

"In general, the patients I see during the course of a day have a medical diagnosis. The referring physician may believe aspects of the patient's psyche are affecting the symptoms or that psychological adjustment is being affected by the diagnosis. The outpatient programs within which I work treat patients with some form of chronic pain (e.g., headaches, neuropathies, back pain, arthritis, fibromyalgia), brain injury (e.g., drug use, traumatic brain injury, stroke, anoxia), or sleep disturbance (e.g., insomnia, sleep apnea, narcolepsy). I may treat these patients alone, but more often I work as part of a multidisciplinary team made up of physicians, nurses, social workers, and occupational, speech, and physical therapists.

"As part of my treatment, I may provide neuropsychological or psychological assessments for treatment or surgical planning. Within the course of treatment, I may offer biofeedback focusing on relaxation therapy and neuromuscular retraining, individual therapy, couples therapy, and family therapy. Additionally, I assist with community support groups for the chronic pain patients and the family members of the brain injury treatment program. In the chronic pain support group, my focus is to offer supportive discussions. I also invite speakers who can educate the group on alternative health care approaches that so many people in pain are willing to try without prior knowledge. For families of the brain injured, I focus on education, troubleshooting behavioral difficulties, and inspiring families to see possibilities for independence where they believe none exist.

"It is essential for these patients that I am part of a team providing treatment. I speak of the patient's emotional adjustment/character style both clinically and in terms of the barriers to treatment the style may pose. Often it seems that psychological diagnoses have served as endpoints, labels upon which other disciplines may justify ending treatment or justify a lack of progress. It is as though the very mention of psychological issues indicates that the patient cannot continue in other treatments until these psychic difficulties are "fixed." In some cases, this may be necessary, as when the person is severely depressed or anxious. However, too often, character styles or acute emotional syndromes are seen as reasons to abandon ship.

"I find it much more challenging and rewarding that, along with the clinical diagnosis, I offer strategies for team members to use to address the patient's defenses or behaviors that may limit progress. Understanding the patient's character defenses in response to his or her illness (e.g., denial, hostility, anger, helplessness, solicitousness, hypervigilance), and communicating how to address these in treatment, helps each team I work with to be more effective in our outcomes. The key is to empower not only the patient to allow change, but also those who are a part of the treating team.

"On the commute home, I often contemplate the hospital as a social context: the relationships between myself, my patients, the members of the treating staff, and how we can all better serve the needs of the patients. So far, I have had no accidents on the drive, just occasional circuit overloads!"

A Day in the Life of Miriam Meyer

Miriam Meyer is in private practice in Washington, Iowa.

"In the morning, I drive past the Black Angus cattle peacefully grazing in our pasture and travel 13 miles to the town of Washington, Iowa (population 7,000). I drop my youngest son off at the Washington Junior High School and proceed to work. I am a counseling psychologist in private practice, and my office adjoins the family practice clinic next to Washington County Hospital in which I began my practice. I am the only licensed psychologist in Washington County and possibly several surrounding counties. I have practiced in the community, located 45 miles south of Iowa City and the University of Iowa, for five and a half years. I began as an employee of a group of family physicians prior to forming a corporation two years ago. My business partner is a licensed social worker. We may be a truly multidisciplinary team in the future since a psychiatrist has expressed interest in joining our practice.

"In my practice, I provide psychological assessment, counseling, consultation, and education workshops. My practice is a general practice of psychology, so I provide services for a wide range of problems and ages, ranging from upper elementary-level age to the elderly. Twenty-three percent of my county's population is over age 65, and we have a growing number of retirement communities; I find I'm receiving more requests for help from family physicians to assess cognitive problems in their elderly patients. I treat people with health-related problems, anxiety and depressive disorders, marriage and family problems, adjustment problems, and abuse-related concerns. I am called to the hospital and to the adjoining nursing home facility to see patients; I also go to other nursing homes.

"My daily routine is punctuated by meetings. Since I am on the medical staff of the local hospital, I attend medical staff meetings and committee meetings to discuss bylaws, ethics, and performance improvement. Organizational involvement includes being a member of the Washington County Mental Health Consortium and the Area Agency Forum. I have been active in the Iowa Psychological Association, including presiding over the division for practicing psychologists in the state. Last, I serve as a member of the clinical advisory committee for the managed care company handling Medicaid mental health benefits in the state.

"A typical day would be similar to the following:

8:00   Preparation for clients, completing paperwork, phone calls
9:00   Clinical assessment interview with a teenage girl who was released from the hospital following a suicide attempt
10:00 Referral of elderly couple, wife has possible Alzheimer's and needs her cognitive functions monitored and her depression assessed
11:00 Psychological assessment referral from Department of Human Services
12:00 Lunch at hospital or noon meeting; phone call to husband on the farm or brief walk with colleague
1:30   Answer mail and dictate notes
2:00   Substance abuse evaluation of teenage boy
3:00   Referral of woman with terminally ill child who is experiencing panic attacks and depression
4:00   Continuing therapy session with middle-aged farmer with marital and career concerns
5:00   Referral of teenage girl with weight concerns
6:00   Do paperwork until son finishes track practice at school

"It is a challenge to practice with such a wide range of problems and ages in a rural health setting, but I learn something new every day. This is a difficult time for psychologists, but I have never had a day I could describe as boring. It is always interesting and very rewarding."

A Day in the Life of Candida Maurer

Candida Maurer is a licensed psychologist and a licensed massage therapist in private practice in Iowa City. She and her husband recently opened the

Eastwind School of Holistic Healing to train practitioners in the field of alternative medicine.

"The day begins with Mary. She has come to me for holistic therapy after two radical mastectomies and a complete hysterectomy two years ago left her depressed and afraid. She has a grown developmentally disabled daughter who lives at home. She and her husband fight almost daily and have not had sex in months. Her list of physical complaints is daunting, including irritable bowel syndrome, fibromyalgia, lymphedema, headaches, chronic pelvic pain, and sciatica. Frighteningly, Mary tells me that her physician has recommended removal of all of her pelvic nerves to relieve the pelvic pain which has become almost debilitating. During her first session, I listened carefully to her list and told her there are several things, including the depression, that I may be able to help her heal. My training in shiatsu has taught me that lymphedema can be lessened with well-placed pressure, and that headaches can have their origin in tense neck muscles. I also know that pelvic pain and sciatica are usually related to an imbalance in the pelvic girdle. I refer her to my husband, who is a psychologist, bodyworker, and a Chinese herbalist. He gives her a decoction of herbs to take on a daily basis.

"Mary and I have spent three sessions doing mind-body therapy. This has involved shiatsu, relaxation therapy, and cognitive-behavioral interventions. At today's session, she tells me that her pelvic pain is virtually gone although her sciatica has continued to bother her. I check her pelvis and find that although it's still rotated, with the left side higher than the right, the rotation is far less severe than previously. I encourage her to breathe deeply while I put pressure on the muscles that hold her pelvis in this awkward position. We talk about her marriage and how the lack of sex with her husband has stressed their relationship. She cries for the first time about her loneliness and shame over her body. Finally, she states that with the lessening of the pelvic pain, she has more energy and feels she may be able to enjoy her husband's sexual attention again. We discuss ways to enhance these sexual feelings, and I send her home with instructions for the use of ice on her inflamed pelvis as well as with an agreement regarding reducing some activity during the week to lessen her stress.

"The next person I see is John. He has problems with low energy, dysthymia, and an inability to complete projects. More importantly, he has come for psychotherapy and energy work regarding a large, benign tumor on the right side of his groin area. His physician has recommended surgery that he wishes to avoid. He believes that there are strong psychological components to his tumor and wishes to explore these, and he also wants to use healing touch and Reiki to accelerate the healing process. We devise a plan in which we alternate weekly sessions between psychotherapy and bodywork. John also begins herbal therapy after our first session.

"In psychotherapy, John comes to realize that he was emotionally abused by his parents. He sees the tumor as an expression of the pain and anger he has avoided dealing with by cutting off all communication with his family. I ask him to find an image for his emotional pain. He sees a gray, slimy cloud around his heart and feels a tight black band constricting his throat. We explore the origins of this cloud in a hypnotic state and he finds that it has been protecting him from the fear of abandonment. I have him ask the image whether it is ready to change its function in his life; while it and he aren't ready now, they will be as he continues to work. I encourage John to talk to this image on a daily basis to get information about his inner state.

"The remainder of my day finds me doing mind-body therapy with one more client as well as more traditional psychotherapy with three other clients. I end the day feeling energized and enthusiastic about my work.

"As I write these words, I can imagine a few of the reactions this description of my work has invoked. Let me answer some of the questions that must come from wondering what all this has to do with counseling psychology.

1. Philosophically, I believe that counseling psychology supports a holistic vision, that mind, body, and spirit are connected, and that we must look to the whole person in order to promote healing.
2. Counseling psychology has always supported the notion of empowering our clients. This notion is central to holistic healing, in that ultimate responsibility for change at any level of functioning lies with the client.
3. As a counseling psychologist trained in the scientist-practitioner model, I look to research to inform my practice. There is a growing body of supportive research in the field of healing touch. Unfortunately, much research remains to be done in alternative healing modalities. I wish that counseling psychology could lead the way in bringing a Western scientific perspective to the exciting and burgeoning field of mind-body medicine."

Primary Care

A key area of application, which is emerging as one of great importance in health care, is that of primary care. The Institute of Medicine (Donaldson, Yordy, Lohr, & Vanselow, 1996) has recently published a volume on the future role of primary care in medicine. The Institute noted that medicine has, for the past several decades, placed more emphasis on specialization, technology, and acute care than on primary care. In hopes of reorienting the practice of medicine toward primary care, the Institute commissioned a committee to examine opportunities for increased attention to primary care. This report contains several provisions of interest to counseling psychologists interested in health care roles.

First, the report defines primary care as follows:

> Primary care is the provision of integrated, accessible health care services by clinicians who are accountable for addressing a large majority of personal health care needs, developing a sustained partnership with patients, and practicing in the context of family and community. (p. 31)

It is interesting to note that this definition broadens primary care beyond a narrow conceptualization that is provider-based to consider the following elements:

- integrated and accessible services
- services provided by primary care clinicians
- systems of accountability for quality and patient satisfaction
- services covering the majority of health care needs
- ongoing partnerships of patients with health care providers and services contextualized in family and community

What do these changes mean for counseling psychologists? There is an explicit recognition by the report's authors that health care providers, while traditionally considered to be physicians, nurse practitioners, and physician's assistants, will involve a broader array of individuals in a primary care team. Thus, there is an explicit role for psychologists. However, it should be noted immediately that psychologists, as well as other team members, will be functioning as exactly that—team members. As will be noted in a later part of this chapter, and expanded on in other chapters, psychologists function on the team in two ways: as practitioners and as researchers. In the practitioner role, psychologists need to develop collaborative skills, since any particular intervention will likely be delivered by a range of practitioners. As researchers, psychologists may have a unique ability to conduct clinically grounded research to provide data for the accountability judgment that is a key aspect of primary care. This aspect of our contribution to health care should not be underemphasized.

Perhaps most importantly, Donaldson and colleagues (1996) define primary care as encompassing six core attributes, three of which are vitally important for counseling psychologists:

1. "Excellent primary care is grounded in both the biomedical and the social sciences" (p. 80). Interestingly, the report noted two areas of psychology as emblematic of this grounding: social support and self-efficacy. Clearly, counseling psychology, with its history of understanding aspects of normal human functioning and decision-making, has critical contributions to make in grounding primary care in the social sciences.
2. Primary care "does not consider mental health separately from physical health." This aspect recognizes the reality that psychological distress often is embedded in a variety of physical symptoms. Patients may resist referral to mental health professionals even when such a referral is clearly indicated; counseling psychologists can assist in the diagnosis of mental distress and disorders within primary care.
3. Primary care provides the best possible opportunity to promote health and prevent disease. Counseling psychology's traditional strengths in prevention within a systemic context are most applicable for this aspect of primary care.

Overall, this section has highlighted a wide array of roles for counseling psychologists. Within the broad domain of research, counseling psychologists can and have made important contributions to the knowledge base concerning the etiology and best treatment of a range of disorders. Within the broad domain of practice, counseling psychologists have demonstrated the efficacy of applying a range of psychological interventions to problems of physical health.

Cautionary Notes

There has been an increase in health care specialization over the past few decades. Similarly, psychologists in health care settings provide numerous, varied types of care ranging from traditional counseling to relaxation training and cognitive rehabilitation. As a consequence, some psychology training programs are adapting to the changes in the health care system by providing specialty "tracks" in which students can begin to develop distinctive skills in addition to core knowledge and abilities. Although increased specialization may keep the counseling psychologist competitive in the marketplace, there are several issues that become paramount as our profession adjusts to the changing needs of society. Three such issues are minimal proficiency versus specialization, identity in counseling psychology, and skill integration: combination or synthesis.

Minimal Proficiency versus Specialization

According to the Ethical Principles (APA, 1992), psychologists are committed to maintaining current knowledge in treatments they use, providing services for which they are qualified, and making appropriate referrals to other professionals as well as to other psychologists. In short, these principles dictate that all practicing psychologists know enough to recognize when to refer to another professional. We are required to sustain minimal proficiency in topics relevant to the practice of psychology as well as to understand and respect specialized competencies of colleagues. These principles may be interpreted to suggest that all psychologists are constrained to obtain minimal knowledge of other subspecialties. Of equal importance, however, is that psychologists recognize the boundaries of their competence and the limitations of their techniques.

Neuropsychology can be an excellent example of this issue. Given that financial rewards for the practice of clinical neuropsychology are above that of the general practitioner of psychology, the marginally ethical or naive practitioner may be tempted to extend his or her perceived sphere of competence to this more lucrative area (Slay & Valdivia, 1988). Just as weekend-workshop attendees can go away thinking they are ready to practice with more competence than they actually have, brief and superficial neuropsychological training in a unidisciplinary setting could invite an exaggerated sense of competence. Training recommendations in neuropsychology include completion of specialized internships and doctoral and postdoctoral programs as well as attainment of the American Board of Clinical Neuropsychology and American Board of Professional Psychology diplomas as evidence of competence for responsible independent professional practice in clinical neuropsychology (APA, 1984, 1987, 1988, 1992; Bieliauskas & Matthews, 1987; Bornstein, 1988; Costa, Matarazzo, & Bornstein, 1986; International Neuropsychological Society, 1981). Thus, the primary goals of neuropsychology training in counseling psychology programs should be (a) to provide minimal proficiency in this area, and (b) to prepare students for competitive neuropsychology training programs at the internship and postdoctoral levels, after which specialization in neuropsychology may be considered.

Some authors have suggested that the integrity and identity of psychology as a discipline are weakened by increasing specialization (Ellis, 1992). Concerns regarding specialization need not be paramount, however, if we adhere to the basic principles stated above. *Minimal proficiency* in various areas can be acquired in counseling psychology programs without jeopardizing core psychology courses. *Specialization,* however, is acquired in addition to core requirements and occurs most commonly in internship and postgraduate training programs. The postgraduate model of specialization is particularly important in health psychology and neuropsychology due to the vast amount of specific information (e.g., anatomy, neurophysiology) required. In medical settings, we are constantly humbled (by our colleagues, patients, and so on) by confrontation with what we do not know or do not understand. A condensed training package, insulated from the challenging realities of real clinical and research work, can be worse than no training at all. The counseling psychologist who wishes to work in health care settings on problems related to health care must consider the issue of minimal proficiency versus specialization and obtain the necessary training if specialized practice is desired.

Identity in Counseling Psychology

To quote a leader in our field, "Some readers may be disturbed that . . . counseling psychology has lost its identity. But is this really important? What matters is that society provides a framework within which persons with specialized knowledge and skills can bring their resources to bear on the needs, problems, and aspirations of people" (Tyler, 1980, p. 21). Nearly two decades later these words remain important for counseling psychologists interested in providing care to persons in health care settings.

It is our strong belief that counseling psychologists can maintain their identity as such while practicing and conducting research in health care settings. Establishing and maintaining identity can be accomplished in several ways.

1. Remember that psychologists define their professional identity based on a multitude of characteristics, such as work setting, clientele, basic philosophy of health and illness, or journals where they primarily publish. Practically speaking, every psychologist may have multiple identities. Developing a new professional specialty and a new professional identity does not imply relinquishing the old ones. Moreover, we do not need to create a new label for each individual psychologist: Larsen's (1992) reference to a counseling neuropsychologist seems cumbersome (and unwieldy) in this respect. It is time to move away from further definition of the ideal counseling psychologist to a more realistic acceptance of diversity within counseling psychology.

2. Maintain currency in the specialty of counseling psychology. For counseling psychologists interested in applying the specialty, there must be a willingness to keep up with the specialty. As an example, many cancer patients experience a dramatic change in their vocational functioning. Counseling psychologists who engage in research or practice with this population must understand the influences of cancer and its treatment on work abilities. The importance of work in the lives of cancer patients remains: Many patients have lost a critical aspect of their identity, and alternate work should be identified that can restore this lost component. Remaining current with theory and research on vocational psychology and career interventions is critical for developing effective interventions and conceptualizing research.

3. Counseling psychologists who work in health care settings have a responsibility to provide the specialty with feedback on the effectiveness or lack thereof of the interventions they apply and the variables they investigate. As an example, a counseling psychologist working with a social psychologist and two orthopedic surgeons (Altmaier, Lehmann, Russell, Weinstein, & Kao, 1992; Altmaier, Russell, Kao, Lehmann, & Weinstein, 1993) demonstrated that a rehabilitation program that included coping skills training and behavioral reinforcement of well behaviors (i.e., exercise) was no more effective than a traditional rehabilitation program emphasizing physical therapy. However, those patients who had their self-efficacy increased in either program improved more than those patients who did not. An implication of this

research was the advisability of investigating the sources of low self-efficacy for patients with back pain and to tailor a program to fit their individual needs. Presentations at conventions and publishing health-related research in traditional counseling psychology journals are two prime communication routes to meet this goal of providing accountability data to the specialty.

Skill Integration: Combination or Synthesis?

In this era of managed, truncated, and capitated health care, competition among health care practitioners has become acute. One response to increased competition has been increased specialization. As a consequence, the counseling psychologist in the health care setting may provide more services, such as relaxation training, smoking cessation groups, and cognitive assessment for ADHD, dementia, and head trauma; however, the caliber of service provision may suffer. That is, it is difficult to maintain excellence when the skills provided vary as greatly as suggested in the example above. There are at least three issues that must be considered when developing a specialization and marketing oneself in the health care arena.

1. Minimal proficiency must be accomplished in all subspecialty areas of health care. That is, neuropsychologists must be familiar with the effects of anxiety, pain, and fatigue secondary to treatment on cognitive performance. Health psychologists must know the difference between delirium and dementia and be able to provide basic mental status and cognitive screening. The bottom line to minimal proficiency in the health care setting is that the psychologist needs to know a little about everything.
2. Boundaries of specialization must be established. The neuropsychologist needs to refer when the patient being tested demonstrates severe depression and/or anxiety that precludes valid assessment of cognition. The health psychologist needs to refer when noncompliance to treatment regimen is secondary to cognitive impairment.
3. The type of specialist the counseling psychologist desires to become should be considered. The models suggested so far have consisted of a combination approach, where the traditional counseling psychologist acquires additional skills for health-related practice and research. Of course, this model works. There are counseling psychologists

working in hospitals, outpatient health care clinics, medical schools, and private nonprofit health care agencies across the United States. An alternate approach, however, may be to determine a unique synthesis of counseling psychology and other specialties to provide a service unparalleled by other health care professionals.

Conclusion

As you read the remaining chapters in this book, we encourage you to keep issues of identity firmly in mind. Be challenged by the excitement and opportunities in health care research and practice that are here now and will grow in the future, but also consider these opportunities with caution and ethical sensitivity. We ask that you believe you can remain a counseling psychologist while applying our profession's traditional strengths and emphases to these new areas.

Suggested Resources

"Health Psychology in the U.S.A." (Wallston, 1993) provides an excellent description of important events in the field of health psychology and in the development of Division 38 of the American Psychological Association. Wallston not only highlights historical trends but also provides interesting anecdotes. He deliberately wrote this chapter to be less of a scholarly work than a "letter to friends," which makes it both informative and fun to read.

For those interested in tracing the debate over the scope and definition of health psychology, a series of articles published in the *American Psychologist* (e.g., Matarazzo, 1980, 1982; Singer & Krantz, 1982) is a good place to start. These articles provide descriptions of why psychologists should consider health-related interventions and provide a foundation for topics such as scope of practice and minimum competency requirements, topics that are still being discussed today.

Belar and Deardorff (1995) have written an excellent text for any psychologist working in a medical setting. *Clinical Health Psychology in Medical Settings* covers history and training issues, provides a comprehensive and helpful consideration of doing assessment and intervention in medical settings, considers ethical and legal issues in practice, and points to future issues. The appendices include listings of relevant journals to read, medical abbreviations and medical problems to know, and professional organizations to join. This text is an essential one to purchase and keep as a reference.

Newsletters of professional organizations are particularly useful reading. *The Health Psychologist* is the newsletter of Division 38 of the APA. It contains a variety of interesting articles; the Winter 1997 issue, for example, covered hurdles involved in conducting a randomized study of a clinical intervention, working with cancer patients, a "day in the life" of a health psychologist, a report from the Division's Committee on Sexuality and Health on the potential of female-controlled methods of HIV prevention for women with mental illness, and a variety of announcements and opportunities.

The American Psychological Association, as part of its Human Capital Initiative, published *Doing the Right Thing: A Research Plan for Healthy Living* (APA, 1995). This report contains summaries of current knowledge and recommendations for needed research in four key areas: understanding chronic illness, promoting health and preventing disease, increasing health among underserved groups, and reshaping the health care system. Recommended readings are included. Counseling psychologists who wish to shape a research agenda in the health area would benefit from reading this report.

Agencies who are multidisciplinary also provide interesting perspectives on our practice. One, in particular, the Agency for Health Care Policy and Research, has a research findings newsletter, *Research Activities,* which highlights recent findings. The Spring 1997 issue contains many summaries of research, several of which (e.g., physician communication, rural health care, and depression among the elderly) would be of interest to counseling psychologists.

For the reader who is specifically interested in neuropsychology applications, *The TCN Guide to Professional Practice in Clinical Neuropsychology* (Adams & Rourke,1992) is a compilation of professional training statements related to the types of training needed for neuropsychology practice. Of particular importance to students are the definitions of and training criteria for neuropsychology as a specialty area of practice.

Discussion Questions

1. Do you agree with the authors' contention that counseling psychologists can retain their identity with the specialty but work in settings traditionally unrelated to counseling psychology?
2. What boundary conditions might define a counseling psychologist apart from his or her work setting?
3. What is your response to the "days in the lives" of the three counseling psychologists presented in this chapter? Which psychologist's life sounds most appealing to you and why?
4. How do you see the increased emphasis on primary care affecting your future work as a counseling psychologist, whether you see yourself in research, training, or practice?
5. Are there ethical principles other than "competence" that might be important in hospital practice? Which principles are they, and how do you see them being tested?

References

Adams, K. M., & Rourke, B. P. (Eds.). (1992). *The TCN guide to professional practice in clinical neuropsychology*. Amsterdam: Swets and Zeitlinger.

Altmaier, E. M., & Johnson, B. D. (1992). Health related applications of counseling psychology: Toward health promotion and disease prevention across the life span. In S. D. Brown, & R. W. Lent (Eds.), *Handbook of Counseling Psychology* (2nd ed., pp. 315–347). New York: Wiley.

Altmaier, E. M., Lehmann, T. R., Russell, D. W., Weinstein, J. N., & Kao, C. F. (1992). The effectiveness of psychological interventions for the rehabilitation of low back pain: A randomized controlled trial evaluation. *Pain, 49,* 329–335.

Altmaier, E. M., Russell, D. W., Kao, C. F., Lehmann, T. R., & Weinstein, J. N. (1993). The role of self-efficacy in rehabilitation outcome among chronic low back pain patients. *Journal of Counseling Psychology, 40,* 335–339.

American Psychological Association. (1984). Report of the Division 40/INS Joint Task Force on Education, Accreditation, and Credentialing. *Division of Clinical Neuropsychology Newsletter, 40,* 3–8.

American Psychological Association. (1987). Resolutions approved by the National Conference on Graduate Education in Psychology. *American Psychologist, 42,* 1070–1084.

American Psychological Association. (1988). Report of the Division 40/INS Joint Task Force on Education, Accreditation, and Credentialing: Subcommittee on Continuing Education. Definition of a Clinical Neuropsychologist. *The Clinical Neuropsychologist, 2,* 22.

American Psychological Association. (1992). Ethical principles of psychologists. *American Psychologist, 47,* 1597–1611.

American Psychological Association. (1995). *Doing the right thing: A research plan for healthy living.* Washington, DC: Author.

Belar, C. D., & Deardorff, W. W. (1995). *Clinical health psychology in medical settings: A practitioner's guidebook* (Rev. ed.). Washington, DC: American Psychological Association.

Bieliauskas, L. A., & Matthews, C. G. (1987). American Board of Clinical Neuropsychology: Policies and Procedures. *The Clinical Neuropsychologist, 1,* 21–28.

Bornstein, R. A. (1988). Guidelines for continuing education in clinical neuropsychology. *The Clinical Neuropsychologist, 2,* 25–29.

Costa, L. D., Matarazzo, J. D., & Bornstein, R. A. (1986). Issues in graduate and post-graduate training in clinical neuropsychology. In S. B. Filskov, & T. J. Boll (Eds.), *Handbook of clinical neuropsychology* (Vol. 2, pp. 652-668). New York: Wiley.

Division of Counseling Psychology. (1994). *What is a counseling psychologist?.* Washington, DC: American Psychological Association.

Donaldson, M. S., Yordy, K. D., Lohr, K. N., & Vanselow, N. A. (1996). *Primary care: America's health in a new era.* Washington: National Academy.

Ellis, H. C. (1992). Graduate education in psychology: Past, present, and future. *American Psychologist, 47,* 570–576.

Engel, G. L. (1977). The need for a new medical model: A challenge for biomedicine. *Science, 196,* 129–136.

Howard, G. S. (1984, August). *Counseling psychology and health psychology: Current status and future directions.* Invited symposium presented at the American Psychological Association, Toronto.

International Neuropsychological Society Task Force (1981). *Report of the task force on education, accreditation, and credentialing of International Neuropsychological Society.* Atlanta, GA: Board of Governors of the International Neuropsychological Society.

Knowles, J. H. (1977). *Doing better and feeling worse: Health in the United States.* New York: Norton.

Krumboltz, J. D., Becker-Haven, J. F., & Burnett, K. F. (1979). Counseling psychology. *Annual Review of Psychology, 30,* 355–402.

Larsen, L. (1992). Neuropsychological counseling in hospital settings. *The Counseling Psychologist, 20,* 556–570.

Matarazzo, J. D. (1980). Behavioral health and behavioral medicine: Frontiers for a new health psychology. *American Psychologist, 35,* 807–817.

Matarazzo, J. D. (1982). Behavioral health's challenge to academic, scientific and professional psychology. *American Psychologist, 37,* 1–14.

Millon, T. (1982). On the nature of clinical health psychology. In T. Millon, C. J. Green, & R. B. Meagher (Eds.), *Handbook of clinical health psychology.* New York: Plenum.

Schofield, W. (1969). The role of psychology in the delivery of health services. *American Psychologist, 24,* 565–584.

Singer, J. E., & Krantz, D. S. (1982). Perspectives on the interface between psychology and public health. *American Psychologist, 37,* 955–960.

Slay, D. K., & Valdivia, L. (1988). Neuropsychology as a specialized health service listed in the National Register of Health Service Providers in Psychology. *Professional Psychology: Research and Practice, 19,* 323–329.

Stone, G. C., Cohen, F., & Adler, N. E. (1979). *Health psychology: A handbook.* San Francisco: Jossey Bass.

Thoresen, C. E., & Eagleston, J. R. (1984). Counseling, health, and psychology. In S. D. Brown, & R. W. Lent (Eds.), *Handbook of counseling psychology* (pp. 930–955). New York: Wiley.

Tyler, L. E. (1980). The next twenty years. *The Counseling Psychologist, 8,* 19–21.

Wallston, K. A. (1993). Health Psychology in the USA. In S. Maes, H. Leventhal, & M. Johnston (Eds.), *International review of health psychology* (Vol. 2, pp. 215–228). New York: Wiley.

2
Training for Health Settings

John D. Alcorn

The evolution of health care into a multidiciplinary field has created enlarged opportunities for counselors and counseling psychologists as health service providers. With this development, there has been a corresponding need to better align traditional training models with those of other health care providers such as physicians and nurses. This chapter provides an overview of the antecedents for current training and practice in health settings and makes specific recommendations for the future training of counselors and counseling psychologists who wish to pursue careers in health service delivery.

Background

The growing involvement of nonmedical service providers in health care has paralleled significant changes in the health care system. As infectious diseases have increasingly been brought under control, attention has shifted to an array of chronic illnesses and health risk factors that interact strongly with habits of living and lifestyle (Department of Health and Human Services, 1990; Gentry, 1984; Syme, 1984). Outcomes of this shift have included the gradual adoption of a biopsychosocial health model (Schwartz, 1982) and the expansion of treatment goals to include prevention, noncurative relief, and improvement of life quality (White, 1988). These changes have paved the way for inclusion of nonmedical service providers, such as psychologists, social workers, and professional counselors within the matrix of health-related professions and have reinforced the addition of health-related content to their training programs. As one example of this growth, the Division of Health Psychology (Division 38) was formed within the American Psychological Association (APA) in 1979 and had attracted 3,000 members by 1997.

Over the past two decades, advances in the application of psychological science to health problems have supported the involvement of psychologists in a growing range of activities, including direct services to patients, consultation-liaison services to physicians and nurses, medical education, and research (Matarazzo, 1980). By the early 1980s, a number of training programs had responded to the growing opportunities for involvement of nonmedical providers in health care delivery by expanding curricula and adding practica in health settings. As this development occurred, professional organizations took steps to outline appropriate training models, promulgate standards of practice, and establish statutory bases for the regulation of practice in health care settings. In a 1981 study, Belar, Wilson, and Hughes (1982) identified 42 psychology programs that offered some form of predoctoral training in health psychology. Most offered specialized curricula within established predoctoral specialty areas such as clinical, counseling, or school psychology, while only six purported to offer a predoctoral specialization in health psychology. In a similar vein, the directories of the Association of Psychology Internship Centers (APIC) for this period revealed a growing number of predoctoral internship programs that offered behavioral medicine or health psychology rotations within their settings. It is noteworthy that the current title of this national organization, Association of Psychology Postdoctoral and Internship Centers (APPIC), reflects the increasing importance given to postdoctoral training in the total preparation of professional psychologists. During an era in which psychologists were becoming more active in health care, graduate programs in professional counseling and doctoral programs in counseling psychology were slow to add health-related curricula and practica for their students. One exception was rehabilitation counseling, which had a long history of association with the medical field.

The reluctance of counseling programs to become involved in training for health settings has stemmed, in part, from philosophical reservations regarding the disease orientation of medical models and counseling psychology's historic ties to prevention-oriented practice in educational settings.

Nonetheless, a small but active group of counseling psychologists and counselor educators have pointed to ways in which traditional emphases in the counseling field align with the goals of comprehensive medical treatment and health promotion (Alcorn, 1991; Altmaier, 1991; Corrigan, 1991; Harris; 1991; Hollandsworth, 1985; Kagan, 1979; Klippel & DeJoy, 1984; Larson & Agresti, 1992; May, 1977; Thoresen & Eagleston, 1985). In particular, traditional emphases on psychoeducation as a treatment modality, communication skills, decision-making, and the integration of career and family issues within a life span developmental perspective have seemed highly correlated with major health goals that included prevention of illness, reduction of health risk factors associated with life style, and the improved management of chronic illnesses that have long-term systemic effects on the lives of patients and their families.

Over the past decade, a growing number of counseling programs have added health-related training components through expanded course offerings and/or practicum/internship placements. Data collected by the Council of Counseling Psychology Training Programs (Kivlighan, 1995) indicate that, nationally, approximately one-third of the predoctoral internships currently accepted by counseling psychology doctoral students are in medical settings (e.g., hospitals, medical schools, Veterans Administration and military medical centers), with about 16 percent of students taking initial postgraduate positions in these settings. The formation in 1996 of a Health Section within the Division of Counseling Psychology (Division 17) of the APA further reflects a growing interest in health applications among graduates of counseling psychology training programs.

While the movement of nonmedical service providers such as counselors and counseling psychologists into health care settings presents many opportunities, there remain a number of important questions and issues. Given the impact of managed care and efforts to contain costs of health care, will there be room for additional providers and, if so, at what levels? What types of curricular content should be required in programs that attempt to prepare students for careers in the health field? What is the core of knowledge and skills that an individual needs to practice in the health setting? Should specialization occur at the predoctoral or postdoctoral level? What types of credentials will be required to practice in health care settings in the future?

Issues related to managed care and the ability of the health care system to support additional health care providers are beyond the scope of this chapter. However, the assumption is made that appropriate roles will be identified for a variety of health care providers and at different levels within managed care systems of the future. As the health care system seeks to contain costs and to operate in a more efficient manner, it seems reasonable that roles will be identified for both master's level and doctoral practitioners. These prospects have implications for the differentiation of service delivery roles as well as for the design of appropriate training programs at all levels. For master's level practitioners, roles are more likely to involve direct and supportive services to specific categories of patients in multidisciplinary settings and will involve working under the supervision of physicians or psychologists. While doctoral providers will continue to have responsibilities for direct service delivery, opportunities will increase in other areas such as consultation-liaison services to primary care physicians, supervision of master's level providers, staff development, and program management and evaluation, as well as clinical research.

The complexity of problems currently being addressed by the health care system and the corresponding explosion of knowledge within the health field have created pressures to increase educational and training requirements for both medical and nonmedical providers. As different disciplines have found niches in the service delivery matrix, multidisciplinary career ladders have evolved. Within this environment, training and credentialing requirements for different groups have been linked to:

1. the complexity of functions performed
2. the degree of risk posed to patients by interventions offered
3. the level of independence sought for practice

Given that physical health concerns override all other considerations in patient care and that physicians ultimately make most of the critical decisions that impact physical status, it is not surprising that they have been assigned leadership roles in most settings. Providers such as clinical dieticians, medical social workers, clinical pastoral counselors, rehabilitation counselors, and psychologists perform valuable services within the overall framework of total patient care but apply interventions that are not physically intrusive or life-threatening and that are typically offered at the request of or under the oversight of physicians. At the same time, as providers such as nurse practitioners and psychologists have sought greater parity with physicians over the past decade, their respective training and credentialing requirements have increased accordingly. It should be noted that exceptions to the physician-led model may exist in some multidisciplinary settings such as obesity clinics, where the focus of treatment is primarily on social and behavioral factors which indirectly influence physical status.

Master's Level Providers

Provider groups such as medical social workers, clinical pastoral counselors, and rehabilitation counselors have established well-identified roles within hospitals and medical clinics, and specialized training programs for these groups have been in place for some time. Although health-related career tracks and training programs for other master's level providers, such as professional counselors, have not been as well developed in the past, many have found places in the health care delivery system. Basic counseling and consultation skills taught in most graduate programs are highly valued and easily adapted to roles that include functions such as program coordination, patient and family support, patient advocacy, staff development, and crisis management. In those settings where some specialized medical knowledge is required in order to work with special categories of patients (e.g., weight loss, pain management, oncology), continuing education opportunities are usually provided for employees as an integral part of ongoing staff development and quality assurance programs. Regardless, master's level counselors usually complete practicum and internship experiences as components of their training program, and most continue to acquire the essential knowledge and skills needed for job performance and professional advancement.

Given current emphases on cost containment, opportunities for master's level providers should increase over time as managed care corporations seek ways to deliver a greater range of services at less cost. Within an integrated system of health care, practitioners at different levels and from different disciplines join treatment teams where everyone is expected to perform functions that complement those of other team members. Team members with less formal training often perform many of the routine functions, freeing doctoral practitioners to perform more highly specialized tasks and/or to concentrate their efforts on more complicated cases. It is possible for master's level counselors to attain the knowledge base and helping skills needed for entry into many health-related positions through completing a well-planned graduate program. As mentioned above, once they are on the job, most counselors continue to develop essential job-related competencies through apprenticeship arrangements and participation in relevant continuing education activities.

Doctoral Psychologists

In recommendations from the Boulder Conference of 1949, psychologists took the stance that education and training for independent practice should include a doctoral program with a one-year predoctoral internship. By the mid-1970s, the National Register of Health Service Providers in Psychology was established, and one year of postdoctoral supervision was included as a registry requirement. Most states require at least one year of postdoctoral supervision in order to be licensed for the independent practice of psychology. Until recently, this additional year of supervision was usually acquired through flexible apprenticeship arrangements or, less frequently, through formal postdoctoral residencies of one or more years. However, guidelines and procedures for the accreditation of training programs in professional psychology were approved by the APA Committee on Accreditation in 1996 to include postdoctoral programs, and the first accreditation site visits for postdoctoral training programs were scheduled in 1997. This move should provide an incentive for increasing both the quality and the numbers of post-doctoral training programs available to psychologists in the future.

Programs that prepare students for health service delivery roles have found it necessary to include health-related content and training experiences within existing discipline-based models in order to expand career opportunities for doctoral graduates and to address service needs in the general society. Such training has been expected to address the broader needs of foundational preparation while also providing the specialized education and training needed to obtain an appropriate internship and to meet the entry and specialty credentialing requirements associated with the discipline. Within a multidisciplinary delivery system, which includes practitioners with varying levels of responsibility and educational requirements, programs have been expected, as a minimum, to offer preparation that was appropriate for entry-level practice while meeting credentialing requirements for the respective field or discipline.

Patterns of Training for Health Settings

It should be noted that counseling and psychological practice in both medical/health settings and mental health settings derives from a common foundation of education and training, and both applications proceed in a similar manner with respect to treatment and research methodologies. At the same time, important distinctions with relevance to specialty training may be drawn. In medical/health settings, biomedical factors will take priority in the diagnosis and treatment of presenting problems while psychological and behavioral dimensions of disease will largely be viewed as moderating or mediating influences on physical disease process. Consequently, the physician-led, medical treatment model will prevail, and concerns for patient morbidity and mortality will serve as bottom lines in treatment decisions (Taylor, 1985). Whereas psychiatry has traditionally maintained a strong role in mental health treatment, primary care physicians in specialties such as family medicine, internal medicine, and pediatrics are more likely to call the plays in physical health settings. Because the training backgrounds of primary physicians have little overlap with that of psychologists and other nonmedical providers, conflicts arising over boundaries of practice tend to occur less often than is the case in mental health settings. The combined efforts of different disciplines can contribute greatly to scope and quality patient care when offered in an climate of mutual respect and collaboration.

Antecedents of Current Training Programs

Prior to the mid-1970s, most psychologists and other nonmedical service providers entered health careers in the absence of structure and guidance from professional organizations and regulatory bodies. While a few programs, largely those that were either a part of or affiliated with medical schools, provided training that was specifically geared to service delivery in medical settings, most offered primarily the generalist preparation embodied in the criteria and standards of the applicable accreditation model. Students seeking careers in the health field often had to assume personal responsibility for locating elective courses and field experiences as they sought to better prepare themselves for a health internship. Following completion of a degree program, graduates were expected to gain additional training and specialized preparation through some type of supervisory arrangement or postdoctoral residency. In addition, there was an expectation that students would engage in an ongoing program of continuing education in response to relevant job or credentialing requirements. In psychology, a number of postdoctoral training positions have been available over the years but have varied widely in terms of content, setting, and quality. In a recent survey, Wiens and Baum (1995) found that this diversity still characterizes postdoctoral training programs for psychologists, particularly with respect to settings, scope, and focus of training provided and in number of residents and staff.

In the early stages of development, most health care professions were permitted entry into specialty practice through a variety of training avenues, including apprenticeships which ranged from informal tutorial arrangements to more highly structured residency programs. However, as these groups sought greater acceptance and support from the public, they found it necessary to adopt more highly structured and formalized patterns of education and training, usually in accordance with uniform standards and guidelines set forth by accrediting and credentialing bodies. As improved standards have been adopted for each level of education and training, the same process of study and revision has proceeded to the next level (e.g., predoctoral, doctoral, and post-doctoral). This pattern of professionalization was characteristic of medical education after the turn of the century, and it has been largely followed by other health care professions following World War II and into the present.

Specialty Practice in Health Psychology

In order to provide structure and direction for the rapidly developing field of health psychology, the Arden House National Working Conference on Education and Training in Health Psychology was held in 1983 under sponsorship of the APA Division of Health Psychology (Stone, 1983). Conference goals included the development of recommendations regarding levels of training, scope and content of curricula, desired training environments, and legal and ethical issues, credentialing, and accreditation (Stone, 1983). Key elements of conference recommendations included the following propositions (pp. 16–17):

1. Training should be offered for both scientist and professional roles.
2. The professional training path should be based on the scientist-practitioner model.
3. Core training should meet APA accreditation criteria.
4. Postdoctoral training is highly desirable for health psychologists; the subgroup working on postdoctoral training recommended a two-year postdoctoral residency in an organized program.
5. The curriculum should provide experiences and content which address cultural and individual diversity, the integration of theory and practice, the research base for practice, skills needed for successful interdisciplinary collaboration, the impact of services on health care settings, patients, and families, and ethical/legal issues.

6. Completion of an internship alone is not viewed as adequate preparation for respecialization in health psychology, and continuing education and/or apprenticeship arrangements are not viewed as appropriate for entry to practice in health psychology.

Although a few clinical psychology programs have continued to offer specialization at the predoctoral level, health psychology increasingly has been viewed as a postdoctoral enterprise (Fox, 1992; Sheridan et al., 1988). This trend toward postdoctoral training has been reinforced by several factors:

1. Pressures to incorporate an expanding knowledge base needed by all professional psychologists has placed severe demands on the curricula of predoctoral training programs and leaves little room for specialized training without increasing the period of time for predoctoral training.
2. Recent revisions to the APA accreditation principles and procedures (APA, 1996) stipulate that "doctoral education and training in preparation for entry-level practice in preprofessional psychology should be broad and professional in its orientation rather than narrow and technical" (p. 3). Thus, substantive specialty preparation in health psychology is better suited to the postdoctoral period and potentially permits entry by graduates from any of the general practice specialties fields accredited by the APA (currently clinical, counseling, and school).
3. While the majority of state and provincial licensing boards in the United States and Canada license or certify applicants for generic practice in professional psychology and about half of 60 jurisdictions include subdoctoral practitioners in the credentialing process, most have provisions for identifying health service providers. The health service provider designation usually requires completion of a predoctoral training program in clinical, counseling, or school psychology plus one to two years of postdoctoral supervised practice in a health setting.

In 1996, the APA Division of Health Psychology (Division 38) submitted a petition for formal recognition of "Clinical Health Psychology" as a psychological speciality to the APA Commission for the Recognition of Specialties and Proficiencies in Professional Psychology (CRSPPP). After review by CRSPPP, the application was approved by the APA Council of Representatives in August, 1997. The petition recognized training in health psychology as occurring at the doctoral, internship, and postdoctoral levels.

Two pathways for entry into health psychology were acknowledged:

1. taking a postdoctoral fellowship, after completing professional psychology preparation in one of the general practice specialties (e.g., counseling psychology), or
2. completing a health psychology predoctoral program, followed by an internship and one year of postdoctoral supervision in health psychology.

The petition emphasized the interrelatedness of biological, psychological, and social aspects of health and disease with behavior and stipulated that these components should be included in the preparation of all health psychologists. With the approval of this new specialty, it is probable that Division 38 will seek separate accreditation status for health psychology in the near future.

In 1996, The APA Division of Counseling Psychology (Division 17) was preparing a CRSPPP petition for recognition of counseling psychology as a predoctoral specialty. While the Division 17 officers were pleased with the postdoctoral training component of the health psychology petition, concerns were registered with CRSPPP regarding the use of terminology that appeared to place health psychology as a subfield of clinical psychology. Although turf issues are obviously involved in this instance and few restrictions seem to be placed on counseling psychologists who wish to practice in health settings, arguments were presented by Division 17 from a philosophical stance that postdoctoral specialities should not be linked in title or otherwise to any of the predoctoral specialities.

The Content of Training for Psychologists

The basic training model for professional psychology has received ongoing review and revision by the psychology profession since the end of World War II. A continuing series of major training conferences since the Boulder Conference of 1949 have strongly influenced the design of curricula for the training of psychologists in general and health psychologists in particular. With regard to training in counseling psychology, the 1964 Greyston Conference on the Professional Preparation of Counseling Psychologists offered little guidance for programs whose graduates projected careers in health settings or for the design of curricula specifically geared to practice in health settings. Two decades later, however, health service roles as psychoeducators, consultants, counselors, and researchers were identified for counseling psychologists in proceedings of the 1987 Georgia Conference on Counseling Psychology (Kagan et al., 1988).

Prior to the 1987 Georgia Conference on Counseling Psychology, participants in the 1983 Arden House Conference (Stone, 1983) had already outlined a training model for health psychologists, which included three articulated stages:

1. a generic or general practice predoctoral program in professional psychology
2. a one-year predoctoral internship which provides a broad exposure to professional practice in a health setting
3. one to two years of specialized postdoctoral residency training in health psychology.

It is worth noting that the conference Work Group on Predoctoral Education/Doctoral Training strongly recommended two years of postdoctoral residency as the minimal training needed for competent practice as a health service provider (Sheridan et al., 1988; Stone, 1983).

Predoctoral Training

The curriculum plan for predoctoral training, of necessity, should adhere to the Guidelines and Principles for Accreditation of Programs in Professional Psychology (APA, 1996). In addition, programs should be informed by the model training program description that was developed through a joint project of the Council of Counseling Psychology Training Programs (CCPTP) and the APA Division of Counseling Psychology (Division 17) and was adopted by the CCPTP in 1997. The CCPTP/Division 17 document conforms to the APA guidelines and principles and is intended to serve as an aid to the application of the parent guidelines and principles. Programs should be appropriately organized with adequate funding to accomplish their mission, and their curriculum and training model should align with their training philosophy and objectives. As a minimum, curriculum content should encompass the following areas:

1. psychological foundations for practice
2. scientific, methodological, and theoretical foundations of practice
3. professional standards, ethics, and legal implications for practice
4. assessment and diagnosis, design of interventions, and evaluation strategies

5. cultural and individual diversity and the characteristics of underserved populations
6. socialization of students as lifelong learners, scholars, and professional problem-solvers
7. opportunities for supervised practice in a sequential pattern which provides exposure to a diverse clientele and is in accordance with student career goals

Consistent with recommendations from the Arden House Conference (Stone, 1983), most health-related internship programs give preference to predoctoral applicants who have been trained in the scientist-practitioner model. Many of these programs reflect biases that endorse training in empirically supported or validated procedures (APA, 1996; Division 12, 1995; Nathan & Gorman, 1998). They are more likely to favor cognitive-behavioral interventions, offered within a data-based, brief therapy model. However, the professional core of preparation for health care practice should include the theoretical and practical training needed to address issues such as compliance to medical regimens, relapse prevention, reduction of risk factors, and assessment of health-related behaviors. In addition, students should receive training and supervised experiences to help them understand the systemic implications of psychological interventions and the impact of cultural and individual diversity on patients' response to health service delivery.

In addition to core requirements embodied in the APA accreditation guidelines and principles, opportunities should be provided for students in a health track to add elective courses and experiences that will enrich their program and better position them to compete for a quality internship. Desired courses may be available within the parent department but often must be taken from other departments across campus. While there are a number of possibilities in the selection of courses for a health concentration, the Working Group on Predoctoral Education at the 1983 Arden House Conference recommended that the following content areas be added to the minimum preparation of psychologists who are preparing for health careers (Stone, 1983, p. 126):

- biological basis of health systems and behavior
- social basis of health systems and behavior
- psychological basis of health systems and behavior
- knowledge and skills regarding health policy and organization.

Additionally, the following courses integrate well with the core curriculum in counseling psychology and will potentially provide students with an edge in the competition for internships:

- introduction to health psychology
- medical aspects of disability
- psychopharmacology
- medical terminology
- neuropsychology
- community health

Such courses often help students to focus research interests and ultimately may set the stage for participation in field-based research projects with faculty members or adjunct faculty members. As one example, core faculty members and students from some programs become regular members of field-based multidisciplinary teams that are engaged in both practice and research activities (Alcorn & McPhearson, 1997). Through such experiences, students are assisted in generalizing their basic preparation to problems and issues arising in the applied health setting. Students who are involved in these activities often identify research topics that become the basis for thesis and dissertation studies.

Practica and Externships

Without exception, well-designed practicum and externship experiences are invaluable in helping students to adapt the knowledge and skills gained from their core program to problems in health settings. As pointed out by Altmaier (1991), nonmedical providers face special challenges in settings that have "been constructed by and for physicians" (p. 358). Preparatory course work that helps students to acquire a basic facility with medical terminology and to gain some understanding of physical disease processes will smooth their transition from the campus to the medical setting. Once there, opportunities for working with physicians and nurses will help students to become familiar with medical protocols, become sensitive to the nuances of consultation-liaison practice, and gain skills in applying principles of interpersonal communications and group dynamics to conflicts that often arise in multidisciplinary team practice. As outlined by Alcorn and McPhearson (1997), advanced practicum or externship placements in health settings may be developed as one option for students during their third or fourth year of graduate study. In these placements, the emphasis should be on quality of patient contacts and related supervision rather than quantity. When core faculty members are on site to provide supervision, the possibilities for achieving an integration of basic scientific knowledge with practice are greatly expanded (i.e., science informs practice and practice informs science). Faculty and student collaboration in multidisciplinary practice settings not only provides insights into the nature of research questions associated with health care but also provides students with the opportunity to gain confidence in the application of research and evaluation skills to health problems as they are encountered in their natural setting.

The Predoctoral Internship

The predoctoral internship is an integral component on the continuum of education and training (Belar et al., 1989). It is a postpracticum experience that serves both as an extension of the on-campus program and a bridge to a postdoctoral training in health psychology. While there are a number of options available for students who project health careers, some internship settings are better suited than others for counseling psychologists. Veterans' Administration hospitals have traditionally provided an excellent source of internship training for counseling psychologists, as well as for other providers, such as clinical psychologists, medical social workers, clinical pastoral counselors, and rehabilitation counselors. Medical schools and hospitals may also provide good training experiences, depending upon the makeup of the staff and the philosophy of the program. Over the years, armed services psychology programs have been an excellent source of internship training for counseling psychologists, and many stations currently have counseling psychologists on staff. Applicants should keep in mind that military appointments obligate participants for enlistment periods that extend beyond the internship year.

Internship experiences should involve students in sequential activities that are graded in complexity and require the application of competencies acquired during the campus phase of the program. Exposure to a broad range of problems and clientele under supervision of competent staff should assist interns to progressively assume more responsibility across the internship year. Rotations of interest to counseling psychologists might include consultation/liaison services for physicians, behavioral medicine, rehabilitation medicine, neuropsychology, pain and eating disorders services, alcohol and substance abuse, and inpatient psychiatry. These experiences should help students to gain professional confidence and to crystalize their interests regarding a postdoctoral training program. Other activities such as participation in colloquia and grand rounds, assisting with staff development and medical education, participation in the admissions triage, and taking turns for "on call" services further enrich the training experience, providing students a sense of what it is like to be a full-fledged professional psychologist. Participation in multidisciplinary team activities can help students to understand better and appreciate the contributions of other providers while developing their own skills as a contributing and respected team member. Depending on the philosophy of the particular setting, students may also be expected to engage in ongoing research and evaluation activities, which can significantly foster their development as scientist-practitioners.

Postdoctoral Education and Training

Since World War II, training beyond the doctoral degree has undergone significant changes. The 1994 conference on postdoctoral education (APA, 1995) culminated the work of a series of committees and conference groups that had sought for almost two decades to formulate standards for professional education in psychology at the postdoctoral level. In particular, recommendations from the National Working Conference on Education and Training in Health Psychology (Stone, 1983), the National Conference on Graduate Education in Psychology (Bickman, 1987), the APA Task Force on Review of the Scope and Criteria for Accreditation (APA Task Force, 1987), the National Conference on Scientist-Practitioner Education and Training for the Professional Practice of Psychology (Belar & Perry, 1990), the Joint Council on Professional Education in Psychology (JCPEP, 1990), and the National Conference on Postdoctoral Education and Training in Psychology (APA, 1995) reflect a growing recognition that specialty practice in psychology requires an integrated program of preparation that extends from the doctoral degree into the postdoctoral period. Summaries of recommendations from these training conference reports are available in Appendix F of the proceedings of the 1994 National Conference on Postdoctoral Education and Training in Psychology (APA, 1995).

In 1996, the APA Council of Representatives approved a taxonomy for the education and training for psychologists which includes postdoctoral education, thereby paving the way for accreditation of postdoctoral training programs. As was true with the accreditation of predoctoral programs and internships, this development will no doubt stimulate the upgrading of training programs as well as bring about the revision of existing credentialing mechanisms to accommodate this expanded structure. Specialty fields such as health psychology will be quick to embrace this model, viewing it as supportive of efforts to achieve recognition for specialized training and ultimately to gain greater parity with medicine.

Increasingly, postdoctoral training is being viewed as a necessary component of the preparation needed for independent practice in any area of applied-professional psychology. Postdoctoral residencies and fellowships provide opportunities for in-depth education and training in an area of specialization and may include training in special proficiencies associated with a given specialty. As an example, one might specialize in health psychology but also add special proficiencies in the treatment of problems such as eating disorders, headaches, or pain. The period of training may, as a minimum, be one year; however, specialization in health psychology will probably require at least two years of formal preparation in the future. Postdoctoral training should culminate with the completion of state or provincial licensing procedures. Increasing numbers of health psychologists will seek board certification in Health Psychology through application to the American Board of Professional Psychology (ABPP). Application for board certification by the ABPP has, in the past, required at least five years of postdoctoral experience; however, this time period has recently been reduced to two years in order to better align the ABPP model with the taxonomy of training adopted in 1996 by the APA. Listing in the National Register of Health Service Providers in Psychology following a year of supervised experience licensure provides an additional credential and potentially increases acceptance of the individual's training for reimbursement purposes.

Counseling psychologists may seek ABPP specialty certification in either counseling or health psychology. Some may pursue both options. Although board certification in psychology has not previously been important to most psychologists in improving employment status, gaining hospital privileges, or qualifying for reimbursement, it is highly probable that health psychology will follow the path of medicine in the near future and board certification in an appropriate specialty will be linked to privileges in certain areas of practice. The viability of ABPP certification in counseling psychology or health psychology will depend, in large part, on the requirements of settings in which counseling psychologists are employed and the degree to which counseling psychology is maintained as a unique specialty field.

Specialization or Special Proficiencies?

As students plan careers in medical and physical health settings, they should anticipate the need for specialty training beyond the doctoral degree as well as lifelong continuing education that may include the addition of special proficiencies. A specialty such as health psychology is broader than a special proficiency but should have unique and differentiating features relative to other specialties with respect to populations served, problems addressed, and the procedures and techniques typically utilized by its practitioners. A special proficiency (e.g., alcohol/substance abuse intervention) is more limited in scope and:

- can be included in its practice by one or more specialties
- can be discriminated by the population, problem, or technology that is its focus
- meets a public need
- is recognized by the psychology profession (JICIRSP, 1995).

Thus, as formalized postdoctoral training is gradually adopted as a prerequisite to the independent practice of health psychology, most practitioners will find the acquision of special proficiences to be helpful in remaining competitive, meeting the needs of specific patient groups, and qualifying for reimbursement in proficiencies that may come under state or agency regulation. (e.g., the regulation of substance abuse counseling and intervention in some jurisdictions). As one response to this need, the American College of Psychology was organized in 1994 by the APA for the specific purpose of providing training and credentialing for the practice of special proficiencies within a continuing education format.

Future Trends and Prospects

A Seamless System of Education, Accreditation, and Credentialing

As the field of health psychology continues to evolve, it is likely to follow the medical model in developing an integrated, seamless system of education, accreditation, and credentialing. Within such a system (figure 2.1), students will be required to complete accredited programs at all levels and complete appropriate examination and credentialing procedures. In many respects, the Examination for Professional Practice in Psychology (EPPP),

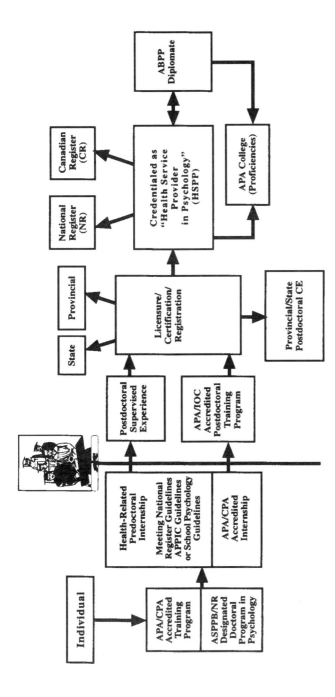

Figure 2.1. Seamless model of training, accreditation, and credentialing. The flow chart illustrates the interrelationships among components that contribute to the training and credentialing of a health psychologist. (Reprinted and modified with permission from the *Register Report* [1997, Vol. 23] published by the Council for the National Register of Health Service Providers in Psychology.)

47

administered by the Association for State and Provincial Psychology Boards, already serves as an exit examination for graduates of professional psychology training programs. As previously stated, the revised procedures of the ABPP now allow application for board examination following two years of postdoctoral training. If postdoctoral practitioners wish to add special proficiencies, additional training and proficiency certification will also be available through the American College of Psychology. As information regarding performance of graduates on various examination procedures is fed back to programs by credentialing bodies (e.g., EPPP scores over eight domains), the entire system should become more highly interrelated and integrated in the future.

Separation of the Predoctoral Program and Internship?

As health psychology has increasingly adopted the medical model of education, questions have been raised regarding appropriateness of maintaining the internship as a part of the predoctoral program versus separating the two components and granting the doctoral degree after all course work, practica, and research/dissertation requirements are completed. Students could then enter an internship with doctoral degrees in hand similar to M.D.s and would potentially be granted more status than would be the case as a doctoral trainee without the degree. The internship program, which is also accredited, would then become totally responsible for continuing the educational process. Recommendations for relocating the internship to the postdoctoral period were made by Practice Group VII of the National Conference on Postdoctoral Education and Training in Psychology (APA, 1995), and a resolution supporting such a move was introduced but not acted upon in the 1997 winter meeting of the American Psychological Association Council of Representatives. Major advantages cited by proponents include the following (APA, 1995, p. 162):

1. The change would effect better alignment of medical and psychology training models with respect to level of practice, status, and title.
2. The awarding of a doctoral degree before entry into internship would facilitate reimbursement for services of interns in an era when managed care companies are refusing to pay for services rendered by subdoctoral, nonlicensed providers.

3. Given the small amount of interaction that typically occurs between campus-based doctoral programs and internship sites once students are placed, the suggested change would place the locus of responsibility on those individuals who are actually providing the training.
4. Students would be more likely to complete their dissertation research in a timely fashion and would be able to devote full attention to the internship experience.

While there presently appears to be little receptivity among training programs for separation of the internship from predoctoral training, the idea is compelling and not likely to go away, at least in health psychology. Given the history of ideas that initially seemed to be revolutionary and impractical (e.g., prescription privileges for psychologists), such innovations often take on a life of their own within professional organizations and, over time, become reality through the efforts and persistence of advocates. As training in health psychology becomes more closely aligned with that of medicine, it seems likely that the notion of separating program and internship will continue to surface in future deliberations of the psychology community as it prepares for the twenty-first century.

Summary

Within the family of health professions in the United States, psychology has arrived on the scene relatively late. While the health field presents many opportunities for nonmedical providers, professional counselors and counseling psychologists have not rushed in large numbers to develop training programs; neither have they developed well established career paths in these settings. At the same time, the recent approval of a Health Section in the APA Division of Counseling Psychology signals a growing interest in health applications among a significant group of counseling psychologists. As counselors and counseling psychologists prepare for health-setting practice in the future, it will be increasingly important to be aware of changes in credentialing and training requirements. In most instances, completion of an accredited program and internship and an appropriate postdoctoral experience will be required for licensure and for gaining health care positions in the future. As factors such as program accreditation and levels of certification become increasingly linked to funding structures, careful attention should be given to the education and training component of career planning.

For counseling psychologists, the development of health psychology as a postdoctoral specialty field is a real plus. Such a structure permits individuals to gain the training offered by a counseling program, accessing specialization in health psychology through the internship and postdoctoral residency. If such a pattern is to prove viable, it is essential that predoctoral training programs in counseling psychology provide appropriate courses and field experiences for those students who choose health careers and that students be assisted in identifying appropriate practica and internships. The combination of traditional emphases in counseling psychology with relevant electives in health-related subject fields can provide a highly attractive training package that will have appeal for internship selection committees.

Finally, the health field is undergoing rapid changes in the face of managed care initiatives and technological advances. Consequences of these changes are increased competition for funds and an increased sensitivity to accountability and cost containment. As nonmedical providers such as counselors and counseling psychologists plan health careers, they should make sound choices in the selection of training programs and internships, maintain a spirit of openness and flexibility in their work with other providers, and exercise patience in locating the right niche in the health system. Those who prepare well and exercise patience coupled with persistence are more likely to be successful!

Suggested Resources

Psychophysiological Disorders: Research and Clinical Applications, edited by Gatchel and Blanchard (1993), provides a current perspective on health psychology and behavioral medicine and then explores the epidemiology and etiology, as well as assessment and treatment, of ten common chronic health problems. This book is styled for the scientist-practitioner and would provide students with an excellent beginning relative to understanding the psychobiological basis for common health disorders.

Healthy People 2000 (U.S. Department of Health and Human Services, 1990) provides an excellent basis for understanding life-span development issues as they relate to physical health and well-being. This publication provides a rationale for the development of prevention programs that are tailored to the peculiar needs of different age groups.

Nicassio and Smith (1995) discuss the biopsychosocial model and examine professional and organizational issues that shape the delivery of health services in *Managing Chronic Illness: A Biopsychosocial Perspective.* This book focuses on clinical issues that are relevant across chronic illnesses rather than dealing with specific conditions. Topics include assessment, stress management, adherence to medical regimens, and ethnocultural considerations of service delivery. It aligns well with counseling psychology training model that tends to take a systemic approach to the understanding of chronic disease.

Tarlow (1989) addresses a number of the chronic health problems that are typically seen by health psychologists in his book *Clinical Handbook of Behavior Therapy: Adult Medical Disorders.* Chapters are written in a parallel form for each disorder. They provide a brief overview of assessment methods and treatment strategies and include a listing of key references. The cognitive-behavioral models presented align well with prevailing treatment in health settings.

Special issues of journals provide an excellent foundation for understanding issues that relate to the training and preparation of psychologists for health settings. Of particular relevance, in chronological order, are the 1983 (2[5]) issue of *Health Psychology* and the 1985 (13[1]), 1991 (19[3]), and 1992 (20[4]) issues of *The Counseling Psychologist.*

Discussion Questions

1. What are the major historical antecedents of nonmedical practice in health care settings?
2. How and in what ways have perspectives from the medical model influenced the developing model of education and training of counselors and psychologist who work in the health field?
3. What major training conferences have shaped the design of training for health psychology programs? What are the major recommendations from the Arden House Conference on Health Psychology?
4. What are some distinguishing features of predoctoral internships and post-doctoral residency programs?
5. What types of special or elective courses and practicum experiences are recommended for the counseling or counseling psychology student who wishes to pursue a health-related career?

6. What is the difference between a specialty and a special proficiency? What are examples of each?
7. What types of credentials would be beneficial for an individual who plans a career as a health counselor or health psychologist?
8. What kinds of education and training will be required in order to obtain a license to practice in a health setting?

References

Alcorn, J. D. (1991). Counseling psychology and health applications. *The Counseling Psychologist, 19*(3), 325–341.

Alcorn, J. D., & McPhearson, R. (1997). Counseling psychology in multidisciplinary health settings: Implications for future training. *The Counseling Psychologist, 25*(4), 637–653.

Altmaier, E. M. (1991). Research and practice roles for counseling psychologists in health care settings. *The Counseling Psychologist, 19*(3), 243–264.

American Psychological Association. (1995). *Education and training beyond the doctoral degree: Proceedings of the National Conference on Postdoctoral Education and Training in Psychology.* Washington, DC: Author.

American Psychological Association. (1996). *Guidelines and principles for accreditation of programs in professional psychology* (Book I). Washington, DC: Author.

APA Task Force on Review of the Scope and Criteria for Accreditation. (1987). *Report no. 4: Recommendations for the future scope of accreditation and for specialty recognition in professional psychology.* Washington, DC: American Psychological Association.

Belar, C. D., Bieliauskas, L. A., Larsen, K. G., Mensh, I. N., Poey, K., & Roehlke, H. J. (1989). National conference on internship training in psychology. *American Psychologist, 44*(1), 60–65.

Belar, C. D., & Perry, N. W. (Eds.). (1990). *Proceedings: National conference on scientist-practitioner education and training for the profession of psychology.* Sarasota, FL: Professional Resource Press.

Belar, C. D., Wilson, E., & Hughes, H. (1982). Health psychology training in doctoral psychology programs. *Health Psychology, 1*(3), 289–299.

Bickman, L. (Ed.). (1987). Proceedings of the national conference on graduate education in psychology [Special Issue]. *American Psychologist, 42*(12).

Corrigan, J. D. (1991). Counseling psychology and health applications: A response. The *Counseling Psychologist, 19,* (3), 382–386.

Department of Health and Human Services. (1990). *Healthy People 2000* (DHHS Publication No. 9150213). Washington, DC: U.S. Government Printing Office.

Division 12 Task Force on Promotion and Dissemination of Psychological Procedures. (1995). Training in and dissemination of empirically validated psychological treatments: Report and recommendations. *The Clinical Psychologist, 48,* 3–23.

Fox, R. E. (1992). Postdoctoral training for the preparation and regulation of professional psychologists. *Psychotherapy in private practice, 10*(1–2), 101–109.

Gatchel, R. J., & Blanchard, E. B. (Eds.). (1993). *Psychophysiological disorders: Research and clinical applications.* Washington, DC: American Psychological Association.

Gentry, W. D. (Ed.). (1984). *Handbook of behavioral medicine.* New York: Guilford.

Harris, J. K. (1991). Evolution of a health focus: Old values-new practices in counseling psychology education and training. *The Counseling Psychologist, 19*(3), 365–375.

Hollandsworth, J. G., Jr. (1985). Counseling psychology, health psychology, and beyond: A reply to Klippel and DeJoy. *Journal of Counseling Psychology, 32*(1), 150–153.

Joint Council on Professional Education in Psychology (JCPEP). (1990). *Report of the Joint Council on Professional Education in Psychology.* Baton Rouge, LA: T. T. Stigall.

Joint Interim Committee for the Identification and Recognition of Specialties and Proficiencies (JICIRSP). (1995). *Principles for recognition of proficiencies in psychology.* Washington, DC: American Psychological Association.

Kagan, N. (1979). Counseling psychology, interpersonal skills, and health care. In G. C. Stone, F. Cohen, & N. Adler (Eds.), *Health psychology: A handbook* (pp. 465–485). San Francisco: Jossey-Bass.

Kagan, N., Armsworth, M. W., Altmaier, E. M., Dowd, E. T., Hansen, J. C., Mills, D. H., Schlossberg, N., Sprinthall, N. A., Tanney, M. F., & Vasquez, M. J. T. (1988). Professional practice of counseling psychology in various settings. *The Counseling Psychologist, 16*(3), 247–365.

Klippel, J. A., & DeJoy, D. M. (1984). Counseling psychology in behavioral medicine and health psychology. *Journal of Counseling Psychology, 31*(2), 219–227.

Kivlighan, D. M., Jr. (1995, August). *1995 survey of doctoral training programs: Report to the Council of counseling psychology training programs.* Report presented at the annual meeting of the American Psychological Association, New York.

Larson, P. C., & Agresti, A. A. (1992). Counseling psychology and neuropsychology: An overview. *The Counseling Psychologist, 20*(4), 549–555.

Matarazzo, J. D. (1980). Behavioral health and behavioral medicine. *American Psychologist, 35,* 8807–8817.

May, E. (1977). Counseling psychologists in general medicine and surgical hospitals. *The Counseling Psychologist, 7*(2), 82–85.

Nathan, P. E., & Gorman, J. M. (Eds.). (1998). *A guide to treatments that work.* New York: Oxford University.

Nicassio, P. M., & Smith, T. W. (Eds.). (1995). *Managing chronic illness: A biopsychosocial perspective.* Washington, DC: American Psychological Association.

Schwartz, G. E. (1982). Testing the biopsychosocial model: The ultimate test facing behavioral medicine? *Journal of Consulting and Clinical Psychology, 50*(6), 1040–1053.

Sheridan, E. P., Matarazzo, J. D., Boll, T. J., Perry, M. W. Jr., Weiss, S. M., & Belar, C. D. (1988). Postdoctoral education and training for clinical service providers in health psychology. *Health Psychology, 7*(1), 1–17.

Stone, G. C. (Ed.). (1983). Proceedings of the national working conference on education and training in health psychology [Special Issue]. *Health Psychology, 2*(5).

Syme, L. S. (1984). Sociocultural factors and disease etiology. In W. D. Gentry (Ed.), *Handbook of behavioral medicine* (pp. 13–37). New York: Guilford.

Tarlow, G. T. (1989). *Clinical handbook of behavior therapy: Adult medical disorders.* Cambridge, MA: Brookline.

Taylor, C. B. (1985). Let's get practical. *The Counseling Psychologist, 13*(1), 105–108.

Thoresen, C. E., & Eagleston, J. R. (1985). Counseling for health. *The Counseling Psychologist, 13,* 23–29.

White, N. F. (1988). Medical and graduate education in behavioral medicine and the evolution of health care. *Annals of Behavioral Medicine, 10*(1), 23–29.

Wiens, A. N., & Baum, C. G. (1995). Characteristics of current postdoctoral programs: Education and training beyond the doctoral degree. In *Education and training beyond the doctoral degree: Proceedings of the American Psychological Association National Conference on Postdoctoral Education and Training in Psychology* (pp. 27–46). Washington, DC: American Psychological Association.

3

Ethical Issues and the Health Care Setting

Sharon E. Robinson Kurpius
Katherine Vaughn Fielder

The wedding of counseling psychology and health care is a natural one, even though counseling psychologists have been slow to discover this. As Klippel and DeJoy pointed out in 1984, the extent to which counseling psychologists assume an important role in health care "depends on counseling psychology's willingness and ability to respond to the challenges associated with studying the relationship of behavior to health" (p. 219). This chapter focuses on the ethics that shape the behavior of counseling psychologists who have chosen to meet this challenge to offer their expertise in the health care arena.

The following discussion of ethical behavior is grounded in five fundamental ethical principles or precepts (Kitchener, 1984):

1. Beneficence, "the principle of benefiting others, of accepting a responsibility to do good, underlies the profession" (Welfel & Kitchener, 1992, p. 180).
2. Nonmaleficence, doing no harm, requires psychologists not to perpetuate physical or emotional harm or to engage in behavior that could result in harm to another.
3. Autonomy is our belief in a client's right to choose.
4. Justice requires psychologists to act fairly and justly, balancing the rights of clients with those of others.
5. Fidelity includes keeping promises and being trustworthy and loyal.

With these five in mind, let us move to a discussion of psychologist responsibilities, patient rights, and business practices.

- Psychologist responsibilities include issues of competence and concerns with dual relationships.
- Patient rights focus on informed consent, confidentiality, and duty to warn.
- Business practices include billing, advertising, and endorsement issues.

Psychologist Responsibilities

Competence

Regarding competence, the initial principle of the *Ethical Principles of Psychologists and Code of Conduct* of the American Psychological Association (APA, 1992), states:

> Psychologists strive to maintain high standards of competence in their work. They recognize the boundaries of their particular competencies and the limitations of their expertise. They provide only those services and use only those techniques for which they are qualified by education, training, or experience. Psychologists are cognizant of the fact that the competencies required in serving, teaching, and/or studying groups of people vary with the distinctive characteristics of those groups. In those areas in which recognized professional standards do not yet exist, psychologists exercise careful judgment and take appropriate precautions to protect the welfare of those with whom they work. They maintain knowledge of relevant scientific and professional information related to the services they render, and they recognize the need for ongoing education. Psychologists make appropriate use of scientific, professional, technical, and administrative resources.

Several areas related to counseling health psychology are subsumed under this principle and defined by specific Ethical Standards:

- education and training
- boundaries and limitations of expertise
- recognition of personal problems that may interfere with professional competency
- provision of services to diverse groups
- use of appropriate assessment strategies

Education and Training

In chapter 2, Alcorn provides an excellent survey of the education and train-ing required to be proficient in providing health care services as a counsel-ing psychologist. As he notes, core training includes not only relevant course work in counseling psychology and health psychology but also practicum and internship experiences in a health or medical setting. Beyond these basic competencies is the responsibility of mental health professionals to be famil-iar with the medical arena. They need to be familiar with both biological and psychological aspects of the illnesses of their patients, available medical interventions, effects of various medications, typical hospital procedures and protocol, and medical terminology. In addition, they need to realize that the medical setting has a long-established hierarchy, with the physician as the final decision-maker with respect to the care of the patient.

Not only are counseling psychologists responsible for ensuring that they are adequately prepared by graduate and postgraduate training to enter the health care field, but they must also maintain their expertise (Ethical Standard 1.05, Maintaining Expertise). This means staying abreast of the evolving knowledge in counseling psychology and in the medical areas in which they practice. This may include taking continuing education courses, reading professional journals in both medicine and psychology, and attend-ing professional conferences such as that of the Society of Behavioral Medicine or sessions for Division 38, Health Psychology, at the APA annu-al convention. As Dubin (1972) suggested, the half-life of a Ph.D. is 10 years when no further postgraduate education is obtained. Belar and Deardorff (1995) suggest that in the area of clinical health psychology this half-life is considerably less.

Boundaries and Limitations of Expertise

Taking into consideration their education, training, and experiences, psy-chologists need to recognize the boundaries and limitations of their exper-tise (Ethical Standard 1.04a, Boundaries of Competence). For example, just because one has extensive knowledge and experience working with individ-uals who have eating disorders does not mean that he or she can transfer that knowledge and experience to working with another medical population. Similarly, a psychologist who has worked exclusively in a private practice or other mental health settings with clients who have not had health-related concerns does not have the expertise to begin offering services as a health psychologist. If a client does seek therapy for psychophysiological problems, the best course would be to refer to a competent colleague or to continue to work with the person while reading related health literature and seeking supervision from a colleague trained in this health care area. Additionally, after seeking the client's permission, it would be essential to talk with his or her physician.

The field of health psychology is extremely diverse, with a variety of practice areas. It is incumbent on mental health professionals to be aware of their own knowledge and skill limitations and take whatever steps are necessary to ensure ethical professional behavior within the boundaries of professional competence.

Personal Problems

In addition to professional competence, we must also be aware of personal competence. When personal problems impact one's ability to provide the highest quality care, according to Ethical Standard 1.13, Personal Problems and Conflicts, psychologists must "recognize that their problems and conflicts may interfere with their effectiveness" (1.13a) and therefore "refrain from undertaking any activity when they know that their personal problems are likely to lead to harm" of others (1.13a). In addition, psychologists need "to be alert to signs of, and to obtain assistance for, their personal problems at an early stage, in order to prevent significantly impaired performance" (1.13b). When personal problems interfere with their ability to provide clients with quality care, they need to "take appropriate measures, such as obtaining professional consultation or assistance, and determine whether they should limit, suspend, or terminate their work-related duties" (1.13c).

Working in health care can be emotionally draining; therefore, health psychologists need to be particularly aware of burnout and work-related stress. As noted by Pope, Tabachnick, and Keith-Spiegel (1987), too often mental health professionals continue to work when feeling too distressed to be effective, and a significant proportion (5.9%) report working while under the influence of alcohol. Clearly, such behavior is not only unethical but it is harmful, violating the tenet of nonmaleficence.

Provision of Services to Diverse Groups

In chapter 15, Ruiz Rodriguez provides an excellent discussion of working with diverse populations. As with the other aspects of competence, mental health professionals must be trained to work with diverse groups either through course work and practica or through work experience with close supervision. Diversity includes racial or ethnic differences, cultural differences, socioeconomic differences, and belief differences, to name only a few.

Based on the precepts of justice and beneficence, competency in working with diverse groups is multidimensional. The foundational issue is conducting cross-cultural counseling ethically. Indeed, our literature is replete with articles related to the knowledge, skills, and awareness necessary to counsel individuals from a culture different from one's own. An aspect of cross-cultural counseling unique to working with medical patients involves their health beliefs. Health beliefs include how patients conceptualize their health concern—as a disease, an illness, or a sickness—and what they believe will make them better—medication, prayer, medical interventions, or doing nothing. Understanding the patient's culture and health beliefs and the perspective of the medical team can help the psychologist to facilitate effective interventions and increase medical adherence by the patient.

Use of Appropriate Assessment Strategies

The final area of competence involves assessment. Many of the authors in this text refer to assessments appropriate for their patient populations. A core concept across all patient categories is that of choosing tests and assessment procedures that take into consideration appropriate standardization procedures for medical patients (Ethical Standard 2.04a, Use of Assessment in General and With Special Populations). Too often tests that have been normed on psychiatric populations are used with health care patients and other mental health clients. In addition, tests and individual test questions designed to assess concepts such as depression, mood, or coping may be assessing aspects of the medical condition or treatment. Knowledge of the components of a disease that may be tapped by particular questions can help psychologists to be more accurate when doing psychological assessments and interpretations.

Another important aspect of assessment is patient confidentiality. Typically, the referring physician will want to know about any assessments that have been conducted with the patient. Before the psychologist gives such information, the patient should have been informed of the potential use of the assessment results and informed consent and release-of-information should have been obtained. It is the psychologist's responsibility to protect test information and to be cautious in how assessment data are shared. Non-mental health professionals are not trained in interpreting psychological assessment data; therefore, the psychologist should interpret the results for them. This allows the psychologist to explain norm groups and any extenuating circumstances surrounding the testing or assessment. The best interests of the patient must be always at the forefront to avoid misuse of assessment data. This is particularly important when medical treatment depends largely on assessment results, as sometimes happens in transplant cases.

In addition to providing feedback to the referring physician, the psychologist must provide feedback to the patient in a manner that is understandable and promotes the patient's welfare. Pope (1992) makes some excellent suggestions for providing test feedback to patients.

A final caveat regarding assessment: Be sure to note the difference between making a psychological diagnosis and arriving at a medical opinion. We need to remember that our domain of expertise is psychology, not medicine, and that to interfere in the medical aspects of a patient's treatment is not only unethical, but also perhaps illegal.

Indeed, the Ethical Principle of Competence should compel mental health professionals to be sensitive to the possibility of negligence and malpractice. Practicing within one's expertise, remaining emotionally healthy, seeking continued education, and consulting and referring as appropriate will be the best defense against incompetence and malpractice.

Dual Relationships

Dual relationships occur when mental health "professionals assume two roles simultaneously or sequentially with a person seeking help" (Herlihy & Corey, 1992, p. 1). These roles may consist of a professional and a nonprofessional role or two professional roles such as therapist, supervisor, consultant, or student. Dual relationships always have a power differential, distort the therapeutic alliance, destroy trust, and compromise therapist objectivity. The patient is the person who is harmed. Although the Ethical Standards strongly discourages dual relationships and states that sexual relationships are unethical, dual relationships are the second most reported ethical dilemma (Pope & Vetter, 1992).

Dual relationships are typically broken into two categories—sexual and nonsexual. "One of the oldest mandates in the health care professions is the prohibition against engaging in sexual intimacies with a patient" (Pope & Vasquez, 1991, p. 101). Although some medical professionals may not have ethical guidelines explicitly prohibiting sexual relationships with patients, Standard 4.05 is quite explicit: "Psychologists do not engage in sexual intimacies with current patients or clients." Nor do they "accept as therapy patients or clients persons with whom they have engaged in sexual intimacies" (Ethical Standard 4.06). The Standards impose a two-year moratorium between termination of therapy and a possible sexual relationship with a client. Even in these circumstances the psychologist must be ready to demonstrate that "there has been no exploitation" of the client (Ethical Standard 4.07b).

Nonsexual dual relationships may be more difficult to recognize than sexual ones for the psychologist in a medical setting. For example, if a patient is a finance broker and casually gives the psychologist information about some stocks and the psychologist acts on this information, a dual relationship has been created. Or if a professional colleague such as a nurse or staff member requests help with a personal problem such as family or work stress, it is unethical for the psychologist to serve in a helping role to that person. Being alert to the possibilities and dangers of dual relationships is the best protection against this ethical violation.

Patient Rights

By entering into a fiduciary relationship, one based on the highest confidence and trust and on the tenet of fidelity, psychologists agree to hold the welfare of the client/patient above all else. This responsibility is directly stipulated in Principles D, Respect for People's Rights and Dignity, and Principle E, Concern for Others' Welfare, and is woven throughout all other Principles and Standards. Principle D specifically states:

> Psychologists accord appropriate respect to the fundamental rights, dignity, and worth of all people. They respect the rights of individuals to privacy, confidentiality, self-determination, and autonomy, mindful that legal and other obligations may lead to inconsistency and conflict with the exercise of these rights. Psychologists are aware of cultural, individual, and role differences, including those due to age, gender, race, ethnicity, national origin, religion, sexual orientation, disability, language, and socioeconomic status.

Protecting the patient's rights within the framework of the medical setting can be challenging. Several patient rights issues are evident in the following case.

A psychologist, employed by the hospital, was asked to consult on the case of a 63-year-old, widowed, Catholic, female, Hispanic patient with end-stage emphysema. The referral came from the attending pulmonologist and nursing staff who had unsuccessfully tried to convince the patient to consent to changing her status from "Full Code," in which no efforts would be spared to save her life in the event of cardiac arrest, to "DNR—Do Not Resuscitate." The patient, who could barely talk because each breath was so labored, stubbornly insisted that her chart not be marked DNR. During the course of therapy, it was revealed by the patient that she had no family other than one son with whom she had unresolved conflicts. She had not had any contact with her son for years, but she spoke with conviction about him visiting her in the hospital soon. All efforts by the nursing staff to reach the son had been unsuccessful. Attempts to discuss the consequences of a Full Code were met with resistance on the part of the patient, who refused to imagine or accept any description of possible negative outcomes. When the psychologist returned for a fourth session with the patient, the chart had been changed to DNR, and the patient refused to talk at all. The nursing staff informed the psychologist that the attending physician had "convinced the patient that she was better off as a DNR than a Full Code."

Clearly, questions regarding patient rights come into play in this scenario. First, who is the client—the referring physician or the patient herself? Whose needs are most important—those of the physician who needed her to consent to the DNR in order to provide what he/she felt was best for the patient or those of the patient who wanted to hang onto life until she talked with her son? Values regarding her right to treatment (psychological as well as physical) also come into play. Further, were her ethnicity and potential religious beliefs taken into consideration by the physician? And finally, did she give informed or coerced consent? Whether on the treatment team or serving as an external consultant, the psychologist has many ethical issues to address in order to facilitate behavior that protects the rights, dignity, and welfare of this patient while respecting the skills and responsibilities of the physician.

As demonstrated in this case, patient rights can easily become at risk in a medical setting. The Ethical Standards related to three patient rights—informed consent, confidentiality, and duty to warn—within the practice of health psychology are reviewed below.

Informed Consent

Mandated by the APA Ethical Standards, informed consent provides clients with sufficient information so that they can evaluate the benefits and risks of psychological treatment before deciding whether to participate in therapy. According to Standard 4.02a, the four basic components of informed consent are:

1. knowledge of significant information regarding treatment
2. capacity to consent
3. voluntary expression of consent
4. appropriate documentation of the consent, preferably in written form

Informed consent is obtained as early as possible and apprises the patient about the course of treatment, fees for services, and limits of confidentiality. The patient should also be told if and by whom the psychologist is supervised and whether the mental health professional is a student or intern. In addition, any questions should be carefully answered to avoid misunderstandings about therapy and the psychologist's role in treatment and to build trust. Regardless of whether the information necessary for informed consent is provided in writing or orally, it is imperative that the language be understandable to the patient (Standard 4.01d).

Before informed consent can be obtained, the counseling psychologist is obligated to determine who the actual client is. This can be difficult in the practice of health psychology in that the request for psychological services can originate from the patient, the patient's family, the attending physician, or the nursing staff. Some medical facilities even dictate routine psychological consultation for patients with certain types of illnesses, such as cancer, which makes the answer to the question, who is the client, more ambiguous. Multiple referral sources create an environment in which the psychologist must carefully explain to patients who referred them for counseling and how this referral will impact the sharing of patient information. This can influence a patient's willingness to give informed consent, particularly if there is information the patient may not want shared with members of the treatment team or with the person who made the referral.

The purposes for a health psychology referral are varied, and each referral brings with it a set of potential informed consent dilemmas. To illustrate, a psychologist may be called by a physician who is frustrated with a patient's noncompliance with medical treatment or by a family in order to mediate different opinions about a dying patient's wishes regarding resuscitation following cardiac arrest. In each of these cases, someone other than the patient has requested psychological intervention; however, the patient is the person who must give informed consent. Therefore, it is the responsibility of the health counseling psychologist to fully inform the patient about the nature of the visit, foreseeable disclosure of information gathered in therapy, who requested the evaluation or therapy, and who will pay for it. At times this may place the psychologist in a difficult position since the person(s) who made the referral may have a goal in mind that is not congruent with the patient's wishes. Belar and Deardorff (1995) refer to this as "coping with competing agendas" (p. 124) in that it is quite possible that the physician's goals do not always coincide with those of the patient.

It should be noted that special circumstances come into play when providing psychological services to minors and people with debilitating physical illnesses. Obtaining informed consent from children, people with brain injuries, or people with end-stage disease can be challenging, if not impossible. The Ethical Standards provide some guidance for these situations: Psychologists are required to "obtain informed permission from a legally authorized person, if such substitute consent is permitted by law" (Standard 4.02b) and to "inform those persons who are legally incapable of giving informed consent about the proposed interventions in a manner commensurate with the person's psychological capacities" (Standard 4.02c-1). Even when the patient is not fully capable of understanding information regarding treatment, the psychologist must seek informed assent (Standard 4.02c-2) and consider the patient's "preferences and best interests" (Standard 4.02c-3). Typically, minors and incapacitated adults give informed assent, while their parent or legal guardian gives informed consent. As Calfee (1997) noted, failure to obtain informed consent is often grounds for malpractice suits.

Informed consent for patients who are minors or mentally incompetent presents the psychologist with special concerns. When the patient is a minor who is at least seven years old, psychologists should get the minor's informed assent for treatment (Lawrence & Robinson Kurpius, 1997), as well as the informed consent of the parents or legal guardian. If an adult patient is incapable of giving informed consent, the consent of a legal guardian is required. Readers are referred to the chapters on rehabilitation (chapter 9) and on pediatric health psychology (chapter 12) for more detailed discussions about these two patient groups.

Issues of informed consent are closely tied to issues surrounding privacy and confidentiality.

Confidentiality

The origins of confidentiality are found in the Fourth Amendment of the United States Constitution, which affords citizens the right to privacy. It is the health psychologist's ethical responsibility to respect a client's legal right to control personal information and others' access to it. Early and continuous discussions of the meaning and limits of confidentiality, as well as information about "foreseeable uses of information generated" (Standard 5.01), provide the standard for ethical practice as well as set the foundation for protection against possible charges of malpractice.

It is important to differentiate between the professional term of confidentiality and the legal concept of privileged communication. Privileged communication is provided between licensed psychologists or other legally credentialed mental health professionals and their patients and varies according to state statutes (Robinson Kurpius, 1997). The privilege belongs to the patient, not to the mental health professional. Generally, four criteria must be met to establish privileged communication (Schwitzgebel & Schwitzgebel, 1980):

1. The communication takes place with the client's understanding that it will not be disclosed.
2. Confidentiality is strictly maintained.
3. The relationship is one which, in the opinion of the community, ought to be fostered.
4. The injury to the relationship by disclosure is greater than the benefit gained by correct disposal of litigation.

To breach privilege without a client's consent is considered an invasion of his or her constitutional right to privacy (Everstine et al., 1980).

Psychologists report that dilemmas involving confidentiality are the most prevalent ethical issue they encounter (Pope & Vetter, 1992). Upholding confidentiality is particularly burdensome in a medical setting, where communication between referral sources, patient's family, nursing staff, quality assurance review boards, and others is critical to the comprehensive care provided within the framework of a multidisciplinary team approach. Hospitals require treatment notes to be charted in the patient's medical record, which is easily accessible by hospital staff and physicians' and psychologists' office staff (Pope, 1990).

Patients must sign a release of information for medical records to be transferred to another party; however, progress notes for psychological care are often kept in the same chart as medical treatment notes. Although releases may not specify psychological information, this information is frequently sent along as part of the complete record (Belar & Deardorff, 1995). In addition, practice guidelines for record keeping (APA Board of Professional Affairs, 1993) note that psychologists are responsible for their staff keeping client information confidential. This raises the question of whether in a hospital setting the psychologist is also responsible for others, such as nurses, aides, and physicians, who may read charted notes maintaining the patient's confidentiality.

Another confidentiality concern arises when one considers that direct communication with the client can be difficult when hospital rooms are occupied by more than one patient and interruptions by medical personnel are commonplace. As Belar and Deardorff (1995) point out, often a patient is not ambulatory and due to the multiple-person hospital room, confidentiality is not possible. In situations where confidentiality cannot be assured, the patient should be given the option of declining psychological intervention without undue coercion to talk with the psychologist.

In spite of the problems inherent in a medical setting, the health psychologist must take meticulous precautions to ensure the confidentiality of his or her clients. Continuous discussion with the patient about the limits of confidentiality from the beginning of the relationship throughout the course of treatment is required by APA Ethical Standard 5.01. In light of the APA Standards, it would behoove any counseling psychologist or mental health professional to obtain written consent to release information even to the referring physician and treatment team.

Duty to Warn/Protect

Exceptions to maintaining confidentiality exist, and Ethical Standard 5.05 presents guidelines for disclosure without the patient's consent. Generally, these exceptions are provided to protect incapacitated adults or children from exploitation and to protect the patient or others from harm. Disclosure of information to obtain fees for service will be discussed later.

In the practice of health psychology it is not unusual to encounter people who struggle endlessly to cope with chronic and/or debilitating illnesses. Within this context, the psychologist is placed in a position where the balance between guarding the welfare of the client and respecting his or her rights to hold different values, attitudes, and opinions (Standard 1.09) must be carefully weighed. There is, perhaps, no other area in which ethical dilemmas emerge with such force. Protecting patients' rights to autonomy and self-determination when they have determined that they no longer wish to live directly conflicts with the psychologist's duty to protect clients from harm (Standard 5.05). The following case clearly exemplifies this ethical dilemma.

The patient is an 81-year-old Caucasian female, self-referred for individual psychotherapy for depression. For the past two years the patient has experienced a rapid decline in her physical health due to a chronic heart condition. She complains of lack of energy, little motivation to accomplish tasks, anger at her "laziness," and guilt about not being able to participate in the active lifestyle to which she was accustomed. She spends much time in therapy reviewing her life, lamenting "mistakes" she has made in raising her children, and resenting the fact that she had not been able to pursue a career in science because of limitations placed on women's career activities when she was younger. She often expresses anger at her physical condition, stating that she has always acted on her desires and that this is the first time in her life that she has been forced to adjust to a situation instead of "fixing" it. As her physical condition deteriorates, she talks openly about suicide, revealing a carefully thought-out plan that she has the means to complete. When discussing the desire to end her life, the patient appears to be calm, objective, and accurate in her assessment of her physical limitations and how suicide might affect her family. The patient conscientiously considers alternatives to suicide and willingly participates in cognitive restructuring activities intended to help her accept her disability. She remains confident in her decision and informs the mental health professional that if her physical condition continues to worsen, the quality of her life is such that life is not worth continuing.

Many issues concerning values and ethics are called into play in this case. The psychologist's personal stance on the right to die, particularly when the patient is elderly and critically ill, is a value that must be seriously examined. In addition, when deciding how to respond to this type of situation, the mental health professional needs to take into consideration legal and ethical guidelines. Our ethical guidelines clearly state that we must prevent individuals from doing harm to themselves or others and to breach confidentiality if necessary to accomplish this (Standard 5.05). In addition, psychologists must be cognizant of the welfare of other persons affected directly or indirectly by their work, and they bear a social responsibility to consider how their behavior may alter both the life of the patient and the lives of the patient's loved ones. Exploration of these complex issues is crucial when patients, such as this 81-year-old woman, are considering self-inflicted or physician-assisted suicide.

In cases such as this one, the primary care physician should be consulted and perhaps other members of the treatment team as well. Of course, it is the psychologist's responsibility to tell the patient that confidentiality will be broken for safety reasons. The psychologist must then be prepared to deal with the consequences of this action on the therapeutic relationship. The mental health professional walks a fine line balancing the patient's right to autonomy and privacy and the responsibility to protect the patient from harm.

In the case of this patient, when the mental health professional discussed her concerns with the physician and treating team, the physician addressed the patient's medical concerns with the patient along with treatment options. As a result, the patient felt as if she had more options and eventually had heart valve surgery. By addressing the problem with the medical team, the patient received optimal care, which positively affected her health on multiple levels.

The dilemmas surrounding duty to warn have escalated with the increasing numbers of HIV+ or AIDS patients (Harding, Gray, & Neal, 1993). The ruling in *Tarasoff v. Regents of the University of California* (1974, 1976) first articulated the responsibility of psychologists to protect third parties from potential harm by their clients. Since that ruling, 14 jurisdictions outside of California have adopted and applied rulings similar to that of *Tarasoff* and in some cases have extended it to include persons who are not directly threatened (Perlin, 1997). What exactly does this mean when you are working with a patient who has a life-threatening communicable illness such as AIDS and refuses to tell his or her sexual partner? In making a decision about duty to protect, mental health professionals need to consider legal and ethical guidelines and what is in the best interests of the patient. It should be noted that each state may differ on what is legally acceptable behavior. For example, Arizona mental health professionals in possession of such information may report this information to the Arizona Department of Health and be immune from civil and criminal liability for making this report (Arizona Revised Statute 32-1457).

APA has taken a leadership role in this area. At the 1991 APA convention, the Council of Representatives passed a resolution that takes the position that psychologists should work with the client to encourage him or her to disclose this information to the partner but that *no* legal duty be imposed to protect third parties. The resolution goes on to state:

> If, however, specific legislation is considered, then it should permit disclosure only when the provider knows of an identifiable third party who the provider has a compelling reason to believe is at significant risk for infection; the provider has a reasonable belief that the third party has no reason

to suspect that he or she is at risk; and the client/patient has been urged to inform the third party and has either refused or is considered unreliable in his/her willingness to notify the third party. (APA, 1991, p. 1)

When balancing all pros and cons of a decision to disclose when working in a medical setting, it is imperative to consult with the attending physician and perhaps with the state psychologist licensing board. In addition, psychologists need to be aware of tort and legislative laws that relate to the area of assessing patient dangerousness and their duty to warn others. This is a area increasingly fraught with lawsuits and court rulings that should guide practice.

By now it should be evident that holding the welfare and rights of the patient above all else can be challenging in the practice of health psychology. Thorough knowledge and careful consideration of all the ethical principles and standards and of relevant state statutes is crucial in order to practice ethically within a health care setting. Beneficence and maleficence must be carefully weighed and decisions regarding disclosure thoughtfully made.

Business Practices

Regard for the patient's welfare is not limited to therapy alone. The psychologist's fiduciary responsibility to the patient continues throughout the business management of a psychological practice. The following discussion examines ethical considerations in the areas of patient/insurance billing, advertising/marketing, and endorsements.*

Third-party payment of fees for psychological services carries with it a direct threat to confidentiality. Before an insurance company will process a claim, a diagnosis and procedure code describing the service and basic rationale for service is required. It is not uncommon for insurance companies to request a more complete description of services in the form of progress notes; therefore, psychologists often find themselves in an ethical bind. Guarantees of confidentiality cannot be given once the records leave the psychologist's care, for it is impossible to know who and how many people have access to the insurance claim while it is being processed. Since the insurance claim becomes part of the health history of the patient, when a person applies for new health or life insurance, the record of prior services can be accessed from a national insurance database.

---

*For a more complete discussion of the business aspects of practice, see "The Business of Psychology" chapter in Bersoff, 1995.

Additionally, psychologists should be aware that some insurance companies provide policy usage summaries to their contracted client organizations and provide the names of, diagnosis codes for, and amounts billed to the employees. This destroys any attempt at patient confidentiality.

Disclosure of patient information is permitted to obtain payment if the patient has consented. However, as Everstine and colleagues (1980) noted, the "blanket" release-of-information form, often signed by the patient when he or she is being checked into the hospital, results in ethical dilemmas when third-party payers demand confidential patient information. Too often the persons requiring this information are clerical workers and not mental health professionals who might have some sensitivity to the confidential nature of the information. Given this potentially broad exposure of patient information, the authors of the APA Standard 5.05a recommend that psychologists submit the minimal amount of information necessary for payment to be made.

A final note regarding insurance companies is in order. It is fraudulent for services of the mental health provider to be submitted to an insurance company as if they had been delivered by the medical provider.

Another business-related issue concerns accurate and appropriate advertisement of services. Ethical Standard 3.03, Avoidance of False or Deceptive Statements, specifies that psychologists must be particularly careful not to guarantee success in the treatment of physical illness or the psychological problems associated with them. Even if advertisements are created by public relations firms or ad agencies, as is increasingly typical for hospitals, psychologists are ethically required to monitor how their names are associated with claims of cure. The use of testimonials of patients who have overcome poor physical health habits is strictly forbidden. In addition, Belar and Deardorff (1995) point out that psychologists must ensure that patients are aware of their professional identity as psychologists: They are not medical doctors.

Other public statements, in addition to advertisements for one's own services, are also covered in the standards for ethical practice. As treatment in health psychology advances and new interventions and techniques are developed, the psychologist must be cautious when endorsing products. Statements about the efficacy of treatments such as relaxation tapes or self-help manuals can be deceptive, if not false. The psychologist is ethically bound to make every effort to ensure the accuracy of statements even when publication rights have been transferred to another party.

Summary

The responsibility for ethical behavior adds to the challenges facing counseling psychologists who wish to offer their expertise in the realm of health care. From the initial consultation through the assessment, intervention, and financial aspects of practice, the psychologist may encounter situations rife with ethical dilemmas. Thorough knowledge of the fundamental ethical principles and their supporting behavioral standards will allow counseling psychologists to practice with competence and confidence that the welfare of their patients is well regarded and vehemently protected. By meeting these challenges the counseling psychologist is rewarded with the personal and professional satisfaction that accompanies their important role in health care.

Suggested Resources

Several sources make significant contributions to our understanding of the ethics involved in the counseling psychologist's practice in the health care arena. Belar and Deardorff (1995), in *Clinical Health Psychology in Medical Settings,* present a comprehensive look at ethical and legal aspects of health-care–related practice as well as a discussion of assessment issues, interventions, and training. In "Ethical and Malpractice Issues in Hospital Practice," Pope (1990) succinctly points out the ethical pitfalls for psychologists working in a hospital setting. The July 1991 issue of *The Counseling Psychologist* was devoted to the roles of counseling psychologists in health care. This is recommended as a starting point for readers who are interested in a global overview.

Three general books on ethics are also recommended. Pope and Vasquez (1991), in their textbook *Ethics in Psychotherapy and Counseling,* provide an excellent coverage of the major ethical issues encountered by psychologists, regardless of practice domain. A compilation of articles written by attorneys, physicians, psychologists, and counselors was published in 1997 by Hatherleigh Press. This work, *Ethics in Therapy,* addresses multiple dimensions of professional practice from a variety of perspectives. Finally, in his work entitled *Ethical Conflicts in Psychology,* Bersoff (1995) has collected an excellent set of readings covering major ethical topics.

Readers are also referred to the American Psychological Association Web site (http://www.apa.org/) for the complete text of APA Ethical Principles of Psychologists Code of Conduct.

Discussion Questions

1. What are the basic issues surrounding competency to offer one's psychological services in a health care setting?
2. In what ways are informed consent, confidentiality, and privileged communication interrelated? How does working in a health care setting influence these ethical considerations?
3. Discuss what is meant by competing agendas and how these can influence the practice of the psychologist in serving patients.
4. How might your personal values and morals come into play when working with a health care team and with patients?
5. How might dual relationships interfere with the psychologist's effectiveness?
6. What aspects of business practice can cause ethical dilemmas to arise and how might these be handled?

References

American Psychological Association. (1991). APA Council of Representatives adopts new AIDS policies. *Psychology and AIDS Exchange, 7,* 1.

American Psychological Association. (1992). Ethical principles of psychologists and code of conduct. *American Psychologist, 47,* 1597–1611.

American Psychological Association Board of Professional Affairs. (1993). Record keeping guidelines. *American Psychologist, 48,* 984–986.

Arizona Revised Statutes 32–1457. *Acquired immune deficiency syndrome; disclosure of patient information; immunity; definition.*

Belar, C. D., & Deardorff, W. W. (1995). *Clinical health psychology in medical settings: A practitioner's guidebook* (Rev. ed.). Washington, DC: American Psychological Association.

Bersoff, D. N. (Ed.). (1995). *Ethical conflicts in psychology.* Washington, DC: American Psychological Association.

Calfee, B. E. (1997). Lawsuit prevention techniques. *Ethics in Therapy.* New York: Hatherleigh.

Dubin, S. S. (1972). Obsolescence or lifelong education: A choice for the professional. *American Psychologist, 27,* 486–496.

Everstine, L., Everstine, D. S., Heymann, G. M., True, R. H., Frey, D. H., Johnston, H. G., & Seiden, R. H. (1980). Privacy and confidentiality in psychotherapy. *American Psychologist, 35,* 828–840.

Harding, A., Gray, L. A., & Neal, M. (1993). Confidentiality limits with clients who have HIV: A review of ethical and legal guidelines and professional policies. *Journal of Counseling and Development, 71,* 297–305.

Herlihy, B., & Corey, G. (1992). *Dual relationships in counseling.* Alexandria, VA: American Association for Counseling and Development.

Kitchener, K. S. (1984). Intuition, critical evaluation and ethical principles: The foundation for ethical decisions in counseling psychology. *The Counseling Psychologist, 12,* 43–56.

Klippel, J. A., & DeJoy, D. M. (1984). Counseling psychology in behavioral medicine and health psychology. *Journal of Counseling Psychology, 31,* 219–227.

Lawrence, G., & Robinson Kurpius, S. E. (1997). *Legal and ethical issues involved when counseling minors.* Manuscript submitted for publication.

Perlin, M. L. (1997). The "Duty to Protect" others from violence. *Ethics in Therapy.* New York: Hatherleigh.

Pope, K. S. (1990). Ethical and malpractice issues in hospital practice. *American Psychologist, 45,* 1066–1070.

Pope, K. S. (1992). Responsibilities in providing psychological test feedback to clients. *Psychological Assessments, 4,* 268–271.

Pope, K. S., Tabachnick, B., & Keith–Spiegel, P. (1987). Ethics of practice: Beliefs and behaviors of psychologists as therapists. *American Psychologist, 42,* 993–1006.

Pope, K. S., & Vasquez, M. J. T. (1991). *Ethics in psychotherapy and counseling: A practical guide for psychologists.* San Francisco: Jossey-Bass.

Pope, K. S., & Vetter, V. A. (1992). Ethical dilemmas encountered by members of the American Psychological Association: A national survey. *American Psychologist, 47,* 397–411.

Robinson Kurpius, S. E. (1997). Current ethical issues in the practice of psychology. *Ethics in Therapy.* New York: Hatherleigh.

Schwitzgebel, R. L., & Schwitzgebel, R. K. (1980). *Law and psychological practice.* New York: John Wiley.

Tarasoff v. Regents of the University of California, 118 Cal., Rptr. 129.529 P.2d 533 (1974).

Tarasoff v. Regents of the University of California, 113 Cal., Rptr. 14.55 P.2d 223 (1976).

Welfel, E. R., & Kitchener, K. S. (1992). Introduction to the special section: Ethics education—An agenda for the '90s. *Professional Psychology: Research and Practice, 23,* 179–181.

II
AREAS OF PRACTICE

4

Working in Medical Settings: Diagnostic, Practice, and Professional Issues

Cheryl Carmin
Sari Roth-Roemer

Counseling health psychologists work in diverse medical settings and face various demands. This second section of the book, Areas of Practice, introduces readers to a number of these different settings, with a focus on the specific problems to be identified and treated. As an introduction to this section, this chapter highlights some of the general issues that must be considered when working with medical patients. We will describe relevant assessment, evaluation, and practice matters and discuss issues such as the importance of differential diagnoses when assessing medical and mental health concerns.

Differentiating between Medical and Psychological Problems

Frequently, psychologists are called upon to assist in determining whether a medical patient is experiencing psychological difficulties. These difficulties may include:

- some form of cognitive deficit
- problems associated with mood (i.e., anxiety or depression)
- substance abuse
- difficulty with pain or symptom management
- difficulty controlling certain behaviors

Any of these issues may complicate medical treatment (Kathol & Wenzel, 1992; Levenson, Hamer, & Rossiter, 1992; Mayou, Hawton, Feldman, & Ardern, 1991). The role of the mental health professional often involves providing an assessment and/or ongoing treatment respective to one or more of these concerns.

Diagnostic Evaluation and Assessment

Since assessment is the first step in differentiating between medical and psychological problems, psychologists working in health care are frequently asked to assess the psychological functioning of medical patients. In a hospital setting this service may be performed under the aegis of a health psychology program, a behavioral medicine service, a consultation liaison psychiatry program, or a medical/surgical service.

The request for consultation or evaluation typically comes from the attending physician, who must write orders in the patient's chart for a consultation by another professional. The report the psychologist generates is ordinarily directed back to the physician who made the original request—not to the patient, as is typical in traditional psychotherapy. This can make a critical difference when the timing of the delivery of difficult information is involved. For example, if there are psychological factors that mitigate against someone receiving an organ transplant, it is critical for the attending physician to receive this information in a timely manner, so he or she can integrate a number of consultants' reports before discussing a treatment plan with the patient.

Generally, it is expected that a consult request will be completed within a brief period of time, often as short as 24 hours, although this varies. If this is not possible, the psychologist is expected to document in the medical record the reason for the delay (e.g., "The patient was unavailable due to a medical procedure"). As part of the consultation, the psychologist is expected to conduct a thorough diagnostic evaluation and to provide a written assessment of the problem and a treatment plan. After the assessment and treatment plan have been discussed with the medical team, it is often up to the medical team, typically led by the attending physician, to assent to further psychological treatment. The counseling health psychologist's role is consultant, not primary decision maker.

The foremost responsibility of the consulted psychologist is to respond to the question or need stated in the consult request. Frequently, however, the request is not clearly stated; in that case it is incumbent upon the consulting psychologist to seek clarification. More often than not, one has to educate medical colleagues that "Please evaluate" is at best a nebulous request. On the other hand, such a request provides an opportunity to get to know a medical colleague while discussing what he or she is hoping to find out. Of course, the psychologist may then be in the uncomfortable position of having to educate the colleague that what he or she is requesting is not possible for a number of reasons. Limitations related to duration of hospital stay, the inherent limits of mental health assessment instruments, or the patient's current mental status may, individually or in concert, affect the mental health professional's ability to provide the requested service.

Assessing Medical versus Psychiatric Conditions

The relationship between medical and psychiatric conditions has been underscored with the fourth edition of the *Diagnostic and Statistical Manual (DSM-IV)* of the American Psychiatric Association (1994). Most of the major diagnostic categories now include the diagnosis of a disorder "due to a general medical condition." This new category highlights the importance of being able to differentiate between psychosocial disorders and medical conditions whose symptoms resemble or mimic psychiatric conditions.

Current epidemiologic studies suggest that 10–15 percent of patients seen in primary care physicians' offices meet criteria for either an anxiety or mood disorder (Eisenberg, 1992). These two categories of disorders by themselves can present challenges when differentiating between medical and psychosocial problems. For example, a patient may describe symptoms of tachycardia, sweating, shortness of breath, and lightheadedness and indicate that these symptoms are paroxysmal and last for approximately 20–30 minutes. Without a medical workup, one could conclude, with a reasonable degree of certainty and based solely on symptom constellation and general epidemiological data, that the most likely diagnosis is panic disorder. However, pheochromocytoma, a serious life-threatening medical condition, can also produce the same symptoms, as can high levels of certain asthma medications (e.g., theophylline) or cardiac conditions (e.g., cardiac ischemia)(Greenberg, 1996). If these medical conditions are left unrecognized, the situation could become life-threatening for the patient and have legal and ethical implications for the counseling health psychologist.

A professional who remains ignorant of competing physical diagnoses can render a psychological intervention that is inappropriate and ineffective.

The mental health professional must be sufficiently conversant with the typical presentation of *DSM-IV* diagnosable conditions and their medical rule-outs in order to avoid potentially endangering a patient's life by providing a psychological intervention when a medical treatment is indicated. In outpatient settings this means encouraging patients to have a complete physical prior to initiating mental health treatment, making sure they are medically cleared for treatment, and maintaining ongoing contact with the patient's primary care physician. When treating hospital patients, interacting with the referring physician as well as becoming familiar with relevant laboratory results and medical conditions and medications that may cause psychiatric symptoms will not only benefit the patient but also aid in interdisciplinary discussions. Asking questions in order to familiarize oneself with the medical setting is the counseling health psychologist's greatest learning tool.

Cognitive Functioning

Consult requests often ask for assistance in determining a patient's level of cognitive function. The rationale behind such a request may be an acute change in a patient's mental status. A previously lucid and alert patient may now appear confused, have difficulty concentrating, be experiencing memory deficits, or even become combative. The task may be to determine if the individual is delirious or demented. A quick response to such a request is crucial, since the patient may be experiencing a rapid change in his or her medical condition due, for example, to a medication interaction or to the early signs of a brain tumor.

Alternatively, chronic problems that the patient may not have mentioned to his or her physician may become apparent. A patient may experience drug or alcohol withdrawal while in the hospital; related cognitive changes may not have been anticipated due to the patient's failure to disclose his or her substance abuse history. Given that psychological assessment is one of the tools available to psychologists, mental status assessment and neuropsychological testing may be necessary to determine whether there is a substance abuse or other problem which is contributing to impaired cognitive functioning. Chapter 10 in this volume provides further detail on this topic.

Besides differentiating between acute and chronic changes in mental status, there are several other reasons why an assessment of cognitive function can be critical. These include determining the etiology of a cognitive deficit and making predictions regarding future level of functioning, ability to adhere to medical treatment regimens, and/or ability to make competent treatment-related decisions.

The patient's ability to comply with what are often complicated medical regimens after being discharged from the hospital can be an important piece of data with respect to medical decision-making and aftercare. During the course of a hospital stay, these problems may not have been apparent since the nursing staff typically manages medication schedules and other health care professionals (e.g., physical and respiratory therapists) manage or monitor their respective areas of patient care. Once hospital treatment is completed, however, the patient is expected to follow a program of home health care. If a patient is not capable of following a complex schedule of which medications to take when, his or her health will be compromised. Illiteracy, intellectual limitations, or cognitive deficits can all influence treatment adherence. Many patients have skillfully hidden these problems throughout their lifetime; the psychologist's role may involve not only discovering these deficits but also assisting patients in using their strengths to comply with treatment and prevent further health problems. For example, suggesting that the patient write down important information or that the patient use a daily or weekly pill container may facilitate medication management in addition to providing a strategy that helps offset mild memory deficits. The psychologist may also recommend home health care to assist the patient in establishing a routine of self-care. Alternatively, the psychologist may have the unfortunate task of determining that a patient's independent lifestyle is no longer feasible and that some type of assisted living situation is needed.

At other times, a mental health professional may be asked to determine whether an individual is able to give informed consent for medical treatment. Typically, this involves assessing whether the patient has the intellectual capacity necessary to understand the nature and side effects of medical treatment, as well as possible outcomes, positive and negative, of the procedure. Thus, the task of assessment includes evaluating intelligence and reasoning skills as well as determining whether the patient is acutely confused or suffering from a thought disorder and, subsequently, unable to give informed consent.

Psychological Assessment

As noted above, there can be a variety of reasons for referring patients to a mental health professional. In many ways, differentiating among symptoms resulting from a medical problem, the side effects of a medication, or a cognitive deficit is relatively straightforward. However, when the treatment difficulties are due to either an acute or longstanding emotional problem, often the counseling health psychologist, the physician, and other members of the health care team have to work collaboratively in order to assist the patient in becoming more proactively and productively involved with his or her treatment.

Among the more common problems medical patients experience are depression and anxiety (Eisenberg, 1992). In addition, patients who have somatoform disorders, while less prevalent, can cause their physicians considerable frustration. This is similarly the case with patients who have personality disorders and other severe psychiatric disorders.

Mental health practitioners use clinical interviewing skills along with psychometric instruments to assess dimensions of personality and how a patient's personality will impact his or her health status. The more psychosocially sophisticated medical providers often consult a psychologist because they "know something is wrong but not exactly what the problem is." This was the case with Ms. M, a young woman who was being considered for a heart transplant. When a repeat episode of congestive heart failure was diagnosed on a recent visit to the clinic, she admitted to not being compliant with her medication regimen and diet. Her cardiologist observed that she seemed somewhat depressed but was unable to elicit any further information and referred her to the psychologist.

During the clinical interview, the psychologist discerned that Ms. M's depression stemmed not only from her medical condition, but also from the way in which she and her family interacted. Although Ms. M was in her mid-twenties and had a child of her own, her parents (with whom she lived due to her health limitations) tended to treat her "like a child." She felt doubly limited by her health and by the unnecessary limitations on her activity imposed by her family. Her parents constantly told her that any given activity could "strain her heart." She was both depressed and anxious.

It is unclear whether the counseling health psychologist's training in interviewing and listening skills allowed this patient to disclose such information or whether it was a matter of having a neutral third party who had the time to listen that made such disclosure safer. Regardless, having strong counseling skills in this area can make an important contribution to the patient's health maintenance.

Mental health practitioners have an array of diagnostic instruments and personality measures available to guide their recommendations. These tools are uniquely part of the training of those in psychology and allied professions. As a plethora of instruments are available, a few guidelines in selecting instruments are essential:

1. When considering the use of any self-report measure, the *reading and general intellectual levels* of the patient must be taken into consideration. There are many individuals who are largely illiterate, for whom English is a second language, or who are not fluent in English. While this may seem obvious, not being sensitive to such issues can create difficulties. Identifying such skill deficits makes an important contribution to patient care, since being unable to read a test is not too different from being unable to read a prescription label.

2. Assessment instruments should always be selected on the basis of *the question being asked and the medical diagnosis indicated.* For example, depression can have a considerable impact on mortality in patients who have had a myocardial infarction (Frasure-Smith, Lesperance, & Talajic, 1993). Clearly, assessing dimensions related to depression, unexpressed hostility, perfectionism, and anxiety or stress would be relevant to patients with ischemic heart disease.

3. The choice of instruments should be guided by *research data.* The more information we have regarding the interaction of personality and illness, the better we can assess who may be at risk and what treatment strategies will work best for whom. Further, it does not enhance the credibility of a mental health professional if the assessment materials he or she relies upon are not well validated in general or, more specifically, for the particular patient population in question. Thus, the use of objective measures having strong psychometric properties is encouraged over the use of less well validated or reliable projective measures.

4. Another factor guiding instrument selection, one that is critical in medical settings, is *time.* Patient burden must also be factored into this equation. Having every patient who is referred complete a Minnesota Multiphasic Personality Inventory-2 (MMPI-2) may be desirable; however, it is not often feasible. Given the weakened physical condition of many medical patients, as well as reduced length of hospital stays, a psychologist may no longer have the luxury of giving a patient an instrument that takes several hours to complete, let alone adminis-

ter an entire test battery. It may be more effective to rely on several shorter instruments that target relevant symptoms and have strong validity, rather than attempt to have the patient take several hours for one instrument or hinge an evaluation on the successful completion of a test battery. Even neuropsychological assessment batteries often need to be carefully selected so as to match the stamina of the patient.

Treatment-Related Issues

Shakin Kunkel and Thompson (1996) recently described the characteristics of an effective *psychiatric* consultant. Interestingly, of the 16 points they made, only one referenced psychotherapy and patient education. Perhaps this serves to underscore the difference in approaches between psychiatry and psychology, as well as the nature of the contribution a counseling health psychologist can make when asked to consult regarding the treatment of medically ill patients. Clearly, as others in this text have noted, the strength of our training is in the areas of listening and communication skills, patient education, and interventions focusing on reducing risk-related behaviors, adaptation, and behavior change.

Role of the Consultant

Perhaps one of the other features unique to counseling psychologists is training in consultation (although this is typically taught in the context of consulting with organizations). In the consultant's role, one may not be the person ultimately providing an intervention. The task of consultation in a health care setting often involves understanding not only what would need to be done if the consultant were providing the intervention, but also how to instruct others in what they may need to do in order to best assist the patient. The consultant must blend knowledge regarding other professionals' roles and functions, the medical milieu, and the patient's capabilities with an understanding of how to best execute an intervention that will answer the referral question and benefit the patient. An example may help to illustrate this.

Mrs. B had a relatively rare progressive lung disease and was being evaluated as a candidate for a transplant. She was having difficulty adhering to a weight loss regimen. In addition, her physician was unclear if Mrs. B was anxious or depressed. Along with several other members of the patient's treatment team, the physician expressed no small amount of frustration with this patient and requested a psychological consultation to clarify what psychological factors might be contributing to her difficulties. During the clinical interview and assessment, the consultant found that Mrs. B had limited intellectual resources (i.e., she fell in the low average range of intelligence) and did not have a clear understanding of respiratory anatomy, physiology, or her illness. Furthermore, she held some superstitious beliefs that were at best unproductive and that she had not related to any of her treatment team. For example, she believed that drinking cooking oil that had been blessed by her minister would heal her lungs. She also disclosed her ambivalence and apprehension about a transplant. During the course of the evaluation, the psychologist reviewed the basics of anatomy with Mrs. B as a means of dispelling her superstition (i.e., things that she swallowed, despite their being blessed, would not go into her lungs). Further, the psychologist also clarified that drinking oil was not helping her reach her weight reduction goal.

The consultant then met with Mrs. B's treatment team and informed them that their interactions with Mrs. B had been geared to a level of sophistication she did not have. This information helped to reduce the team's frustration. Recommendations to the patient's physician and team included:

1. Provide the patient with ongoing education about respiratory anatomy and physiology.
2. Communicate information in small increments.
3. Demonstrate using anatomic models.
4. Repeat information as frequently as possible in order to reinforce the patient's understanding.
5. Use concrete examples when drawing analogies.
6. Have the patient prepare at least one question every time she visits the clinic.

Psychological follow-up was offered to assist the patient in dealing with issues of weight management and her emotional response to her illness and eventual surgery.

Intervention Strategies

Subsequent psychological treatments are often of considerable benefit to patients with a range of medical problems. Again, time is often limited and interventions may need to be completed within the scope of only a few days.

Further, medically compromised patients may be less interested in long-term, insight-oriented psychotherapy than in learning methods to facilitate their recovery. As Hollandsworth (1985) aptly noted over a decade ago, "behavior change, not insight, is the preferred goal" (p. 151). While this is not to say that insight-oriented treatment may not be effective, there is little research to support its use with medical patients. As hospital stays have become progressively shorter and managed care allows fewer outpatient and inpatient sessions, interventions that are brief, directive, and focused on the problem at hand may best serve the patient's immediate, if not long-term, needs.

As with assessment instrument selection, the counseling health psychologist is best guided by empirical data when selecting an intervention strategy. Outcome research has demonstrated that cognitive-behavioral interventions are successful in treating a variety of medical problems, including:

- reducing Type A behavior in ischemic heart disease patients (Nunes, Frank, & Kornfeld, 1987; Powell & Thoreson, 1987)
- weight reduction (Brownell, Stunkard, & McKeon, 1985)
- hypertension (Chesney et al., 1987)
- smoking cessation (Schwartz, 1987)
- nausea and vomiting resulting from chemotherapy (Andrykowski, 1990)
- pain management in cancer patients (Syrjala, Cummings, & Donaldson, 1992)
- improving blood cell counts in HIV+ patients (Antoni et al.,1991)
- anxiety and depression which are often comorbid with medical illness (See Giles, 1993 for reviews of effective treatments)
- treatment compliance (Hegel, Ayllon, Thiel, & Oulton, 1992)

The patient's response to psychological intervention must also be considered. When, for example, the pulmonologist suggests that the patient see a mental health professional for help with asthma, the patient may become suspicious and respond by pointing out that he or she is asthmatic, not crazy. Agreeing with the patient and then explaining that coping with illness and speeding recovery are the goals may be an effective way to respond to the patient's skepticism.

When called upon to see a patient for the first time, the counseling psychologist may encounter considerable animosity if the patient has not been prepared for the meeting. In such a situation, the mental health provider should first listen to the patient's concerns and then seek to clarify how he or she can help the patient overcome or more comfortably adjust to illness. If, as sometimes happens, the patient asks the psychologist to leave, the clinician should do so, cordially thanking the patient for his or her time.

In some cases, patients are right; their symptoms are not psychological in origin. An example of such a situation involved a patient, Mr. C, who had recently undergone lung surgery and was readmitted to the hospital for chest pain and shortness of breath. Mr. C's surgeon became quite irate at not being able to find anything medically awry and told him that he was ordering a "psych" consult because his symptoms were "all in his head." Needless to say, Mr. C was less than enthusiastic about seeing a psychologist. Prior to the consult, the psychologist had received no information other than the patient was having chest pain that was not of medical origin. After responding to Mr. C's interrogation about training, background, credentials, etc., and then reassuring the patient that he was not crazy, the psychologist suggested that they meet again after the patient had seen his pulmonologist the following day. Mr. C agreed. By the next day, this patient had been diagnosed with costochondritis, a painful inflammation of the cartilage joining the sternum and ribcage, had received appropriate medication, and was feeling much better. The psychological intervention consisted of wishing the patient well upon his discharge from the hospital.

Clearly, diagnostic assessment, listening, and therapy skills that are included in the training of counseling psychologists can make a significant contribution to better understanding patient functioning. Although seemingly obvious, it is critically important not to lose sight of the patient in the process of his or her treatment. The fact that the patient is an independent, knowledgeable contributor to his or her treatment should not to be overlooked in the morass of information that is accumulated over the course of a patient's hospital stay.

Referring to and Collaborating with Other Professionals

As Altmaier, Johnson, and Paulsen, have observed (see chapter 1), establishing one's autonomy in a medical setting can involve a battle that is hard fought and not easily won. Mental health professionals are sometimes categorized as ancillary staff or as technicians rather than as members of the medical staff or treatment team. Further, they may be struggling with psychiatrists for equal recognition.

What may help to solidify psychologists' position in the medical community, as well as to reduce the turf issues with other similarly trained professionals, is knowing when and how to make a referral. If psychologists attempt to function beyond the scope of their training or alienate professional colleagues with inappropriate referrals, there can be grave legal and ethical consequences.

Psychopharmacologic Referrals

Often, in medical center settings where mental health professionals enjoy a strong collaborative relationship with physician colleagues, they may be asked, either formally or informally, to make a recommendation regarding medications. How should one respond? Given that many counseling health psychologists have years of specialization in particular areas (e.g., working with pain or cardiology patients, specializing in the treatment of anxiety disorders), they may be quite current with regard to the psychopharmacology of certain medications and their utility in the treatment of certain disorders. Psychologists with such experience may feel comfortable making recommendations regarding medication.

However, this practice has its pitfalls. Making a specific recommendation regarding a medication and its dosage could potentially jeopardize a patient's health, if not his or her life. Knowledge about medication interactions is virtually exploding; what was true last month may no longer be applicable today. Further, to make a recommendation in writing in the medical record puts the psychologist at risk for malpractice and/or the loss of his or her license, as this type of advice is out of the psychologist's scope of practice. Given that the patient population we are addressing includes individuals who are medically ill, it is likely that these patients are already being prescribed medications for their condition(s). The complexity of psychopharmacologic treatment of medically compromised patients cannot be emphasized strongly enough. Suffice it to say that even physicians are relying more on individuals with doctorates in pharmacology to provide advice and guidance when treating patients for whom polypharmacy is the only option.

Complicating the issue of medication management even further is the suggestion that nonpsychiatric physicians tend to undermedicate their patients and to not continue medication long enough for patients to benefit fully

(Simon & Walker, 1996). Even acting as the initial consultant for the nonpsychiatric physician may make subsequent psychiatric treatments more difficult if medication trials or treatment have been unknowingly inadequate. Thus, it may make greater sense to refer questions specific to medication to colleagues in psychiatry. For example, a psychologist was asked to evaluate a woman on an oncology unit with a longstanding history of anxiety. Diagnosis of her symptoms revealed she had a generalized anxiety disorder that was notably interfering with her daily functioning and compliance. While cognitive-behavioral intervention was indicated, so was psychopharmacologic intervention. By being able to evaluate the need for psychopharmacologic intervention and consulting a psychiatrist to assist with the psychopharmacologic management of her anxiety, the psychologist was able to collaborate effectively in the treatment of this woman's psychological distress.

Medical Referrals

As we often remind our medical colleagues, a patient who has a medical condition can also have an emotional problem. Medical team members often normalize the emotional response of their patients. It is not uncommon to hear, "Of course he's depressed, he has cancer!" Reminding the physician and medical team that just as it is normal for a patient to bleed following a car accident and that we are responsible for stopping that bleeding and treating the injury, it is also normal for a patient to have an emotional response to his or her medical condition and that it is important to treat that patient's suffering.

The reverse also holds. Emotional problems can sometimes mask serious medical illness. To illustrate, a woman with a history of coronary artery disease was being treated as an outpatient for panic symptoms and an acute traumatic response to having been in a car accident. She described feeling short of breath and lightheaded, both symptoms she associated with her panic attacks. She also reported that she was experiencing an unrelenting and severe headache, a symptom not typically associated with panic but, rather, one often associated with hypertension. The psychologist referred her back to her cardiologist and encouraged her to call her physician that day. She was subsequently admitted to the hospital for coronary artery bypass surgery.

While it is impossible to have expertise in every area relevant to a patient's functioning, the treating mental health professional needs to develop an acute sense of what seems "normal" for a given patient. In addition, one should not hesitate to forcefully encourage a patient to have a problem medically assessed if it seems unrelated to his or her psychological presentation. Alternatively, having a physician colleague one can call to ask a few pointed questions in support of making such a referral acts to enhance one's credibility with a patient and one's willingness to work collaboratively with colleagues.

Learning the Language

One of the most critical factors for a counseling health psychologist working in a medical setting is acculturation. In order to effectively interact with or to function as effective members of a treatment team, psychologists must be familiar with the settings in which they work. This means not only knowing about the patient population, the diseases, and the medical treatments, but also learning the hierarchy, knowing to whom one can go to find out needed information, and being able to "speak the language" of the particular setting. Being conversant in medical terminology and being able to translate psychological phenomenon into operational and behavioral descriptions are essential for a counseling health psychologist to be effective in health care settings.

Suggested Resources

A number of excellent comprehensive texts explore the practice of psychology in medical settings. Resnick and Rozensky (1996), in their edited text, *Health Psychology Through the Life Span: Practice and Research Opportunities,* address not only some of the specific areas within which psychologists provide service, but political issues as well. There are excellent examples of how to develop a service delivery program and how research and practice complement one another.

The *Textbook of Consultation-Liaison Psychiatry* (Rundell & Wise, 1996) is a compendium of information whose target audience is psychiatrists. It is, however, valuable to the psychologist who is working on an interdisciplinary team or interested in the differences in how psychologists and psychiatrists practice within similar settings.

The *Handbook of Clinical Psychology in Medical Settings* (Sweet, Rozensky, & Tovian, 1995), provides a comprehensive overview of general and professional issues, practice management issues, clinical concerns, and program development. The book is directed to clinical psychologists but has much to offer counseling psychologists as well.

A number of professional organizations provide a forum for the advancement of practice and research in health psychology.

Health Psychology Section, Division 17, Counseling Psychology, American Psychological Association (750 First Street, N.E., Washington, DC 20002-4242, phone: 202/336-5500) reflects the interest and career path of many counseling psychologists. The Division of Counseling Psychology has recently formed the Health Psychology Section. The Section publishes a newsletter as well as supports the interests of its members by sponsoring programs at the annual APA convention.

Society of Behavioral Medicine (SBM; 401 E. Jefferson St., Suite 205, Rockville, MD 20850-2617, phone: 301/251-2790, Web site: http://socbehmed.org/sbm/sbm.htm) is a multidisciplinary organization that integrates behavioral and biomedical science to assist in the understanding of health and illness. *Annals of Behavioral Medicine* is the organization's official publication.

Association for the Advancement of Behavior Therapy (AABT; 305 Seventh Avenue, 16th fl., New York, NY 10001, phone: 212/647-1890) is a multidisciplinary organization whose unifying interest is the advancement of cognitive and behavioral approaches to research and treatment. Their annual meeting, which occurs in November, includes paper and poster sessions and symposia on health-related topics as well as on treatment of specific disorders (e.g., anxiety, depression). Preconference institutes are offered and may be of particular interest to individuals who wish to build their skills in these areas.

Discussion Questions

1. Why is it important for counseling health psychologists to be knowledgeable about both the psychological and medical symptoms common to the setting in which they work?
2. What is the role of the counseling health psychologist in a medical setting?
3. What are some of the guidelines that need to be considered in selecting an appropriate assessment instrument?

4. Why is knowing when to refer to another specialty an important skill for a counseling health psychologist to have?

5. What factors should be taken into consideration when planning a treatment intervention?

References

American Psychiatric Association. (1995). *Diagnostic and Statistical Manual* (4th ed.). Washington, DC: Author.

Andrykowski, M. A. (1990). The role of anxiety in the development of anticipatory nausea in cancer chemotherapy: A review and synthesis. *Psychosomatic Medicine, 52,* 458–475.

Antoni, M. H., Bagget, L., Ironson, G., LaPerriere, A., August, S., Klimas, N., Schneiderman, H., & Fletcher, M. A. (1991). Cognitive-behavioral stress management intervention buffers distress responses and immunologic changes following notificication of HIV-1 seropositivity. *Journal of Consulting and Clinical Psychology, 59,* 906–915.

Brownell, K. D., Stunkard, A. J., & McKeon, P. E. (1985). Weight reduction at the work site: A promise partially fulfilled. *American Journal of Psychiatry, 142,* 47–52.

Chesney, M. A., Agras, W. S., Benson, H., Blumenthal, J. A., Engel, B. T., Foreyt, J. P., Kaufmann, P. G., Levenson, R. M., Pickering, T. G., & Randall, W. C. (1987). Nonpharmacologic approaches to the treatment of hypertension. *Circulation,* 76(Suppl. I), 104–109.

Eisenberg, L. (1992). Treating depression and anxiety in primary care: Closing the gap between knowledge and practice. *New England Journal of Medicine, 326,* 1080–1084.

Frasure-Smith, N., Lesperance, F., & Talajic, M. (1993). Depression following myocardial infaction: Impact on 6-month survival. *Journal of the American Medical Association, 270,* 1819–1825.

Giles, T. R. (Ed.). (1993). *Handbook of effective psychotherapy.* NY: Plenum.

Greenberg, D. B. (1996). Internal medicine and medical subspecialties. In J. R. Rundell, & M. G. Wise (Eds.), *Textbook of consultation-liaison psychiatry* (pp. 548–607). Washington, DC: American Psychiatric.

Hegel, M. T., Ayllon, T., Thiel, G., & Oulton, B. (1992). Improving adherence to fluid restrictions in male hemodialysis patients: A comparison of cognitive and behavioral approaches. *Health Psychology, 11,* 324–330.

Hollandsworth, J. G., Jr. (1985). Counseling psychology, health psychology, and beyond: A reply to Klippel and DeJoy. *Journal of Counseling Psychology, 32,* 150–153.

Kathol, R. G., & Wenzel, R. (1992). Natural history of symptoms of depression and anxiety during inpatient treatment on general medicine wards. Journal of *General Internal Medicine, 7,* 287–293.

Levenson, J. L., Hamer, R. M., & Rossiter, L. F. (1992). A randomized controlled study of psychiatric consultation guided by screening in general medical inpatients. *American Journal of Psychiatry, 149,* 631–637.

Mayou, R., Hawton, K., Feldman, E., & Ardern, M. (1991). Psychiatric problems among medical admissions. *International Journal of Psychiatry in Medicine, 21*(1), 71–84.

Nunes, E. V., Frank, K. A., & Kornfeld, D. S. (1987). Psychologic treatment for the Type A behavior pattern and coronary artery disease: A meta-analysis of the literature. *Psychosomatic Medicine, 48,* 158–173.

Powell, L. H., & Thoreson, C. E. (1987). Modifying the Type A behavior pattern: A small group treatment approach. In J. A. Blumenthal, & D. C. McKee (Eds.), *Applications in behavioral medicine: A clinician's source book* (pp. 171–207). Sarasota, FL: Professional Resource Exchange.

Resnick, R. J., & Rozensky, R. H. (Eds.). (1996). *Health psychology through the life span: Practice and research opportunities.* Washington, DC: American Psychological Association.

Rundell, J. R., & Wise, M. G. (Eds.). (1996). *Textbook of consultation-liaison psychiatry.* Washington, DC: American Psychiatric.

Schwartz, J. L. (1987). *Review and evaluation of smoking cessation methods: The United States and Canada, 1978–1985* (DHHS Public Health Service, NIH Publication No. 87-2940). Washington, DC: U.S. Government Printing Office.

Shakin Kunkel, E. J., & Thompson, T. L., II. (1996). The process of consultation and organization of a consultation-liaison psychiatry service. In J. R. Rundell, & M. G. Wise (Eds.), *Textbook of consultation-liaison psychiatry* (pp. 12–23). Washington, DC: American Psychiatric.

Simon, G. E., & Walker, E. A. (1996). The consultation-liaison psychiatrist in the primary care clinic. In J. R. Rundell, & M. G. Wise (Eds.), *Textbook of consultation-liaison psychiatry* (pp. 947–955). Washington, DC: American Psychiatric.

Sweet, J. J., Rozensky, R. H., & Tovian, S. M. (Eds.). (1995). *Handbook of clinical psychology in medical settings.* NY: Plenum.

Syrjala, K. L., Cummings, C., & Donaldson, G. (1992). Hypnosis or cognitive behavioral training for the reduction of pain and nausea during cancer treatment: A controlled clinical trial. *Pain, 48,* 137–146.

5

Coronary Heart Disease: A Psychosocial Perspective on Assessment and Intervention

Carl E. Thoresen
Jennifer Hoffman Goldberg

Recently, in an editorial for a special issue of *Science* devoted to heart disease, two eminent biologists predicted the end to heart attacks by the year 2000 and to diseases of the heart early in the twenty-first century (Brown & Goldstein, 1996). The basis of this highly upbeat prediction was data demonstrating that drugs that lower serum cholesterol (called statins) sharply reduce coronary mortality over several years. Completely ignored in this editorial, however, were two major points:

1. Cardiovascular diseases are multidimensional and chronic, influenced by a host of factors; any one factor, such as serum cholesterol, accounts for only a portion of coronary disease and death.
2. The prevention and the treatment of coronary diseases require a variety of interventions, some medical, some educational, some psychosocial, and some sociocultural; unlike many infectious diseases, there is no single cure or magic bullet.

We note this *Science* editorial because it poignantly reveals a fundamental flaw in the biomedical model that often permeates cardiovascular research and clinical practice: the focus on selected biological processes to the exclusion of other human processes (e.g., cognitions, behaviors) that powerfully contribute to cardiovascular diseases (CVD) and, indeed, to all chronic if not infectious diseases.

Cardiovascular diseases, specifically diseases of the heart, remain the leading cause of death and disability in men and women in the United States and other industrialized countries (American Heart Association, 1995). Cardiovascular diseases encompass a wide spectrum of diseases, from congenital and structural disorders to end-stage congestive heart failure to the immune disorder of rheumatic heart disease. Coronary heart disease (CHD), often called coronary artery disease (CAD), and stroke are the two most common and preventable cardiovascular diseases (please see Colantonio, Kasl, Ostfeld, & Berkman, 1993, and Thompson, Sobolew-Shubin, Graham, & Janigian, 1989, for a discussion of the psychosocial components of stroke).

In this chapter we provide a selective introduction to social and psychological factors (referred to collectively as psychosocial or lifestyle factors) related to CHD and to CHD physiology, primarily in terms of diagnosis/assessment and intervention. In doing so we introduce readers to different conceptual models used in research on CHD. Because diagnostic and intervention issues cut sharply across several specialty areas within cardiology and medicine and several areas of psychology (e.g., counseling, social), a comprehensive discussion is well beyond the scope of this chapter. We will, however, suggest resources for those interested in further exploring this highly prevalent and important topic.

Some of the causes of CHD are immutable, such as age, family history, and gender, but most can be ameliorated by psychosocial intervention. Research has revealed a number of factors that have predicted increased risk for CHD. The current major established risk factors are smoking, elevated serum cholesterol, high blood pressure, sedentary behavior, and diabetes, as well as age, family history, and gender. Several additional risk factors exist but are less well accepted by cardiologists and others.

While the death rates for CVD have declined dramatically—roughly 40 percent—over the past 30 years, the prevalence of CHD still remains high. For example, almost 25 percent of the American population (roughly 60 million people) has some form of CVD (American Heart Association, 1995). This means that more people are staying alive with the clinical indicators of CHD, including atherosclerotic (plaque) build-up and a myocardial infarction (MI or heart attack). Even at the most advanced stages of CHD (tertiary prevention), psychologists and others can help with quality-of-life issues as well as death and dying.

We believe that CHD is a particularly salient area for psychologists and others interested in promoting health and fostering prevention. Research is needed to identify, explore, and clarify the role of current, possible, and new psychosocial risk factors. We need to further refine the degree or threshold level of risk factors that contribute to CHD (e.g., When does a risk factor, such as perceived stress, become a major risk factor?). In addition, we need to identify more clearly which individuals are at risk and which interventions can best help them reduce both physiological and psychosocial risk as well as improve quality of life.

Background of Coronary Heart Disease

Coronary heart disease is a disease of the coronary arteries that supply the heart itself with oxygen and various nutrients carried by the blood. Coronary heart disease can present itself as clinical syndromes of angina (chest pain), arrhythmias (interruption of the heart's electrical rhythm), MI (fatal and nonfatal heart attack), and sudden cardiac death (sudden and unexpected onset of symptoms and death within one hour).

The major cause of CHD is atherosclerosis, a gradual thickening of the heart's arterial walls from plaques composed of lipids, cholesterol, and other substances that over time gradually block arterial blood flow. The most prevalent consequence of atherosclerosis is an MI. During an MI, one of the arteries within the heart muscle supplying blood becomes completely blocked. When the tissue of the heart in that area ceases to receive vital blood and oxygen, the tissue begins to die within minutes. Quick action is needed to resume blood flow and prevent heart muscle tissue from dying— a permanent consequence (American Heart Association, 1995).

The causes of MIs are still not fully understood, although several theories exist. Some research suggests that social and emotional stress/distress and the physiological arousal that occurs in chronic sympathetic nervous system hyperarousal play a role, either directly or more likely as a moderating variable. For example, a study of serum cholesterol levels in certified public accountants found dramatic increases around the April tax deadline, even when other risk factors remained constant, thus contributing to increased CAD (Friedman, Rosenman, & Carroll, 1958). Catecholamines, the so-called "stress-hormones" released in response to stressful situations, have been shown to increase blood pressure, and may play a role in thrombosis, possibly by irritating the intima (inner lining) of the coronary arteries (Parker et al., 1995). Autopsies of young soldiers (age < 35 years) killed in both the Korean and Vietnam Wars revealed that over 75 percent showed some signs of atherosclerosis; 20 percent showed more than a 50 percent occlusion rate (Joseph, Ackerman, Talley, Johnstone, & Kupersmith, 1993). Recently, a five-year follow-up study of patients with CAD who suffered from exercise-induced myocardial ischemia (deficiency of oxygen supply to the heart) found that the ischemia caused by mental or emotional stress significantly predicted increased fatal and nonfatal cardiac events, even more so than exercise-induced ischemia and other risk factors (Jiang et al., 1996).

The primary causes of death in the United States have changed dramatically since 1900. Although the majority of deaths in 1900 were caused by infectious agents (e.g., influenza) or acute events, the ten leading causes of death today are almost all from chronic disease conditions, such as CHD and cancer. This dramatic change for the first time in history from acute to chronic diseases requires a very different model for conceptualizing and treating disease (Thoresen & Eagleston, 1985). An acute or infectious disease model—the biomedical model—emphasizes a relatively rapid onset, often with the invasion of a specific bacterial or viral agent, and seeks a cure by destroying that particular agent. This acute model, however, fails to fit most chronic diseases in which the onset emerges gradually over time, often many years, because the causes cannot be pinpointed to one external factor such as a virus. Furthermore, while chronic diseases are treatable, they are not curable. Thus, the biopsychosocial or chronic disease model places much more emphasis on biological, developmental, psychological, and social/environmental risk factors that contribute to disease onset, and structured, often long-term interventions.

CHD Risk Factors: Positive, Possible, and Plausible Types

Several factors increase the risk of CHD; these risk factors also appear to overlap substantially with other diseases and disorders, such as stroke, elevated blood pressure, and perhaps some cancers (Booth-Kewley & Friedman, 1987; Everson et al., 1996). Most attention to date has been given to well-established or "positive" risk factors that can be changed: cigarette smoking, elevated serum cholesterol, and higher blood pressure (hypertension). Recently, physical inactivity has achieved positive status. These risk factors focus more on physiological or behavioral variables than on social, emotional, and cognitive variables.

Almost 50 percent of the variance that accounts for CHD still remains unknown, even after considering all established or positive risk factors, including genetic risk factors of age, gender, and family history. Unquestionably, other factors now considered "possible" or "plausible" need to be looked at carefully. Several have been associated in studies spanning several years with a much greater risk of CHD: anger and hostility, depression, lack of social support, obesity (excessive body fat and body fat distribution), perceived stress and anxiety, Type A behavior pattern, and vital exhaustion. Figure 5.1 (Allan, 1996) graphically depicts many of these positive, possible, and plausible risk factors, although not all of these risk factors contribute equally to CHD. Cigarette smoking, for example, contributes about 20 percent of the variance. Note that two recent possible risk factors, vital exhaustion and depression, were not included in this graph but could be added. Undoubtedly, other possible factors will emerge in future research.

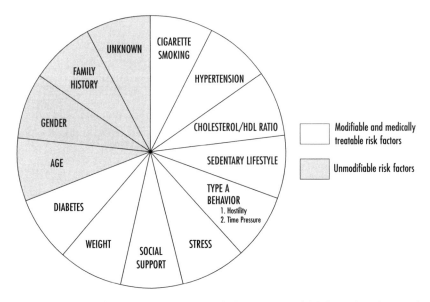

Figure 5.1. Risk factors for coronary heart disease (CHD). A number of risk factors have been established. Cigarette smoking, elevated serum cholesterol (and cholesterol-HDL [high-density lipoprotein] ratio), hypertension, and sedentary lifestyle are considered the standard, positive, risk factors. Psychosocial risk factors are still tentative and sometimes controversial. The degree of risk sometimes depends on the degree to which the risk factor occurs in a person's life (e.g., the risk from cigarette smoking varies with the amount smoked). Similiarly, the higher the serum cholesterol or cholesterol-HDL ratio, the greater the risk. Risk factors combine synergistically, that is, their total effect is greater than the sum of the parts. From "Introduction: The Emergence of Cardiac Psychology" by R. Allan in R. Allan and S. Scheidt (Eds.), *Heart and Mind* (p. 4). Copyright 1996 by the American Psychological Association. Reprinted with permission.

Unfortunately, the magnitude or level of a psychosocial risk factor, rather than just its presence or absence, has not received enough attention. The acute biomedical model too often emphasizes dichotomous thinking, that a risk factor is either present or absent, in the same sense that a person is considered either diseased or healthy, with healthy defined as the absence of disease signs and symptoms (Thoresen & Eagleston, 1985). Attention to critical threshold levels and possible curvilinear as well as linear relationships between risk factors and CHD outcomes is needed. For example, in most people, the risk for CHD increases linearly as the rate of smoking increases. CHD risk, however, may not increase linearly with total serum cholesterol levels, especially if the ratio of high-density lipoproteins (HDL, the "good" cholesterol) to low-density lipoproteins (LDL, the "bad" cholesterol) or to total cholesterol is not considered. Alcohol offers a beneficial effect for many at very low consumption levels (the "one drink per day with a meal" guideline) but quickly becomes detrimental with higher consumption, while greatest relative benefits on mortality for physical activity come from changing a very sedentary lifestyle to a moderately physical one (Blair et al., 1996).

Women and CHD

We consider the women-and-CHD relationship separately because in CHD research women have so often been ignored or assumed to be comparable to men. Clearly CHD is not just a men's disease (American Heart Association, 1995). Until the late 1980s, CHD was commonly seen as a men's middle age problem, yet CHD ranks as the leading overall cause of death in women as well as men, killing more women than the combined total for cancer, AIDS, osteoporosis, and domestic violence. In 1991, 479,358 women died from CVD (25 percent from CHD) compared to 446,792 men. The onset of CHD in women, however, trails men by about 10 years. While men under 55 have two to three times more MIs than women, women under 55 are two to three times more likely to die from an MI.

Wegner, Speroff, and Packard (1993) summarized the findings of gender differences for CHD:

- The prognosis for women who have had an MI is worse than for men (women die earlier).
- The prognosis for women who have undergone conventional medical and surgical procedures for CHD is worse than for men.

- Women have an excess of silent ischemia and undetected MIs, although frequency and consequences are still unclear.
- Women with the same degree of disease pathology receive fewer invasive (mostly surgical) procedures than men.
- Women benefit as much as men do from aspirin, beta-blocking drugs, and thrombolytic therapy. Some data suggest this may also be true for coronary artery bypass surgery and several heart medications.
- Women's benefit from longer-term cardiac disease management programs remains unknown (too few women have been involved).
- Women participate much less often in cardiac rehabilitation programs, drop out more often, but may benefit as much as men if they participate.

In terms of CHD risk factors, women are similar to men. For example, of women between the ages of 20 and 74, 23 percent smoke (28 percent of men), 29 percent have high serum cholesterol (26 percent of men), 36 percent have hypertension (45 percent of men), and 34 percent are overweight (32 percent of men) (Higgins & Thorn, 1993). Generally, prediction of CHD with established somatic risk factors is comparable to men. Women at lower socioeconomic status and education levels are, however, at greater risk for CHD than men at similar levels. Graff-Low, Thoresen, King, Patillo, and Jenkins (1995) recently compared two groups of women, a post-MI group and a physically sedentary group, on several psychosocial measures, including the videotaped structured Type A interview (VSI). Both had comparable total scores on Type A behavior pattern (TABP) but the post-MI women were significantly more hostile and more depressed. The failure of the VSI to predict cardiac events in the post-MI women was noteworthy. In fact, those who had lower overall scores tended to be at higher risk of cardiac recurrence. The authors point out that such results illustrate the problems of using diagnostic assessments with women that are based on men. Unfortunately, few psychosocial measures used in CHD research have been adequately designed in terms of providing valid and reliable information for women.

A recent review (Brezinka & Kittel, 1996) of studies on women, psychosocial factors, and CHD (1980–1994) suggested the following profile of a woman at higher CHD risk:

- comes from a lower social class
- has little formal education
- smokes
- consumes higher levels of dietary fat and cholesterol

- engages in little physical exercise
- experiences higher levels of perceived stress and physical tension
- is typically a homemaker who feels unsupported socially
- if she works outside the home, she still does all the home tasks
- seldom has vacations
- if a widow, is at higher risk and may experience considerable loneliness and hopelessness

See Burell (1996) for an excellent description of women's experiences in treatment for changing lifestyle after an MI or coronary bypass surgery.

Diagnosis and Assessment

Diagnosis and assessment of CHD center on two main areas: the medical condition and the psychosocial factors related to the development and maintenance of CHD. In many ways what you as a professional decide to diagnose or assess concerning CHD reveals what you believe to be the critical and perhaps causal components of the disease. Furthermore, diagnosis and assessment are intimately connected to intervention. The decision of what to assess or diagnose becomes the basis for intervention and often the means of measuring how well an intervention is working.

We now better understand the need for multiple measures and modes of assessment and the need for tailoring them for cultural, racial, ethnic, gender, and language factors, although in practice we still too often lapse into "uniformity myths" about patients and treatments (Kiesler, 1966). The often dominating belief that "one size fits all" when it comes to assessing and treating people has started to yield to more contextualized approaches (e.g., Kopta, Howard, Lowry, & Beutler, 1994). This change reflects an "it all depends on . . ." mindset and avoids the dichotomizing limitations of the biomedical model mentioned earlier (Engel, 1977). Our discussion of stepped care intervention models later in this chapter speaks to the need to provide a range of interventions suited to individual needs.

Medical Diagnosis and Assessment

Because medical assessment, diagnoses, and interventions usually happen concurrently with psychosocial assessment and intervention, and because the medical components of the disease are often very salient in the patient's life, psychologists need to understand medical procedures to effectively address psychosocial issues. Space limitations prevent a full discussion of medical terms and procedures here, but we offer an abbreviated glossary of major CHD-related medical terms and procedures (table 5.1). In composing this glossary we have drawn heavily on the following references and direct the reader to them for a more in-depth discussion: Achuff, 1996; American Heart Association, 1994, 1995; Guerci, 1996; Scheidt, 1996; and Traill, 1996.

Psychosocial Diagnosis and Assessment

We focus here very selectively and briefly on weight, physical activity, waist-to-hip ratio, and smoking, as well as six promising psychosocial factors. Doing so allows us to illustrate some major assessment problems shared by all risk factors. These psychosocial factors include: Type A behavior pattern (TABP), anger and hostility, vital exhaustion, depression, social isolation/social support, and psychosocial stress/anxiety. We especially focus on the TABP because the diagnostic and assessment issues involved have been widely studied, are related to assessment and diagnostic issues of other psychosocial factors, and reflect the extensive experience of the first author.

Despite the evolving and at times impressive evidence that psychosocial factors clearly play a role in cardiac health and disease, we remain in "early adolescence" when it comes to psychosocial diagnosis and assessment. Unlike many physiological assessments that are developed to the point where there is consensus about assessment protocols to measure a factor (e.g., ECG, blood pressure), diagnosis and assessment of psychosocial factors commonly lack adequate standardization. Scores of measures have been used, for example, to assess psychological stress or distress, as well as anger and hostility, anxiety, and depression. Seldom has a particular measure in the psychosocial world been officially sanctioned by means of a nationwide consensus conference, as commonly happens in medicine (e.g., with ECG). The failure of researchers to use more standardized assessments has contributed to inconsistent, ambiguous, and at times invalid findings within psychosocial research. The problems of research in the Type A area, to be discussed, well illustrate this failure. Reasons for this lack of consensus are many.

1. Psychologists and others are often dealing with more ill-defined and less readily observable phenomena that typically overlap. Seldom does any psychological, social, or behavioral factor, such as distress or

Table 5.1
Glossary of Major CHD-Related Medical Terms and Procedures

Acute myocardial infarction. The death of a portion of heart muscle usually caused by sudden occlusion of a previously narrowed coronary artery.

Beta blockers. A class of drugs that block the beta-adrenergic branch of the sympathetic nervous system. This branch controls heart rate, blood pressure, strength of cardiac contraction, and various other automatic functions, so that blocking that portion of the autonomic nervous system causes heart rate, blood pressure, and strength of heart contraction to fall.

Cardiac catheterization. Cardiac catheterization involves inserting a small catheter (tube) into an artery under local anesthesia (usually into the femoral artery in the groin) and feeding it up through the aorta to the coronary arteries. A radioactive dye is injected and films are taken to reveal the extent and location of coronary artery blockage. It is considered the definitive measure of CAD.

Cardiac enzyme evaluation. Diagnosing a heart attack in part evaluates the presence of cardiac enzymes in the bloodstream, such as creatine phosphokinase (CK), an enzyme a normal heart leaks into the blood when heart muscle tissue dies.

Congestive heart failure. A clinical syndrome in which the pumping ability of the heart is insufficient for the needs of the body and as a result fluid accumulates in the lungs and elsewhere in the body.

Electrocardiogram (ECG). The ECG is a noninvasive procedure in which electrical recordings are taken at 12 different sites (or leads). These leads record different areas of heart function. ECGs taken at rest can show evidence of current or previous myocardial infarction. Changes in the ST segment (part of the electrical wave pattern of a heartbeat) can be a sign of ischemia (lack of oxygen to the heart).

Ejection fraction (EF). The proportion of the total blood volume in the heart at the beginning of a contraction that is ejected with each beat. The EF is a powerful predictor of prognosis, with lower EF after an MI correlating with higher mortality in subsequent months and years.

Holter monitoring. Because changes in ECG readings often do not occur during resting ECG testing or stress testing, a Holter monitor can be worn over a 24-hour period to assess a partial ECG.

Silent infarction. An MI that occurs without chest pain or other clinical symptoms. This is surprisingly common and is often only discovered on routine ECGs in many people; perhaps 25–30 percent of all infarcts are silent.

Stress testing. The stress test for CHD involves taking ECG recordings of a person exercising on a treadmill or stationary bicycle. The level of physical difficulty is gradually increased and is terminated when any symptoms occur, such as major changes in the ECG readings, or when the heart rate is at 85 percent of the maximum for the person's age group.

anger, exist independent of other factors or of the social context in which the person is involved. As a result these psychosocial factors are usually interrelated, and a variable like anger may be a component of psychological stress or depression or it may interact with one's social exchanges and thus affect levels of social isolation.

2. A construct like anger can be seen as representing an interrelated number of processes, each quite complex: physiological, cognitive, social, emotional, gender, social-environmental, and psychomotor-behavioral (Williams & Williams, 1993). Because of this complex mix of processes, a particular diagnosis or assessment of anger can tap any one or more of the above mentioned processes while neglecting others (e.g., just observing facial expression or only asking about feeling frustrated of aggravated) (Levenson, Ekman, & Friesen, 1990).

3. Adding to the ambiguity of psychosocial assessment are sociocultural factors. Appels (1996) illustrates the impact of culture on CHD and why psychologists and other behavioral scientists focusing on personality and behavior patterns "should never forget that these personality characteristics are formed and shaped by the culture in which people live." Appels demonstrated a marked positive relationship ($r=0.60$, $p<.05$) between CAD mortality and a culture's focus on "individualistic achievement." Several authors (e.g., Henry & Stephens, 1977; Thoresen & Ohman, 1987) have voiced concern about the need to contextualize ("culturalize") our psychosocial assessment and intervention efforts.

Weight, Physical Activity, and Waist-to-Hip Ratio

Obesity, or excess body fat, has been linked to increased risk for CHD, both directly and because of its association with other CHD risk factors such as high blood pressure and lower HDL levels (Manson et al., 1990; Willett & Manson, 1995). The role of obesity as a direct risk factor has been debated when other risk factors for CHD, such as high blood pressure, are controlled statistically. Controlling for these other factors is controversial, however, because these risk factors are often the result of excess weight (see Miller, Turner, Tindale, Posavac, & Dugoni, 1991, for a discussion of the "indirect restriction of range" problem). Some prospective studies have shown that obesity directly increases the risk for CHD (Pi-Sunyer, 1995). Obesity often occurs in conjunction with a sedentary lifestyle, another risk factor for CHD. In addition to general obesity, a greater abdominal pattern of body fat (measured by the ratio of waist size to hip size) is associated with increased risk for cardiovascular disease (Bjorntorp, 1990) (for additional information see Brownell & Fairburn, 1995; Brownell & Wadden, 1992).

Smoking

The major impact of smoking on CHD is so crucial that it deserves an entire chapter itself. Here we can only allude to the problems. Cigarette smokers have a risk of CHD at least two to four times greater than that of nonsmokers, and in the event of a myocardial infarction are more likely to die. Smoking also moderates the effects of other risk factors; for example, the combination of smoking with higher cholesterol produces a greater risk than adding the two risk factors alone (Perkins, 1985). The CHD risk is greater for heavy smokers and those who began smoking as early as adolescence. That is why the recent upsurge of young smokers is alarming. Assessment is often done via self-report. Because self-report is often unreliable, evidence of smoking, such as CO_2 breathalator and blood serum, is often used in controlled studies. Please see Lichtenstein and Glasgow (1992), as well as references cited in the Intervention section of this chapter (p.115), for a more complete discussion of diagnostic and assessment issues in smoking.

Type A Behavior Pattern

The problems with how TABP has been diagnosed and assessed can help us understand the problems and issues facing psychosocial assessment in CHD generally (Friedman et al., 1986; Thoresen & Powell, 1992). The TABP was first conceptualized by two cardiologists, Meyer Friedman and Ray Rosenman, as a clinical syndrome, a collection of observed qualities and characteristics of persons that cluster together consistently and relate to a disorder that has an unclear etiology and treatment. The hallmark of this syndrome is the chronic struggle consistently observed in most male coronary patients to accomplish more and more, often vaguely defined goals, in less and less time. Two qualities seem to capture this struggle: an excessive level of time urgency, characterized by impatient thoughts and behavior, and easily aroused, excessive hostility, including a quickness to experience anger.

To diagnose this multidimensional syndrome, Friedman and Rosenman devised a structured 15-to-20-minute interview protocol. They used an interview rather than a questionnaire because much of the diagnosis for Type A was based not so much on what people said but on how they expressed themselves verbally and nonverbally. Several psychomotor signs, such as facial signs of hostility and repetitive hand or foot movements, were also assessed. Over the past 25 years the structured interview has evolved, given the experience of using it with thousands of cardiac patients as well as noncoronary adults (see Friedman, Fleischman, & Price, 1996, for a detailed description of TABP assessment using the videotaped clinical examination).

Friedman and Rosenman conducted the kind of diagnostic assessment that allowed them to observe directly a number of selected behavioral and psychomotor characteristics in addition to self-reported signs and symptoms. This process of observing the patient's behavior in a structured context to make the diagnosis is consistent with good medical practice but is seldom used for psychosocial diagnosis in controlled CHD studies. Why might this kind of observation be important? The answer lies in the multidimensional nature of this clinical syndrome: There is too much complexity involved to capture it all in a brief self-report questionnaire, especially when issues of social desirability and poor self-awareness are involved (e.g., many do not see themselves as hostile or deny feeling angry or having hostile thoughts).

As with almost all CHD risk factors, the evidence demonstrating a relationship between TABP and CHD risk is often inconsistent, if not ambiguous. Simply put, the relationship between any risk factor is not always linear nor is it predictive under all conditions for all people. We do not know, for example, why some people with the same degree of coronary artery disease (stenosis), the most prevalent type of CVD, suffer acute MIs, others experience angina pectoris, others have silent ischemia, and still others die suddenly (Scheidt, 1996).

Three meta-analyses of TABP and CHD (Booth-Kewley & Friedman, 1987; Matthews, 1988; Miller et al., 1991) have concluded that TABP is predictive of CHD risk, doubling the risk compared to those who are not Type A, but only under certain conditions:

1. when white males are involved
2. when participants are sampled from the general population, not from those already with advanced CHD
3. when a structured interview, not a questionnaire, is used

The relationship for women and nonmajority males remains unclear. We suspect, however, based on clinical experience and current research in

Sweden (Burell, 1996), that women high in TABP characteristics may indeed be at risk, as well as men of color, especially those with more education and higher socioeconomic status.

Several studies failing to demonstrate a predictive relationship of TABP with CHD used a questionnaire and not a structured interview (see Booth-Kewley & Friedman, 1987). Other studies that used the structured interview, such as the multiple risk factor intervention trial (MRFIT) with over 3000 persons, failed to use it appropriately. Scherwitz (1988) analyzed these interviews and found they were not validly conducted (e.g., interviewers often cut the interview short to less than eight minutes and did most of the talking). When these interviews were rescored by other researchers to focus on the hostility components of TABP, the results showed that hostility significantly predicted MIs over several years, but only for men under 47 years old (Dembroski, McDougall, Costa, & Grandits, 1989). Others have also shown that when the global structured interview assessment failed to predict CHD, reanalyses of the interviews focusing on the hostility component of TABP did predict CHD (Hecker, Chesney, Black, & Frautschi, 1988; Shekelle et al., 1985).

The multidimensional if not complex nature of psychosocial factors, such as TABP and hostility, in influencing CHD was recently demonstrated by Houston, Babyat, Chesney, Black, and Ragland (1997). Prompted by the impressive results of animal studies showing that social dominance in males produced dramatically higher CHD, they rescored interview tapes of 750 healthy men 22 years after they had been initially interviewed for TABP to assess "pressured social dominance" (e.g., verbal competitiveness, immediateness of response, and fast speaking) (see discussion of Kaplan, Manuck, Williams, & Straun, 1993, on social dominance and psychosocial stress/anxiety in this chapter, p. 113). Results from multivariate analyses indicated that what could be called an "impatient effort to socially control the interview" (pressured social dominance) led to 1.6 times more deaths even when all standard risk factors were controlled ($p=.02$). Furthermore, hostility also independently predicted death (1.5 times higher, $p=.02$), as did what they called Type A content (1.5 times higher, $p=.059$). Those who evidenced a "placid pattern" had almost 40 percent fewer deaths ($p=.04$). What is particularly interesting about these data is the fact that a much publicized earlier study (Ragland & Brand, 1988) of these same men at 22 years had shown that TABP, when assessed globally as a single category (either Type A or Type B), was not at all predictive of death. These results speak clearly to the value of looking much more carefully and specifically at psychosocial factors and avoiding the use of single global measures of multidimensional concepts. They also point more clearly at what might be the focus of interventions to help prevent coronary events.

Following are some general conclusions about TABP:

1. Exclusive use of self-report questionnaires may seriously misrepresent the often complex psychosocial construct being assessed. Combining such self-reports with a different mode of assessment (e.g., interview, behavior ratings by others) seems essential, given the limits of only using questionnaire data due to, for example, social desireability, limited self-awareness, and lack of motivation.

2. Diagnosis and assessment that lead to a global, categorical rating (e.g., person is either Type A or Type B) can seriously confound and confuse results, since considerable heterogeneity typically exists among people who are globally labeled (e.g., Type A, depressed, socially isolated).

3. Using persons with advanced CHD to assess the TABP/CHD relationship and only using death as the CHD outcome seriously underestimate the power of TABP, or any psychosocial factor, to predict CHD or other major diseases. This problem comes from the severe "indirect restriction of range," a statistical issue. A factor used to select participants in a study, (e.g., only persons with advanced CHD) can be highly related to the health outcome being predicted (e.g., cardiac death). Because of this strong relationship between severe CHD and cardiac death, other factors such as a psychosocial factor like TABP have little power to predict (see Miller et al., 1991, for extended discussion).

4. Diagnosis and assessment in studies with TABP (and other psychosocial factors) have been almost exclusively based on white, middle to upper-middle class males. Socioeconomic status and gender, however, clearly present diagnostic and assessment issues that have been ignored. These issues deserve immediate attention given the fact that CHD is the leading cause of death in women (as well as men) and that CHD mortality is significantly higher among less educated and lower socioeconomic groups.

5. Two general approaches are needed: (a) refining conceptualizations of TABP (and other psychosocial risk factors), making them more specific and situationally sensitive, and (b) examining how TABP overlaps with other psychosocial factors such as depression, anxiety, and perceived stress.

Anger and Hostility

The diagnoses and assessment of anger and hostility closely parallel the experience with TABP. Williams and others started exploring the hypothesis that the pathogenic or virulent core of TABP might be hostility (Williams, 1987). Several prospective studies using the Cook-Medley Hostility Scale (Ho), a 50-item scale based on the MMPI, found that higher Ho scores predicted all-cause mortality over 20- to 25-year periods (e.g., Barefoot, Dodge, Peterson, Dahlstorm, & Williams, 1989). A revised 27-item version of the Ho, using three subscales (aggressive responding, hostile affect, and cynical attitude) found that these scales predicted survival better than the total Ho score. These three Ho scales have also predicted physiological impairment in how the heart functions (Helmers et al., 1993). As is usually the case, however, some studies using the Ho scale have failed to predict increased mortality over several years (see Thoresen & Powell, 1992).

Barefoot (1992) more recently found that when assessing hostility a variation of the Type A structured interview is more effective than Ho self-report scales. Called the Interpersonal Hostility Assessment Technique (IHAT), this interview captures more sensitively the cognitive, affective, and behavioral components of hostility. Four style-related types of hostility have been identified from the interview: evading questions in hostile manner, irritation in voice, confronting interviewer, and indirectly challenging by criticizing questions asked in the interview.

Barefoot, Patterson, Haney, and Cayton (1994) found that IHAT scores were significantly higher for commercial pilots with CAD assessed by coronary angiography compared to healthy pilots. They also found drastically higher mortality rates for "hostile smokers" than for smokers low on hostility, possible evidence that the physiologic component of hostility mediates the impact of smoking on health. Goodman, Quigley, Moran, Meilman, and Sherman (1996) found that if patients undergoing balloon angioplasty (an intervention that squeezes the plaque back in the coronary arteries) displayed hostile TABP during the structured interview, they were twice as likely to require another angioplasty intervention within six months.

These mixed findings closely resemble results of earlier unsuccessful TABP studies in that the specific situations in which assessments were conducted varied widely (e.g., taking the MMPI—from which the Ho scale is derived—for admission to graduate school compared to taking it while in medical school). Further, the multidimensionality of the Ho scale, as with all measures of TABP, makes the validity of a single total score or category label highly questionable. Steinberg and Jorgensen (1996) found, for example, that the shortened Ho scale (27 items) had at least five different significant factors, indicating considerable multidimensionality. Given this heterogeneity, the interpretation of what a single total hostility score means remains clouded.

Others have found similar results with anger (Allan & Scheidt, 1996). For example, self-reported anger predicted a three times higher risk of fatal and nonfatal MIs in older men over seven years when compared to men with lower anger (Kawachi, Sparrow, Spiro, Vokonas, & Weiss, 1996). Recent studies also suggest that repeated episodes of anger may increase CHD risk. Ironson and colleagues (1992) had participants with CHD recall a situation within the last six months that resulted in being "frustrated, angry, irritated, or upset" (note the synonyms used for anger). They also had them imagine being falsely accused of shoplifting and talk about their reactions, do mental arithmetic, and do physical exercise on a bicycle ergometer. Of all these tasks, recalling the angry episode caused the heart's left ventricle to pump significantly less blood—a major indication of a diseased heart. Boltwood, Taylor, Burke, Grogin, and Giacomini (1993) also demonstrated similar effects of anger on the heart in a highly controlled study using state-of-the-art assessment of the heart's functioning during anger recall. It is highly significant that these studies clearly demonstrate that the cognitive features of negative emotions, such as anger, can powerfully impact the heart's physiology. The impact of anger and hostility when experienced in vivo, not just by recall, may be even more powerful.

Many studies loosely use the terms anger and hostility as if they were identical in what they mean and how they are assessed (see Siegmen & Smith, 1994, for a comprehensive discussion of anger). The benefits of direct observation versus paper/pencil self-reports also emerge in the anger literature, particularly the value of assessing facial expressions of anger (e.g., Levenson, et al., 1990). Again, when it comes to assessing negative emotional states, given their multidimensionality, the power of directly observing persons in terms of validity seems quite apparent.

Vital Exhaustion

In the months preceding their MI, people will often report they feel unusually tired, irritated, and demoralized. Some have described this experience as "flu-like," since it shares some of the symptoms of a viral infection. Appels and others (e.g., Appels & Schouten, 1991) have reported a consistent predictive relationship between what they call vital exhaustion (VE) and CHD risk. For example, Kop, Appels, Mendes de Leon, de Swart, and Bar (1994) found in 127 patients undergoing successful angioplasty for CAD that of those scoring high on the Maastricht VE Questionnaire, 35 percent suffered a new cardiac event within 18 months after surgery, compared to only 17 percent not exhausted; this impressive difference was not explained by standard risk factors or other psychosocial factors. Appels (1996) also studied vital exhaustion in healthy adults (N=3877) over 4 years, finding that an age-adjusted risk for an MI is 2.28 times greater for those higher in vital exhaustion.

Until recently, vital exhaustion was only measured by a 21-item questionnaire, with questions like, "Have you experienced a feeling of hopelessness recently?" "Do you have the feeling that you can't cope with everyday problems as well as you used to?" and "Do you ever wake up with a feeling of exhaustion and fatigue?" Appels recently developed the Maastricht Interview for Vital Exhaustion (MIVE), noting that it is significantly more powerful in discriminating MI patients from healthy control subjects than the questionnaire (Appels & Meester, 1996). Evidence of the psychometric qualities of the MIVE (e.g., internal consistency, concurrent validity) is also impressive. Note that several MIVE items seem conceptually related to TABP, hostility, depression, and low social support: "more irritated lately . . . feel dejected . . . blow up more easily . . . sometimes cry or feel like crying . . . wake up repeatedly during the night." Appels and Meester found that vital exhaustion assessed by interviews was related to TABP and hostility. This seems to be another example of how different psychosocial risk factors overlap with one another, probably because people's experiences of anger and hostility, TABP, depression, and anxiety often share common elements.

Depression

Compared to TABP and hostility/anger, diagnostic and assessment procedures for depression are well established and widely used (e.g., *DSM-IV* criteria). Health professionals have long observed that patients commonly suffer from depression in the months after the MI (see Fielding, 1991, for review). Several recent studies suggest that depression is not only a consequence of suffering an MI or other cardiac problem, but it may also be a cause or risk factor for CHD. Barefoot and Schroll's (1996) 27-year study of almost 900 participants showed that higher depressive symptoms on the MMPI depression scale were related to a 70 percent higher risk of an MI and a 60 percent greater risk of death from all causes. Women in this study were also at higher risk for an MI and death than men. To explore the risk of death for post-MI patients, Frasure-Smith, Lesperance, and Talajic (1993) followed patients for six months after their MI. Of those with major depression (16 percent of the total sample), 17 percent died within six months, compared to only 3 percent without depression, a fivefold difference in death. In a prospective study, Pratt and others (1996) reported that of 1500 participants followed for 13 years, those initially depressed on self-report scales were six times more likely to suffer an MI, even after controlling for age, gender, blood pressure, and smoking.

Social Support

A relative newcomer to the list of possible CHD risk factors is lack of social and emotional support, also referred to as social isolation. People appear much more likely to die from all causes, including CHD, if they feel disconnected or isolated from others, experiencing an absence of emotional support as opposed to informational or instrumental support. Generally, men and women lacking social support, especially emotional support, have a two- to three-times-higher mortality from all causes than those with good support, with men being somewhat at higher risk than women. In their excellent review of five major prospective studies, each spanning almost a decade (N=37,000), House, Landes, and Umberson (1988) concluded that strong evidence exists for a relationship between social support, disease risk, and mortality.

To date, there are no generally accepted diagnostic guidelines or measurement of social support, although numerous questionnaires and some interviews have been developed. The overall emerging picture, at least as related to CHD risk, emphasizes the importance of functional or process measures of social support (e.g., perceived quality of emotional support, depth of intimate contacts). Structural or more quantitative features of social support (e.g., the number of friends, the frequency of contacts) may be less relevant. For example, Seeman and Syme (1987) looked at differences in functional and structural social support among patients receiving angiography to diagnose possible CHD. They found that "feeling loved" was related to much less coronary artery disease. Some studies, however, have found that both types of support are related to reduced CHD (e.g., Orth-Gomer, Rosengren, & Wilhelmsen, 1993). Interestingly, in this study a lack of emotional support (functional) and a lack of an extended network of people created a risk for CHD that was as great as cigarette smoking.

Berkman, Leo-Summers, and Horwitz (1992) followed almost 200 men and women who survived an acute MI and found that, even when a number of other factors were controlled for, the lack of emotional support predicted significantly higher CHD death rates. In a large (N=1234) study of hospital-ized MI patients, Case, Moss, Case, McDermott, and Eberly (1992) found cardiac recurrence (fatal and nonfatal) was twice as high (15.8 percent ver-sus 8.8 percent) for patients living alone, compared to those living with a partner. Williams and colleagues (1992) also reported in another major study (N=1368 over five years) that people living without a close friend had 3.34 times more deaths than those married or having a close friend.

Social support seems clearly related to other psychosocial factors. Understandably, people lacking social support, especially emotional support, may also be at greater risk of feeling more angry and depressed, thinking more pessimistically, becoming more sedentary, and living with more hope-lessness and despair. Social support may also moderate other risk factors for CHD. For example, Orth-Gomer and Uniden (1990) followed over 200 men assessed for TABP (structured interview) for 10 years. Type A men lacking social support suffered a 69 percent death rate, compared to 17 percent for Type A men who lived more socially connected lives. Conceivably, social support may also mediate the impact of other risk factors, such as smoking or serum cholesterol levels, on CHD (e.g., hostile versus nonhostile smokers).

Psychosocial Stress and Anxiety

While we will only briefly discuss the broad topic of psychosocial stress, we do want to mention several impressive studies. (For a more extensive dis-cussion of the cognitive, emotional, and social dimensions of stress and dis-tress, see Allan and Scheidt, 1996, and Cohen and Williamson, 1991.) In an impressive series of experimental animal studies (e.g., Kaplan et al., 1993), substantial CAD was actually produced in male and female macaque mon-keys by placing them in a new living group of "stranger" monkeys every few weeks—the psychosocial stressor. These monkeys have coronary systems very similar to human systems. These studies have controlled for all known physical and behavioral risk factors including heredity, and the results have been consistently replicated. Interestingly, the monkeys at highest risk of CAD are dominating males who continually struggle for control of the social groups when change occurs (e.g., an "outside" male shows up); for females, those of lower social status suffer the highest risk.

In a recent study illustrating how psychosocial stress in humans may lead to serious cardiac events, Jiang and colleagues (1996) found that 126 CAD patients who showed silent ischemia (partial and temporary asymptomatic constrictions of coronary arteries, which reduces blood flow to the heart) during a laboratory task (e.g., talking with strangers about a very personal concern) were almost three times more likely to suffer a fatal or nonfatal cardiac event over five years. These patients also demonstrated higher rates of silent coronary ischemia in daily life situations, as assessed by ambulatory heart monitoring equipment. Ruberman, Weinblatt, Goldberg, and Chaudbury (1984) found an almost five-times-higher death rate (4 percent versus 15 percent) for post-MI patients who scored high on stressful life events and/or social isolation. Such data strongly suggest that psychosocial stress, if chronically experienced, may be contributing to physiological changes that, in turn, increase cardiac disease and events. From a clinical viewpoint, we believe it is very important to educate clients about this possible stress-CHD risk, since silent ischemia is not felt by the person. This process is particularly salient for those already evidencing some clinical CAD, as is the case with many people as they grow older.

Although anxiety represents a distinct topic in the psychological literature, the manifestations of state anxiety overlap perceived psychological stress in many ways. A just-published study (Moser & Dracup, 1997) found a 4.9 times greater risk for post-MI patients of major cardiac complications, including reinfarction and death, if they showed higher state anxiety within 48 hours of being hospitalized. These data are consistent with those of Frasure-Smith (1991), who also found higher anxiety levels while hospitalized predictive of coronary death. An obvious intervention is suggested by these results: Provide some type of immediate anxiety/distress reduction while hospitalized and in the weeks following discharge from the hospital.

Additional Comments on Diagnosis and Assessment

We have selectively discussed some psychosocial risk factors for CHD and in each case have mentioned a few studies. While a fuller discussion of the interdependence of psychosocial risk factors for CHD is not possible here, we want to emphasize that psychosocial risk factors are seldom freestanding, independent factors as described in most research studies. More often than not, coronary-prone people suffer from a collage of shared psychosocial disruptions and disorders. Variations of depression, anger, and fear may be the most common. We also have not considered a number of sociocultural factors deserving attention, especially since psychologists and other health professionals are most likely to work with individuals and small groups. Economic, political, and cultural factors can exert tremendous influence on how we think about CHD and how we diagnose, assess, and intervene. The recent advent of managed care illustrates the economic and political influences on who receives what kind and how much care in different sociocultural settings.

A recent monograph by Pincus and Callahan (1995) on socioeconomic and educational influences in chronic disease merits mention. They argue that the major reason why poorer and less educated people suffer more disease and death (CHD as well as other diseases) is not so much because they are denied the full range of medical services (which they often are), but because they are uninformed and unskilled in understanding how one's beliefs, thoughts, emotions, behavior, and social network influence health status. Pincus and Callahan present extensive data on this point and discuss the personal health behaviors and the psychological and cognitive constructs that people of lower educational and socioeconomic status levels often lack, such as how to alter behavior and how to use cognitive skills to manage, for example, diet and nutrition, exercise, and smoking. Such persons may also have fewer coping and problem-solving skills. Lacking these behavioral and cognitive competencies can increase the onset and level of CHD risk factors. We believe that sociocultural and psychosocial factors are intimately related to psychosocial risk factors and need to be seen as highly related issues in efforts to diagnose, assess, and intervene.

CHD Interventions

We first discuss briefly some major medical interventions because patients or clients often ask about them, expecting the psychologist (or nonphysician) to know what they are and what they do. Our major focus, however, will be the results of well-controlled CHD-related psychosocial interventions, with selective mention of a few specific studies and discussion of the findings of systematic reviews of CHD interventions. We will also note some methodological issues. We strongly encourage readers to consult the actual studies and reviews since we can only mention highlights here.

Medical Interventions

Several pharmacological, medical, and surgical procedures are available to treat CHD. During acute myocardial infarction and ventricular arrhythmia (electrical irregularities of the heart), which can lead to sudden cardiac death, a variety of pharmacological interventions are commonly implemented (e.g., beta blockers, calcium channel blockers). Thrombolytic agents, usually streptokinase or tPA (tissue plasminogen activator) are administered to dissolve clots blocking coronary arteries; they are especially effective when administered in the early hours after symptoms of an MI begin. Anticoagulants, like aspirin and heparin, help to dissolve clots and prevent clots from reforming in the arteries.

PTCA (Percutaneous Transluminal Coronary Angioplasty)

PTCA, commonly called angioplasty, is a procedure to decrease the blockage of a coronary artery. During this procedure, a catheter with a small balloon attached to the end is inserted into an artery (in much the same way as cardiac catheterization) and passed up through the aorta to the area of blockage. The balloon is then inflated to condense the plaque and reopen the artery. Angioplasty can be performed only when an artery is partially blocked, as complete blockage prevents placement of the balloon. Success rates for the procedure are high (over 90 percent) and complication rates are low. The largest drawback, however, is that the blockage reappears in at least 30–35 percent of patients within a three- to six-month period following the procedure. Newer PTCA procedures cut the plaque away as well as use lasers to obliterate plaque. Another catheterization procedure to reopen a blocked area of the artery uses stents, small metal devices inserted into the artery to expand it and hold the change in place (Fischman et al., 1994).

CABG (Coronary Artery Bypass Graft Surgery)

CABG surgery is used to bypass the blocked area in the artery and allow for continued blood flow. An artery or vein from the patient's own body is used for the procedure. In most cases, multiple grafts are done when several coronary arteries are blocked. Mortality rates from CABG are approximately 1–2 percent. Patients who have undergone CABG report significantly less angina and greater activity ability than patients treated with other medical procedures. Controversy exists over whether these patients live longer, have fewer myocardial infarctions, and have increased work ability when compared to other treatments (Cameron, Davis, Green, & Schaff, 1996; King et al., 1994; Yusuf et al., 1994).

Psychosocial Interventions

The past two decades have seen impressive increases in well-controlled CHD-related psychosocial interventions, although they are still few in number (Williams & Chesney, 1993). The vast majority of studies examining CHD in the psychosocial area remain descriptive in nature, typically comparing persons with CHD (or with one of the CHD risk factors) with those without CHD (case-control designs) and, in some cases, following persons over several months or years (prospective designs) to see what factors predict CHD.

When it comes to psychosocial or lifestyle interventions, some have been dramatically effective in reducing CHD-related disease (morbidity) and, in some cases, death. But we do not yet understand which psychosocial factors are most predictive of CHD nor which interventions are the most powerful and most cost-effective. We know that not everyone benefits from any particular intervention, and we do not know enough about which persons need which intervention. Furthermore, we do not yet understand which physiological mechanisms responsible for CHD relate to lifestyle factors. Allan and Scheidt (1996) cite 14 possible physiological mechanisms. They suggest the leading candidate may be chronically elevated sympathetic nervous system activity, both neural and hormonal. Examples of how excessive sympathetic nervous system activity might cause CHD include:

- increased atherosclerosis from higher activation of macrophages and "clumping" or aggregation of blood platelets, thus contributing to build-up of arterial plaque
- increased ischemia caused by needing more myocardial oxygen due to elevated heart rate, blood pressure, and heart contractions, prompted in part by psychosocial risk factors
- reduced threshold level for ventricular fibrillation leading to sudden coronary death and possibly related in some cases to excessive anger and hostility

Following is a discussion of interventions with weight and physical activity, cigarette smoking, and other psychosocial factors, including specific examples of effective psychosocial interventions as well as a discussion of the stepped care approach.

Weight Reduction and Physical Activity

Health benefits, including reduced blood pressure and reduced cholesterol levels, accompany even modest weight loss (10 percent or less reduction)

(Goldstein, 1992). Likewise, even moderate levels of exercise produce substantial health benefits, such as reduced mortality (Blair et al., 1996). Physical activity has its own benefits in decreasing the risk for CHD, such as increasing HDL ("good" cholesterol), and it also plays a role in weight loss. Physical activity also acts as a means to reduce weight and is the strongest factor in being able to maintain weight loss. Numerous interventions exist to promote weight reduction, weight maintenance, and increased physical activity as discussed in Brownell and Fairburn (1995) including commercial, self-help, educational and cognitive-behavioral approaches.

Cigarette Smoking Cessation

Numerous studies indicate that smoking cessation reduces the risk for CHD, even in chronic smokers. A prospective study of registered nurses showed that quitters had a 24 percent reduction in risk compared to ongoing smokers after two years, and following 10 to 14 years of abstinence the risk was nearly identical to those who never smoked (Kawachi et al., 1993). For patients with CHD, smoking cessation has been shown to increase levels of HDL (Gottlieb, 1992). Readers interested in smoking cessation programs may refer to The Agency for Health Care Policy and Research Smoking Cessation Clinical Practice Guideline (1996), Curry (1993), and Lichtenstein and Glasgow (1992).

Reducing CHD Risk in Cardiac Patients

What is the evidence that psychosocial interventions significantly reduce CHD disease in those already afflicted? We believe the evidence is now promising enough to justify controlled use of psychosocial interventions as a part of cardiac health care policy and practice. Our recommendation is based primarily on meta-analytic and narrative reviews of psychosocial interventions with CHD patients (e.g., Davidson, Gidron, & Chaplin, 1996; Ketterer, 1993; Linden, Stossel, & Maurice, 1996; Nunes, Frank, & Kornfeld, 1987), with the caveat that interventions need to be carefully tailored to those being served, mindful of cultural, ethnic, racial, and gender differences as well as the type and severity of CHD. Above all, careful evaluation is mandatory using appropriate diagnostic and assessment procedures.

Results of Controlled Interventions

Interventions have targeted various outcomes, some focused on changes in blood pressure, smoking, or diet, others on intrapersonal and interpersonal issues (e.g., chronic stress, TABP) and still others on cardiac morbidity and mortality. Linden and colleagues (1996) sought evidence from 23 studies that reduced "psychological distress" (mostly depression, anxiety, anger/hostility, and TABP) could reduce cardiac morbidity and mortality as well as improve quality-of-life-related factors. Using meta-analysis they found that various psychosocial interventions, such as group counseling to reduce TABP, reduced cardiac mortality 40 percent over two years, and nonfatal cardiac events (most by new infarctions) 46 percent, compared to those receiving some combination of medication and physical exercise treatment. These differences were still significant at the four-year follow-up but were not as dramatic.

Other reviews of psychosocial interventions with post-MI patients (e.g., Ketterer, 1993) have also reported differences in the 30–40 percent range for reducing CHD events favoring psychosocial intervention compared to usual care (i.e., taking medications and seeing their physician). An earlier meta-analysis (Nunes et al., 1987) based on fewer studies also found comparable results. With two or three exceptions, most of the studies reviewed have been based on sample sizes of less than 150 participants; furthermore, all interventions have used small groups to provide treatment (Bracke & Thoresen, 1996).

Outcomes of these same psychosocial studies were examined recently by Davidson and colleagues (1996). They cited serious limitations of basing conclusions about psychosocial interventions solely on statistical null hypothesis testing, a practice that has been sharply criticized (see Cohen, 1994; Rosenthal & Rubin, 1982). To gain a more clinical or practical perspective on what differences actually mean, other than not being due to chance, these authors compared psychosocial interventions in CHD to common medical interventions, such as medications or surgical procedures. They asked the question: How many lives were saved or MIs prevented by various interventions? They compared eight randomly selected medication (drug) interventions with eight randomly selected psychosocial interventions. They used a weighted version of the Binomial Effect Size Display procedure which uses a 2 x 2 contingency table (Rosenthal & Rubin, 1982). They found that medication treatments prevented an average of 0.3 reinfarctions and 0.5 deaths per 100 persons; however, psychosocial interventions prevented 2.9 reinfarctions and 1.7 deaths per 100. This represents a nearly tenfold difference in nonfatal recurrences and a threefold difference in cardiac deaths. While the same drug interventions reported much more impressive P values (all $p<.001$) compared to the psychosocial treatment ($p<.05$), this was due to their much larger sample sizes (20 times larger than psychosocial interventions). Thus, when comparing two active interventions, not just a no-treatment control, these psychosocial approaches proved to be much more powerful in terms of preventing major cardiac events. Are these psychosocial interventions more costly than medical ones? Surprisingly, they were not more costly and, indeed, appear to be more cost effective when compared to costs of medical interventions (see Linden et al., 1996; Yates, 1996).

Examples of Psychosocial Interventions

We briefly mention these CHD interventions to give readers a better sense of what they are and how they work.

1. The first and largest study, called *MRFIT (Multiple Risk Factor Intervention Trial)*, was conducted in the 1970s with over 12,000 males at high risk for CHD (smokers, those with high blood pressure and serum cholesterol) (Shekelle et al., 1985). Usual care was compared to brief group counseling for smoking, stepped care for high blood pressure (to be described), and dietary advice about lowering cholesterol. Results were dramatic for those at highest risk (top 12.5 percent) over seven years, with 57 percent fewer cardiac deaths among group counseling patients, compared to those receiving usual care. Differences, however, for most participants were not significant because usual care and intervention participants both made improvements over the seven years. This study demonstrated that brief, relatively inexpensive psychosocial treatments (e.g., self-instructional manuals, brief small group seminars) could be cost effective for those with much higher overall CHD risk.

2. *The Recurrent Coronary Prevention Project (RCPP)* involved over 1000 post-MI patients in group counseling over 4.5 years and compared these patients to those in group discussion meetings with cardiologists. The focus was primarily on reducing TABP using a variety of techniques and procedures, including social modeling, behavioral rehearsal, self-efficacy enhancement, cognitive restructuring, and physical relaxation training coupled with structured homework assignments ("behavioral drills" workbook with such daily tasks as to practice smiling, expressing affection, listening without interruption). The counseling group intervention had 44 percent fewer cardiac recurrences over 4.5 years than the cardiac discussion group (Friedman et al., 1986). A four-year follow-up revealed 30 percent fewer fatal and nonfatal cardiac events for those in the counseling group

(Thoresen, 1990). Differences favoring group counseling were also found for subgroups of patients, such as fewer sudden cardiac deaths and fewer cardiac events for those with less physical damage to the heart from the MI. Results were also impressive for patients undergoing CABG and receiving group counseling (e.g., Powell & Thoresen, 1988); they had over 50 percent fewer cardiac events than CABG patients in cardiac discussion groups. Burell and colleagues (1994) recently replicated these RCPP results in Sweden, and Burell (1996) and others have also shown this type of group counseling to be effective in reducing cardiac events with post-MI and post-CABG women. Another replication of RCPP is currently underway in the Republic of South Africa (Wolff & Thoresen, 1996) with white and black South Africans who have suffered an MI. To date, preliminary results are encouraging in terms of reducing some risk factors (e.g., TABP, blood pressure, anger).

3. Significantly, *Frasure-Smith* (1991) reported an innovative intervention consisting of one brief contact with patients while they were in the hospital recovering from an MI followed by monthly 30-minute telephone interviews conducted by trained nursing aides. If necessary, nurses made a home visit to further clarify a problem and provide support. Frasure-Smith found that patients with elevated perceived stress scores while hospitalized for an MI who received this intervention had 50 percent fewer fatal cardiac events over five years. Patients who were less stressed while hospitalized, however, showed no differences compared to those receiving usual care.

Psychosocial interventions are particularly needed to help people change coronary-prone behavior, such as smoking, chronic stress, Type A behavior, depression, hostility, sedentary behavior, exhaustion, and social isolation. We strongly suspect that these psychosocial lifestyle patterns are intimately involved in creating the physiological changes that, in turn, lead to CHD. We also realize that medications and surgeries, while often life saving, seldom change the causes leading to CHD. It is in this domain where the preparation and training of psychologists and other mental health professionals, in what Allan and Scheidt (1996) have called cardiac psychology, can make the kind of difference in people's lives that has too often been neglected.

The Most Effective Psychosocial Treatments

So far, use of a greater number of intervention procedures over longer periods of time appears to be the most effective. Nunes and colleagues (1987) compared eight types of treatment (e.g., relaxation training, cognitive restructuring) on how much lifestyle changed and found that the strongest positive relationship (r=0.48, $p<.05$) was for interventions that used a greater variety of treatment procedures. This finding was also echoed by Linden and others (1996) in their review as well as by Thoresen and Powell (1992). The value of using several procedures is probably due to the great heterogeneity among cardiac patients as to what each perceives as needed and as useful, as well as to differences in the specific types of lifestyle problems each is experiencing (e.g., hostility problems with spouse or anxiety problems with return to work).

Stepped Care Interventions

Providing the best treatment for each person has long been a dilemma for health professionals. The logic of a stepped approach model to intervention starts with the assumption that some patients need minimal treatment while others, along a continuum, need more treatment of different kinds over a longer time. The logic also considers cost effectiveness: Do not provide more treatment than is needed. In managing high blood pressure, for example, stepped care is commonly used. The patient is asked first to increase physical activity, reduce or eliminate smoking, and reduce excessive body fat. After four to six weeks, if their blood pressure remains consistently high, an antihypertension medication is often prescribed. Many people can be successful with the first step; all people with elevated blood pressure do not need medication.

Black (1996) describes a generic model with five steps plus a pre-step recruitment phase:

1. minimal intervention, brief education focused on self-instruction
2. media-assisted intervention, adding print, videotape, computer, or audiotape media to the first step
3. minimal contact counseling: one or two brief sessions with a trained person to overcome specific barriers
4. structured group counseling over several sessions
5. individual counseling, supplementing group counseling

Brownell and Wadden (1992) offer a variation of the stepped approach model that often fits better when dealing with a more heterogeneous problem in terms of disease severity. Their model of obesity treatment, for example, suggests using individual client factors and program factors as part of the stepped care decision to classify individuals, matching them to a particular treatment step or level. For example, a person who is 5–20 percent overweight would begin treatment at step 1 or step 2, while a person who is 40–100 percent overweight and is more likely to have already tried step 1 or 2 unsuccessfully would begin treatment at step 3 or step 4. Black's stepped approach model seems especially relevant to primary prevention focused interventions, while the Brownell and Wadden strategy appears well suited for those with more advanced problems.

To date, few CHD interventions have been designed and evaluated explicitly with a stepped approach model in mind. Currently, a National Heart, Lung, and Blood Institute clinical trial with 3000 depressed and/or socially unsupported post-MI patients (50 percent of whom are women and minority members) is using two steps, individual counseling and group counseling, and, if needed, a third step, antidepressive medication. Between 4 and 12 individual sessions are being used, depending on need, followed by 8 to 12 group sessions over the six months immediately following the MI. This is a population that has been poorly served because their depression and social isolation typically have been ignored in cardiac rehabilitation programs.

Many post-MI patients who are not significantly depressed or socially isolated can benefit from a more minimal "step" intervention. For example, some might benefit from working on their own with a structured manual designed to promote lifestyle change for cardiac patients, with the possibility of a troubleshooting session or two, if needed, with a trained lay counselor (American Heart Association, 1990; Miller & Taylor, 1995) or participating in peer-led structured group counseling for six to eight sessions (Lorig, 1997). Another example for post-MI patients is a nurse-based case management program (DeBusk et al., 1994), which uses telephone contact, computers, limited individual meetings, and medications if needed, to help reduce smoking and serum cholesterol and to improve more heart healthy diets. These projects using variations of a stepped care approach offer promising directions and some evidence that treatment can be better tailored to the needs of people, often at reduced costs. When it comes to interventions, one size simply does not fit all.

Some Forgotten Factors: Religiousness and Spirituality

Earlier we noted that no one technique or method has yet been shown to account for the success of small group interventions in reducing disease and improving quality of life. Cited techniques often include various kinds of relaxation training, self-monitoring, behavioral skills training, cognitive restructuring, and moderate exercise focused on risk factors. Other factors, however, seldom receive recognition in helping persons with CHD to make needed life changes and to cope effectively with CHD.

Ornish and his colleagues, in helping those with severely advanced CAD slow and, in some cases, reverse the CAD, acknowledge that spiritual concerns and issues of faith can play a powerful role in making drastic lifestyle changes, such as using meditation and yoga daily, following strict vegetarian diets, listening with compassion, and having intimate group discussions about meaning and purpose in life (Ornish et al., 1990). A recent study (Oxman, Freeman, & Manheimer, 1995) highlighted the power of these forgotten factors in how we think about and provide care for those with CHD. Oxman and his colleagues followed more than 150 patients who had coronary surgery (CABG or aortic valve replacement) and found a tenfold difference in death over six months; those who reported gaining considerable comfort and strength from their religious beliefs and who spent time regularly with others in group activities had very few deaths (2–3 percent), compared to an almost 25 percent mortality rate for those who did not. Several demographic, medical, and psychosocial risk factors failed to account for these dramatic differences in mortality.

How might we explain these kinds of results? Perhaps those who report a belief in a higher power have a more optimistic outlook, engage in more healthy behaviors, have more social support, are less hostile, or are less depressed. They, therefore, could experience less chronically elevated sympathetic nervous system arousal, which in turn could reduce the physiological changes associated with CAD and sudden cardiac death. At this point we do not know why, but we are starting to realize that spiritual and religious factors can make a difference in medical and psychosocial outcomes. We often forget that many Americans are spiritually or religiously minded: 94 percent believe in God, 76 percent believe that prayer or meditation is an important part of their life, and 60 percent indicate that faith is the most important influence in their life (Gallup, 1990, 1996). We do not, however, know much about what it means when people say they are spiritual or religious. Yet given the results, we need to take seriously questions about spirituality and religion in the lives of people seeking help (see chapter 17 in this book).

Based on their extensive clinical experience leading post-MI groups of men and women, Bracke and Thoresen (1996) have suggested that helping patients look at their unexplored and unresolved spiritual, religious, and existential issues can play a crucial role in making the kind of lifestyle changes that reduce morbidity and mortality (also see Burell, 1996; Thoresen & Bracke, 1997). Such a suggestion is hardly new, given the long-standing and often ignored history in medicine and psychology. Hippocrates, for example, noted over 2500 years ago that "You ought not to attempt to cure the body without the soul" (Plato, 1953/1871, p. 103). Sir William Osler (1987), a major founder of cardiology in the late nineteenth century, admonished physicians to ask, "What kind of person has the disease?" rather than "What kind of disease does the person have?" William James (1961/1902) admonished psychologists to consider ways to promote more spiritually enriching lives. In helping people make lifestyle changes, we may provide more effective interventions if we offer the opportunity to examine issues of life's meaning and purpose, of what is held to be divine or sacred, and by what principles one chooses to live. Not all patients are necessarily interested in these issues, but many are and yet have little opportunity to explore them in current health care programs.

Some Current Controversies

As with any evolving field of knowledge and practice, some controversies exist. Within the area of cardiovascular health and disease, continuing debate seems inevitable given the multidisciplinary nature of the topic (e.g., it's more than just medicine) and the multidimensionality of the problems (e.g., it's more than physiology). We see three interrelated areas of controversy, which are both broad and basic:

1. issues of the etiology of CHD and the "mechanisms issue" (i.e., How does CHD actually develop in people?)
2. issues of diagnosis, assessment, and evaluation (i.e., What is the best way to find out what specific problems and processes are involved?)
3. issues of intervention or treatment (i.e., Who needs how much of what kinds of treatment?)

One issue concerning the etiology of CHD, with implications for assessment and treatment, centers on the importance of psychosocial factors in the etiology of CHD. Some have been reluctant to consider psychosocial or lifestyle factors because the evidence, in their view, is yet not compelling.

But, as Allan and Scheidt (1996) recently noted, "There are substantial data supporting the relationship between modifiable psychosocial risk factors and coronary heart disease" (p. 443). The conflict involves how much and what kinds of substantiation are needed. One need only recall the reluctance of many for decades to acknowledge cigarette smoking as a CHD risk factor. We believe the evidence of a psychosocial-CHD connection is now promising enough to warrant psychosocial assessment and to offer treatment programs under well-controlled conditions in order to determine what works well with whom. The controversies surrounding the etiology of CHD will continue as the scientific process involves skepticism and challenge. We suspect that one currently popular model for the mechanism of psychosocial influence—excessive sympathetic nervous system activity—will be further refined, but will continue to prove useful in directing assessment and treatment efforts.

Another issue of contention involves the validity of theory, intervention, and assessment techniques for women and ethnic minorities. Many now acknowledge that research based on upper-middle-class white males, the backbone for almost all CHD research and intervention, may not be valid for women and minorities. Research on these other groups is, however, still lacking.

An additional question concerns the applicability of the brief therapy model for psychosocial intervention with CHD. It is conceivable that some patients could benefit from a brief, structured program as part of a stepped care model approach. Others, however, may require longer program participation, particularly those who require greater help with psychological and social functioning.

A final controversy centers on how to best diagnose and assess psychosocial factors. Much research has relied heavily on paper-and-pencil, self-report questionnaires. Some researchers feel, however, that such measures lead to an impoverished picture or still photograph of the person that barely scratches the surface of who the person is and how he or she experiences everyday life. For example, McAdams (1993) suggests a more "in-depth" qualitative perspective in which various measures can be used to assess the person's story (personal myth), describing how the person constructs meaning in his or her life. Our hunch is that assessment pictures will be supplemented by narrative methods. We all know that everyone will not benefit equally from the same treatment, just as we know that all people do not develop CHD from the same type and level of risk factors. How best to improve assessment remains debated, but this additional data could be used to tailor interventions more effectively.

Conclusion

Although deaths from cardiovascular and cerebrovascular diseases have diminished impressively since the 1960s, the marked prevalence and incidence of these diseases still remain. CHD alone is the greatest single cause of death and disability in all Americans, men and women, regardless of ethnicity, race, gender, or socioeconomic status level. Essentially, more people with CHD are surviving, but typically under restricted conditions, often requiring continuous medication and expensive surgeries. They are alive but do not necessarily have an adequate quality of life. The economic costs of CHD remain exorbitant and for many the psychosocial costs are tragic. We still cannot account for almost 50 percent of the variance in what predicts and presumably causes CHD, yet we can do a great deal. We now know enough about what helps reduce death and disability to justify expansion of a variety of cost-effective interventions coupled with appropriate assessment and evaluation. While the stampede to embrace managed care has created serious problems for many in providing the kind of medical and psychosocial care that people need, this dramatic change has also created a climate that is increasingly receptive to addressing psychosocial issues in CHD. If we continue to clearly document that addressing psychosocial or lifestyle issues makes a difference in preventing and reducing chronic and acute health problems, then support for providing the kind of psychosocial assessment and intervention mentioned in this chapter will grow. We hope you will participate in creating more effective ways to help people from all walks of life reduce their risk of CHD and increase their quality of life. The need is great and the time is right for doing so.

Suggested Resources

Heart and Mind: The Practice of Cardiac Psychology, edited by Allan and Scheidt (1996), is an excellent up-to-date collection of chapters, including a thorough description of cardiology (written for a nonmedical audience), an overview of the basics of empirical research on cardiac psychology, and several chapters on various clinical techniques and interventions to alter psychosocial factors and reduce coronary events such as group therapy for coronary patients. The glossary of medical terms and procedures is very useful.

Heart and Stroke Facts (American Heart Association, 1994) is a helpful guide, with annual statistical updates, covering basic information on CHD and stroke, including cardiac physiology, major disorders, risk factors, risk reduction, and some treatment information.

Spira (1997) has written a useful guide to psychological treatment of people in groups who are suffering from chronic diseases, such as CHD, breast cancer, eating disorders, and substance abuse. *Group Therapy for Medically Ill Patients* provides detailed information on various group approaches to helping people change lifestyle-related factors.

A group of medical experts prepared *An Active Partnership for the Health of Your Heart* (American Heart Association, 1990), a workbook for those suffering from CHD or those seeking to reduce their risk of CHD. Sections on the basics of CHD, food, exercise, stress, and smoking include self-assessments and suggestions for developing plans to make changes and for dealing with setbacks. Readers will find this a helpful resource, as it provides a brief but informative summary of CHD-related problems and ways of helping patients make needed changes. Videos are available to use in conjunction with the workbook.

Every ten years, a special edition of the *Journal of Consulting and Clinical Psychology* is devoted to behavioral medicine, including articles on cancer, CHD, chronic disease, obesity, smoking, and other topics. The August 1992 volume includes numerous key articles cited in this chapter.

Discussion Questions

1. What are the differences between positive, possible, and plausible risk factors? Describe at least one of each type.
2. What role, if any, does gender play in the assessment and treatment of CHD?
3. What is a major limitation in using only the biomedical model in assessing and treating CHD?
4. Describe at least two major issues in diagnosis and assessment of TABP that also apply to other psychosocial risk factors for CHD.

5. What are some advantages and disadvantages of using a stepped approach model in the treatment of CHD?

References

Achuff, S. C. (1996). Angina pectoris. In J. D. Stobo, D. B. Hellmann, P. W. Ladenson, B. G. Petty, & T. A. Traill (Eds.), *The principles and practice of medicine* (pp. 9–15). Stamford, CT: Appleton & Lange.

The Agency for Health Care Policy and Research Smoking Cessation Clinical Practice Guideline. (1996). *Journal of the American Medical Association, 275,* 1270–1280.

Allan, R. (1996). Introduction: The emergence of cardiac psychology. In R. Allan, & S. Scheidt (Eds.), *Heart and mind: The practice of cardiac psychology* (pp. 3–14). Washington, DC: American Psychological Association.

Allan, R., & Scheidt, S. (Eds.). (1996). *Heart and mind: The practice of cardiac psychology.* Washington, DC: American Psychological Association.

American Heart Association. (1990). *An active partnership for the health of your heart.* Dallas, TX: Author.

American Heart Association. (1994). *Heart and stroke facts.* Dallas, TX: Author.

American Heart Association. (1995). *Heart and stroke facts: 1995 statistical supplement.* Dallas, TX: Author.

Appels, A. (1996). Personality factors and coronary heart disease. In K. Orth-Gomer, & N. Scheiderman (Eds.), *Behavioral medicine approaches to cardiovascular disease prevention* (pp. 149–160). Manwah, N J: Erlbaum.

Appels, A., & Meester, C. (1996). An interview to measure Vital Exhaustion II: Reliability and validity of the interview and correlation with personality characteristics. *Psychology and Health, 11,* 573–581.

Appels, A., & Schouten, E. (1991). Waking up exhausted as a risk indicator of myocardial infarction. *American Journal of Cardiology, 68,* 395–398.

Barefoot, J. C. (1992). Developments in measurement of hostility. In H. Friedman (Ed.), *Hostility, coping, and health* (pp. 13–31). Washington, DC: American Psychological Association.

Barefoot, J. C., Dodge, K. A., Peterson, B. L., Dahlstorm, W. G., & Williams, R. B. (1989). The Cook-Medley Hostility Scale: Item content and ability to predict survival. *Psychosomatic Medicine, 51,* 46–57.

Barefoot, J. C., Patterson, J. C., Haney, T. L., & Cayton, T. C. (1994). Hostility in asymptomatic men with angiographically confirmed coronary artery disease. *American Journal of Cardiology, 74,* 439–442.

Barefoot, J. C., & Schroll, M. (1996). Symptoms of depression, acute myocardial infarction, and total mortality in a community sample. *Circulation, 93*(11), 1976–1980.

Berkman, L. F., Leo-Summers, L., & Horwitz, R. I. (1992). Emotional support and survival after myocardial infarction: A prospective, population-based study of the elderly. *Annals of Internal Medicine, 117*(12), 1003–1009.

Bjorntorp, P. (1990). "Portal" adipose tissue as a generator of risk factors for cardiovascular disease and diabetes. *Arteriosclerosis, 10,* 493–496.

Black, D. R. (1996). *Stepped approach model: Emergence of a social science framework for service delivery.* Unpublished manuscript, Purdue University, Department of Health, Kinesiology, and Leisure Studies, West Lafayette, IN.

Blair, S. N., Kampert, J. B., Kohl, H. W., Barlow, C. E., Macera, C. A., Paffenbarger, R. S., Jr., & Gibbons, L. W. (1996). Influences of cardiorespiratory fitness and other precursors on cardiovascular disease and all-cause mortality in men and women. *Journal of the American Medical Association, 276*(3), 205–210.

Boltwood, M. D., Taylor, C. B., Burke, M. B., Grogin, H., & Giacomini, J. (1993). Anger reports predict coronary artery vasomotor response to mental stess in atherosclerotic segments. *American Journal of Cardiology, 72,* 1361–1365.

Booth-Kewley, S., & Friedman, H. (1987). Psychological predictors of heart disease: A quantitative review. *Psychological Bulletin, 101,* 342–362.

Bracke, P. E., & Thoresen, C. E. (1996). Reducing Type A behavior patterns: A structural group approach. In R. Allan, & S. Scheidt (Eds.), *Heart and mind: The practice of cardiac psychology* (pp. 255–290). Washington, DC: American Psychological Association.

Brezinka V., & Kittel F. (1996). Psychosocial factors of coronary heart disease in women: A review. *Social Science and Medicine, 42,* 1351–1365.

Brown, M. S., & Goldstein, J. L. (1996). Heart attacks: Gone with the century? *Science, 272*(5262), 629.

Brownell, K. D., & Fairburn, C. G. (Eds.). (1995). *Eating disorders and obesity: A comprehensive handbook.* New York: Guilford.

Brownell, K. D., & Wadden, T. A. (1992). Etiology and treatment of obesity: Understanding a serious, prevalent, and refractory disorder. *Journal of Consulting and Clinical Psychology, 60*(4), 505–517.

Burell, G. (1996). Group psychotherapy in Project New Life: Treatment of coronary-prone behaviors for patients who have had coronary artery bypass graft surgery. In R. Allan, & S. Scheidt (Eds.), *Heart and mind: The practice of cardiac psychology* (pp. 291–310). Washington, DC: American Psychological Association.

Burell, G., Ohman, A., Sundin, O., Strom, G., Ramund, B., Calhed, I., & Thoresen, C. E. (1994). Modification of Type A behavior patterns in post-myocardial infarction patients: A route to cardiac rehabilitation. *International Journal of Behavioral Medicine, 1,* 32–54.

Cameron, A., Davis, K. B., Green, G., Schaff, H. V. (1996). Coronary bypass surgery with internal-thoracic-artery grafts—effects on survival over a 15-year period. *New England Journal of Medicine, 334,* 216–219.

Case, R. B., Moss, A. J., Case, N., McDermott, M., & Eberly, S. (1992). Living alone after myocardial infarction: Impact on prognosis. *Journal of the American Medical Association, 267*(4), 515–519.

Cobb, S. (1976). Social support as a moderator of life stress. *Psychosomatic Medicine, 38,* 300–314.

Cohen, J. (1994). The earth is round (p < .05). *American Psychologist, 49,* 997–1003.

Cohen, S., & Williamson, G. M. (1991). Stress and infectious disease in humans. *Psychological Bulletin, 109*(1), 5–24.

Colantonio, A., Kasl, S. V., Ostfeld, A. M., & Berkmn, L. F. (1993). Psychosocial predictor of stroke in an elderly population. *Journals of Gerontology, 48,* S261–S268.

Curry, S. J. (1993). Self-help interventions for smoking cessation. *Journal of Consulting and Clinical Psychology, 61,* 790–803.

Davidson, K. W., Gidron, Y., & Chaplin, W. F. (1996). *Statistical significance versus clinical significance and the evaluation of medical and psychological interventions for post-MI patients.* Unpublished manuscript, Dalhousie University, Department of Psychology, Halifax, Nova Scotia, Canada.

DeBusk, R. F., Miller, N. H., Superko, H. R., Dennis, C. A., Thomas, R. J., Lew, H. T., Berger, W. E. I., Heller, R. S., Rompf, J., Gee, D., Kraemer, H. C., Bandura, A., Ghandour, G., Clark, M., Fisher, L., & Taylor, C. B. (1994). A case-management system for coronary risk factor modification after acute myocardial infarction. *Annals of Internal Medicine, 120,* 721–729.

Dembroski, T. M., McDougall, J. M., Costa, P. T., & Grandits, G. A. (1989). Components of hostility as predictors of sudden death and myocardial infarction in the Multiple Risk Factor Intervention Trial. *Psychosomatic Medicine, 51,* 514–522.

Engel, G. L. (1977). The clinical application of the biopsychosocial model: A challenge for biomedicine. *Science, 196,* 129–136.

Everson, S. A., Goldberg, D. E., Kaplan, G. A., Cohen, R. D., Pukkala, E., Tuomilehto, J., & Salonen, J. T. (1996). Hopelessness and risk of mortality and incidence of myocardial infarction and cancer. *Psychosomatic Medicine, 58,* 113–121.

Fielding, R. (1991). Depression and acute myocardial infarction: A review and reinterpretation. *Social Science and Medicine, 32,* 1017–1027.

Fischman, D. L., Leon, M. B., Baim, D. S., Schatz, R. A., Savage, M. P., Penn, I., Detre, K., Veltri, L., Ricci, D., Nobuyoshi, M., et al. (1994). A randomized comparison of coronary-stent placement and balloon angioplasty in the treatment of coronary artery disease. *New England Journal of Medicine, 331,* 496–501.

Frasure-Smith, N. (1991). In-hospital symptoms of psychological stress as predictors of long-term outcome after acute myocardial infarction in men. *American Journal of Cardiology, 67,* 121–127.

Frasure-Smith, N., Lesperance, F., & Talajic, M. (1993). Depression following myocardial infarction: Impact of 6-month survival. *Journal of the American Medical Association, 270,* 1819–1825.

Friedman, M., Fleischmann, N., & Price, V. A. (1996). Diagnosis of Type A behavior pattern. In R. Allan, & S. Scheidt (Eds.), *Heart and mind: The practice of cardiac psychology* (pp. 179–198). Washington, DC: American Psychological Association.

Friedman, M., Rosenman, R., & Carroll, V. (1958). Changes in the serum cholesterol and blood-clotting time in men subjected to cyclic variation in occupational stress. *Circulation, 17,* 852–861.

Friedman, M., Thoresen, C. E., Gill, J., Ulmer, D., Powell, L. H., Price, V. A., Brown, B., Thompson, L., Robin, D., Breall, W. S., Bourg, W., Levy, R., & Dixon, T. (1986). Alteration of Type A behavior and its effects on cardiac recurrences in post-infarction patients: Summary results of the Recurrent Coronary Prevention Project. *American Heart Journal, 112,* 653–665.

Gallup, G., Jr. (1990). *Religion in America: 1990.* Princeton, NJ: Princeton Religious Research Center.

Gallup, G., Jr. (1996, December). *Epidemiology and spirituality.* Paper presented at the Sprituality and Health Conference, Harvard Medical School, Cambridge, MA.

Goldstein, D. J. (1992). Beneficial effects of modest weight loss. *International Journal of Obesity and Related Metabolic Disorders, 16,* 397–415.

Goodman, M., Quigley, J., Moran, G., Meilman, H., & Sherman, M. (1996). Hostility predicts restenosis after percutaneous transluminal coronary angioplasty. *Mayo Clinic Proceedings, 71*(8), 729–734.

Gottlieb, S. O. (1992). Cardiovascular benefits of smoking cessation. *Heart Disease and Stroke, 1,*173–175.

Graff-Low, K., Thoresen, C. E., King, A., Pattillo, J., & Jenkins, C. (1995). Anxiety, depression and heart disease in women. *International Journal of Behavioral Medicine, 1,* 305–319.

Guerci, A. D. (1996). Unstable angina and acute myocardial infarction. In J. D. Stobo, D. B. Hellmann, P. W. Ladenson, B. G. Petty, & T. A. Traill (Eds.), *The Principles and Practice of Medicine* (pp. 16–27). Stamford, CT: Appleton & Lange.

Hecker, M. H., Chesney, M. A., Black, G. W., & Frautschi, N. (1988). Coronary-prone behaviors in the Western Collaborative Group Study. *Psychosomatic Medicine, 50*(2), 153–164.

Helmers, K. F., Krantz, D. S., Howell, R. H., Klein, J. Bairey, C. N., & Rozanski, A. (1993). Hostility and myocardial ischemia in coronary artery disease patients: Evaluation by gender and ischemic index. *Psychosomatic Medicine, 55,* 29–36.

Henry, J., & Stephens, P. (1977). *Stress, health and the social environment.* New York: Springer-Verlag.

Higgins, M., & Thorn, T. (1993). Cardiovascular disease in women as a public health problem. In N. K. Wegner, L. Speroff, & B. Packard (Eds.), *Cardiovascular health and disease in women* (pp. 15–19). Greenwich, CT: Le Jacq Communication.

House, J. S., Landes, K. R., & Umberson, D. (1988). Social relationships and health. *Science, 241,* 540–545.

Houston, B. K., Babyat, M. A., Chesney, M. A., Black, G., & Ragland, D. R. (1997). Social dominance and 22-year all-cause mortality in men. *Psychosomatic Medicine, 59,* 5–12.

Ironson, G., Taylor, C. B., Boltwood, M., Bartzokis, T., Dennis, C., Chesney, M., Spitzer, S., & Segall, G. M. (1992). Effects of anger on left ventricular ejection fraction in coronary artery disease. *American Journal of Cardiology, 70*(3), 281–285.

James, W. (1961/1902). *The varieties of religious experience.* New York: Macmillan. (Original work published 1902)

Jiang, W., Babyak, M., Krantz, D. S., Waugh, R. A., Coleman, R. E., Hanson, M. M., Frid, D. J., McNulty, S., Morris, J. J., O'Connor, C., & Blumenthal, J. A. (1996). Mental stress-induced myocardial ischemia and cardiac events. *Journal of the American Medical Association, 275,* 1651–1656.

Joseph, A., Ackerman, D., Talley, J. D., Johnstone, J., & Kupersmith, J. (1993). Manifestations of coronary atherosclerosis in young trauma victims—an autopsy study. *Journal of the American College of Cardiology, 22,* 459–467.

Kaplan, J. R., Manuck, S. B., Williams, J. K., & Straun, W. (1993). Psychosocial influences on atherosclerosis: Evidence for effects and mechanisms in non-human primates. In J. Blascovich, & E. Katkin (Eds.), *Cardiovascular reactivity to psychological stress and disease* (pp. 3–26). Washington, DC: American Psychological Association.

Kawachi, I., Colditz, G. A., Stampfer, M. J., Willet, W. C., Manson, J. E., Rosner, B., Hunter, D. J., Hennekens, C. H., & Speizer, F. E. (1993). Smoking cessation in relation to total mortality rates in women. A prospective cohort study. *Annals of Internal Medicine, 119,* 992–1000.

Kawachi, I., Sparrow, D., Spiro, A., Vokonas, P., & Weiss, S. (1996). A prospective study of anger and coronary heart disease: The Normative Aging Study. *Circulation, 94,* 2090–2095.

Ketterer, M. W. (1993). Secondary prevention of ischemic heart disease. The case for aggressive behavioral monitoring and intervention. *Psychosomatics, 34*(6), 478–484.

Kiesler, D. J. (1966). Some myths of psychotherapy research and the search for a paradigm. *Psychological Bulletin, 65,* 110–136.

King, S. B., III, Lembo, N. J., Weintraub, W. S., Kosinski, A. S., Barnhart, H. X., Kutner, M. H., Alazraki, N. P., Guyton, R. A., & Zhao, X. Q. (1994). A randomized trial comparing coronary angioplasty with coronary bypass surgery. *New England Journal of Medicine, 331,*1044–50.

Kop, W. J., Appels, A. P., Mendes de Leon, C. F., de Swart, H. B., & Bar, F. W. (1994). Vital exhaustion predicts new cardiac events after successful coronary angioplasty. *Psychosomatic Medicine, 56*(4), 281–287.

Kopta, S. M., Howard, K. I., Lowry, J. L., & Beutler, L. E. (1994). Patterns of symptomatic recovery in psychotherapy. *Journal of Consulting and Clinical Psychology, 62*(5), 1009–1016.

Levenson, R. W., Ekman, P., & Friesen, W. V. (1990). Voluntary facial action generates emotion-specific autonomic nervous system activity. *Psychophisiology, 27*(4), 363–384.

Lichtenstein, E., & Glasgow, R. E., (1992). Smoking cessation: What have we learned over the past decade? *Journal of Consulting and Clinical Psychology, 60,* 518–527.

Linden, W., Stossel, C., & Maurice, J. (1996). Psychosocial interventions for patients with coronary artery disease: A meta-analysis. *Archives of Internal Medicine, 156*(7), 745–752.

Lorig, K. (1997). *Chronic disease self-management program.* Unpublished manuscript, Stanford University, Stanford School of Medicine, Stanford, CA.

Manson, J. E., Colditz, G. A., Stampfer, M. J., Willett, W. C., Rosner, B., Monson, R. R., Speizer, F. E., & Hennekens, C. H. (1990). A prospective study of obesity and risk of coronary heart disease in women. *New England Journal of Medicine, 322,* 882–888.

Matthews, K. (1988). CHD and Type A behaviors: Update on and alternative to the Booth-Kewley and Friedman quantitative review. *Psychological Bulletin, 104,* 373–380.

McAdams, D. P. (1993). *Stories we live by.* New York: Guilford.

Miller, N. H., & Taylor, C. B. (1995). *Lifestyle management for patients with coronary heart disease.* (Monograph Number 2). Champaign, IL: Human Kinetics.

Miller, T. Q., Turner, C. W., Tindale, C. W., Posavac, E. J., & Dugoni, B. L. (1991). Reasons for the trend toward null findings in research on Type A behavior. *Psychological Bulletin, 110*(3), 469–485.

Moser, D. K., & Dracup, K. (1997). Is anxiety early after myocardial infarction associated with subsequent ischemic and arrhythmic events? *Psychosomatic Medicine, 58,* 395–401.

Nunes E. V., Frank, K. A., & Kornfeld, D. S. (1987). Psychological treatment for Type A behavior pattern and for coronary heart disease: A meta-analysis of the literature. *Psychosomatic Medicine, 48,* 159–173.

Ornish, D., Brown, S. E., Scherwitz, L. S., Billings, J. H., Armstrong, W. T., Ports, T. A., McLanahan, S. M., Kirkeeide, R. L., Brand, R. J., & Gould, K. L. (1990). Can lifestyle changes reverse coronary artery disease? *Lancet, 336,* 129–133.

Orth-Gomer, K., & Uniden, A. L. (1990). Type A behavior, social support, and coronary risk: Intervention and significance for mortality in cardiac patients. *Psychosomatic Medicine, 52,* 59–72.

Orth-Gomer, K., Rosengren, A., & Wilhelmsen, L. (1993). Lack of social support and incidence of coronary heart disease in middle-aged Swedish men. *Psychosomatic Medicine, 55*(1), 37–43.

Osler, W. (1897). *Lectures on angina pectoris and allied states.* New York: Appleton-Century-Crafts.

Oxman, T. E., Freeman, D. H., & Manheimer, E. D. (1995). Lack of social participation or religious strength and comfort as risk factors for death after cardiac surgery in the elderly. *Psychosomatic Medicine, 57,* 5–15.

Parker, S. D., Breslow, M. J., Frank, S. M., Rosenfeld, B. A., Norris, E. J., Chrisopherson, R., Rock, P., Gottlieb, S. O., Raff, H., & Perler, B. A. (1995). Catecholamine and cortisol responses to lower extremity revascularization: correlation with outcome variables. Perioperative Ischemia Randomized Anesthesia Trial Study Group. *Critical Care Medicine, 23,* 1954–1961.

Perkins, K. A. (1985). The synergistic effect of smoking and serum cholesterol on coronary heart disease. *Health Psychology, 4,* 337–360.

Pi-Sunyer, F. X. (1995). Medical complications of obesity. In K. D. Brownell & C. G. Fairburn (Eds.), *Eating disorders and obesity: A comprehensive handbook* (pp. 401–405). New York, London: Guilford.

Pincus, T., & Callahan, L. F. (1995). What explains the association between socioeconomic status and health: Primarily access to medical care or mind-body variables. *Advances, 11*(3), 29–39.

Plato. (1953/1871). The dialogues of Plato (B. Jowett, Trans.). Oxford, England: Jowett Copyright Trustee. (Original work published 1871)

Powell, L. H., & Thoresen, C. E. (1988). Effects of Type A behavioral counseling and severity of prior acute myocardial infarction on survival. *American Journal of Cardiology, 62,* 1159–1163.

Pratt, L. A., Ford, D. E., Crum, R. M., Armenian, H. K., Gallo, J. J., & Eaton, W. W. (1996). Depression, psychotropic medication, and risk of myocardial infarction: Prospective data from the Baltimore ECA follow-up. *Circulation, 94*(12), 3123–3129.

Ragland, D. R., & Brand, R. J. (1988). Type A behavior and mortality from coronary heart disease. *New England Journal of Medicine, 318*(2), 65–69.

Rosenthal, R., & Rubin, D. B. (1982). A simple, general purpose display of the magnitude of experimental effects. *Journal of Educational Psychology, 74,* 166–169.

Ruberman, W., Weinblatt, E., Goldberg, J., & Chaudbury, B. S. (1984). Psychosocial influences on mortality after myocardial infarction. *New England Journal of Medicine, 311,* 552–559.

Scheidt, S. (1996). A whirlwind tour of cardiology for the mental health professional. In R. Allan, & S. Scheidt (Eds.), *Heart and mind: The practice of cardiac psychology* (pp. 15–62). Washington, DC: American Psychological Association.

Scherwitz, L. (1988). Interviewer behaviors in the Western Collaborative Group Study and the Multiple Risk Factor Intervention Trial Structured Interviews. In B. K. Houston, & C. R. Snyder (Eds.), *Type A behavior pattern: Research, theory and intervention* (pp. 146–167). New York: Wiley.

Seeman, T. E., & Syme, S. L. (1987). Social networks and coronary artery disease: A comparison of the structure and function of social relations as predictors of disease. *Psychosomatic Medicine, 49*(4), 341–354.

Seigman, A. W., & Smith, T. W. (1994). *Anger, hostility, and the heart.* Hillsdale, NJ: Erlbaum.

Shekelle, R. B., Hulley, S. B., Neaten, J. D., Billings, J. H., Borhani, N. O., Gerece, T. A., Jacobs, D. R., Lasser, N. L., Mittemark, H. B., & Stamler, J. for the Multiple Risk Factor Intervention Trial Research Group. (1985). The MRFIT Behavior Pattern Study II: Type A behavior and the incidence of coronary artery disease. *American Journal of Epidemiology, 122,* 559–570.

Spira, J. L. (Ed.). (1997). *Group therapy for medically ill patients.* New York: Guilford.

Steinberg, L., & Jorgensen, R. S. (1996). Assessing the MMPI-based Cook-Medley Hostility Scale: The implications of dimensionality. *Journal of Personality and Social Psychology, 70*(6), 1281–1287.

Thompson, S. C., Sobolew-Shubin, A., Graham, M.A., & Janigian, A. S. (1989). Psychosocial adjustment following a stroke. *Social Science and Medicine, 28,* 239–247.

Thoresen, C. E. (1990, June). *Long-term effects of Type A group treatment in the Recurrent Coronary Prevention Project.* Paper presented at the First International Society of Behavioral Medicine, Uppsala, Sweden.

Thoresen, C. E. (1996). *Effects of reducing coronary-prone behavior in post-myocardial infarction patients: A four year follow-up.* Unpublished manuscript, Stanford University, School of Education, Stanford, CA.

Thoresen, C. E., & Bracke, P. (1997). Reducing coronary recurrences and coronary-prone behavior: A structured group treatment approach. In J. Spira (Ed.), *Group therapy for medically ill patients* (pp. 92–129). New York: Guilford.

Thoresen, C. E., & Eagleston, J. R. (1985). Counseling for health. *The Counseling Psychologist, 13,* 15–87.

Thoresen, C. E., & Ohman, A. (1987). The Type A behavior pattern: A person-environment interaction perspective. In D. Megnussen, & A. Ohman (Eds.), *Psychopathology: An interaction perspective* (pp. 325–346). San Diego, CA: Academic.

Thoresen, C. E., & Powell, L. H. (1992). Type A behavior pattern: New perspectives on theory, assessment, and intervention. *Journal of Consulting and Clinical Psychology, 60*(4), 595–604.

Traill, T. A. (1996). Approach to the patient with cardiovascular disease. In J. D. Stobo, D. B. Hellmann, P. W. Ladenson, B. G. Petty, & T. A. Traill (Eds.), *The principles and practice of medicine* (pp. 3–8). Stamford, CT: Appleton & Lange.

Wegner, N. K., Speroff, L., & Packard, B. (1993). *Cardiovascular health and disease in women.* Greenwich, CT: Le Jacq Communication.

Willett, W. C., & Manson, J. E. (1995). Epidemiologic studies of health risks due to excess weight. In K. D. Brownell, & C. G. Fairburn (Eds.), *Eating disorders and obesity: A comprehensive handbook* (pp. 396–400). New York, London: Guilford.

Williams, R. B. (1987). Refining the Type A hypothesis: Emergence of hostility complex. *American Journal of Cardiology, 60,* 27–31.

Williams, R. B., Barefoot, J. C., Califf, R. M., Haney, T. L., Saunders, W. B., Pryor, D. B., Hlatky, M. A., Siegler, I. C., & Mark, D. B. (1992). Prognostic importance of social and economic resources among medically treated patients with angiographically documented coronary artery disease. *Journal of the American Medical Association, 267*(4), 520–524.

Williams, R. B., & Chesney, M. A. (1993). Psychosocial factors and prognosis in established coronary artery disease: The need for research on interventions. *Journal of the American Medical Association, 270*(15), 1860–1861.

Williams, R. B., & Williams, V. (1993). *Anger kills: Seventeen strategies for controlling the hostility that can harm your health.* New York: Harper/Perennial.

Wolff, E., & Thoresen, C. E. (1996, September). *The Recurrent Coronary Prevention Project: A South African replication.* Paper presented at the Tenth European Health Psychology Society Conference, Dublin, Ireland.

Yates, B. T. (1996). *Analyzing costs, procedure, process, and outcomes in human services.* Thousand Oaks, CA: Sage.

Yusuf, S., Zucker, D., Peduzzi, P., Fisher, L. D., Takaro, T., Kennedy, J. W., Davis, K., Killip, T., Passamani, E., Norris, R., et al. (1994). Effect of coronary artery bypass graft surgery on survival: Overview of 10-year results from randomised trials by the Coronary Artery Bypass Graft Surgery Trialists Collaboration. *Lancet, 344,* 563–570.

6

Chronic Illness: Promoting the Adjustment Process

Cynthia McRae
Charlie H. Smith

Chronic illness has emerged as the leading cause of death and the principal source of health care expenditure in the United States (National Center for Health Statistics, 1992). This development is in sharp contrast to previous generations, when infectious diseases such as pneumonia, tuberculosis, measles, and influenza represented the greatest threats to health. As advances in modern medicine have diminished the potential lethality of most acute illnesses in the developed countries of the world, life expectancy has increased and we have become vulnerable to a broad range of diseases that may be acquired over a lifetime. One of the greatest challenges facing health care professionals today is how to help individuals cope with chronic conditions and live as fully as possible.

The Problem

Chronic illnesses are present in approximately 50 percent of the working population and nearly 80 percent of the geriatric population in the United States (Pope & Tarlov, 1991). Included among these relatively common medical problems are musculoskeletal disorders such as rheumatoid arthri-

Support for completion of this chapter was provided by Grant #R29 NS32009-03 from the National Institute of Neurological Disorders and Stroke.

tis and osteoporosis, lung diseases like asthma and chronic obstructive pulmonary disease (COPD), neurologic diseases such as Parkinson's disease, multiple sclerosis (MS), and epilepsy, as well as diabetes mellitus, hypertension, chronic liver disease, and renal failure. These conditions are often characterized as having:

- a noncontagious origin
- obscure etiology
- multiple risk factors
- a prolonged degenerative course
- functional impairment
- incurability

Although physicians can often treat many of the symptoms of chronic illness and provide palliative care, the underlying pathophysiology of these diseases cannot be resolved.

It is clear that adjustment to chronic illness involves coping not only with the debilitating physical aspects of disease, but also with the accompanying psychosocial changes and limitations. For patients, the general course of chronic disease results in a series of losses leading to changes in independence, sense of well-being, and quality of life. Persons with MS, for example, must initially adjust to the confirmation of diagnosis, which may be met with shock and denial, or relief that at last an unknown condition has a name and can be addressed. As the disease progresses, their focus shifts to the interrelated physical, social, and cognitive changes that occur. Life roles often change, medical treatments are modified, ambulation vacillates between fair and poor, and the financial burden of the disease increases as patients are forced to rely on expensive treatments and home health care. Finally, issues of grief and loss emerge and the possibility of extended suffering and dying becomes a frightening reality.

In addition to the issues just described in the scenario for MS, there are many other psychosocial concerns associated with chronic conditions. For instance, medical treatment, such as dialysis or insulin injection, can often be stressful, adding to the adjustment demands of the situation. Changes in sexual functioning are perplexing and frustrating. Adherence to prescribed medical regimens is often a problem for both patients and health care providers. The unpredictable nature of many chronic illnesses contributes to the stress and uncertainty of the future. Concerns about genetic predisposition may be salient for family members of patients with Huntington's disease, Parkinson's disease, or other conditions of uncertain etiology.

Chronic illness does not affect patients alone. Spouses and family members are also touched by the effects of disease. For example, family caregivers often experience prolonged stress, depression, burnout, changes in life roles, and increasing helplessness as the disease progresses (Bodnar & Kiecolt-Glaser, 1994; Haley, West, Wadley, & Ford, 1995; Zarit, Reever, & Bach-Peterson, 1980). Therefore, it is important to consider the needs of the family and caregivers, not only because their own well-being will be affected but also because the patient's level of adjustment is often directly related to the physical and emotional health of the spouse and family.

Clearly, there is a need for psychological consultation and intervention in the area of chronic illness. There are numerous issues for psychologists and counselors to address that can contribute to the welfare of the patient and family as they face the ongoing challenges that are part of chronic conditions. Fortunately, the field of counseling psychology is well qualified to address many of these issues. For example, counseling psychologists are trained to view individuals from a developmental perspective, which is especially helpful when considering the long-term course of chronic illness and the interaction of disease with normal developmental processes. Psychologists are also able to structure learning experiences designed to facilitate change. These activities may be very important in terms of prevention and health promotion as we work to reduce behavioral risk factors and change unhealthy behaviors that can exacerbate chronic diseases (e.g., instituting a smoking cessation program that may decrease the incidence of COPD). Further, psychologists recognize the importance of understanding individual patients within the context of their cultural background (Young & Zane, 1995) and unique health beliefs that contribute to the perceived significance, cause, and prognosis of their disease.

In addition, counseling psychologists provide such services as individual, family, and group counseling, psychological assessment, consultation regarding treatment adherence (Dunbar-Jacob, Burke, & Puczynski, 1996), interventions such as relaxation training or treatment of eating disorders, and liaison work with other health care professionals (Alcorn, 1991; Altmaier, 1991). Finally, with an emphasis on building strengths and utilizing unrecognized resources, psychologists and mental health professionals help patients and families develop effective coping strategies for optimizing the adjustment process in patients who are chronically ill (Thoresen & Eagleston, 1985; Tucker, 1991).

Following this introduction of some of the psychosocial issues associated with chronic illnesses, we will provide an overview of assessment issues and techniques, a discussion of interventions designed to make the ongoing adjustment process as positive as possible, and a brief look at considerations for the future. Recognizing that counselors who work with persons with chronic illnesses are based in a variety of settings, we will approach this chapter with a broad view of mental health professionals who are in a number of consultation environments.

Diagnosis and Assessment

Psychological assessment information is often combined with data from other disciplines to develop a more complete picture of the patient, which then aids all members of the health care team in determining the most appropriate interventions.

Fundamentals of Assessment

There are a number of issues to consider before assessing a person with a chronic illness. These issues are outlined below.

1. It is important to *understand the question being asked by the referring physician.* In some situations the information requested is related to emotional or cognitive status, for example, "Is this person depressed or anxious?" or "Can this patient learn the skills needed to perform home dialysis?" At other times psychologists are asked to assess personality variables or styles that suggest whether one medical treatment may be more effective than another (Christensen, Smith, Turner, & Cundick, 1994). Information provided by psychologists may also be used to determine the most appropriate candidates for organ transplantation (Olbrisch & Levenson, 1995).

2. When first meeting the client, it is important to *establish rapport* in order to obtain cooperation and the best possible results from the assessment session (Belar & Deardorff, 1995; DeGood, 1983). Patients are often referred to the psychologist without their being informed of the reasons. For example, pain is a possible though uncommon symptom of Parkinson's disease. When a person with Parkinson's disease complains repeatedly about pain, and his or her physician, who may not specialize in this disease, can

find no obvious explanation for pain (e.g., arthritis), the physician may refer patient to a psychologist for pain management. If the physician does not discuss this referral with the patient, it may create a challenging situation for the psychologist. If the patient or family members assume the physician thinks the pain is "all in the patient's head," they will be defensive and less cooperative.

3. The *quality of assessment data* will be influenced by the length of the assessment battery or period of testing. Because of diminished stamina and concentration span in many persons with chronic diseases, the accuracy of information and effort to produce the best results will decline over time (Derogatis, Fleming, Sudler, & DellaPietra, 1996). For example, expecting persons who are chronically ill to complete the entire Halstead-Reitan battery (Reitan & Davidson, 1974) in one day seems unreasonable. A prolonged assessment battery puts the client at risk for providing information that reflects the effects of fatigue rather than what one wants to accurately assess. For this reason, psychologists may choose to use abbreviated or more focused instruments and test batteries.

4. Prior to assessment it is also important to consider that persons with chronic illnesses may have some *psychopathology* that keeps them from adhering to treatment or cooperating with medical personnel (Levenson, 1992). An interesting example is a client who came several hundred miles every six months for a reevaluation of chronic pain. He had received intensive inpatient treatment 18 months earlier but seemed not to be benefiting from the follow-up program. A psychosocial update of this young man revealed that he lived in his car, had not been able to keep a job, and was experiencing auditory and visual hallucinations. After the psychologist reported these findings to the physician, the client was diagnosed with schizophrenia and treated accordingly. Recognizing and treating coexisting psychiatric factors enabled the patient to benefit from prescribed interventions.

5. Before selecting assessment instruments to be administered to persons with chronic illnesses, *appropriate norms* must be considered. What norms are available? Do they provide a suitable comparison for this person or chronic illness group? If norms do not exist for particular groups, this does not mean the instrument cannot be used. However, results must be interpreted cautiously in light of the clinical utility of the information and the question being asked.

Practical Aspects of Assessment

There are a number of practical issues to consider when assessing persons with chronic illness. Due to the space limitations of this chapter, we will consider only three: time of assessment, sources of information, and types of data that may be collected. What is important to know in order to understand the patient and his or her environment most comprehensively? How can we assess most thoroughly, help the medical team with treatment planning, and consider the future most efficiently?

Time of Assessment

Clearly, the issues at various stages of illness are different. Recalling our earlier example of the MS patient, overwhelming concerns at time of diagnosis are different from those during the process of adjustment five years later. Therapeutic interventions, as well as the progression of the disease, may have introduced new concerns and stresses that interfere with previously effective coping strategies. Therefore, it is important to collect baseline data to monitor the improvements effected by interventions as well as the deterioration experienced as part of the disease process. Because MS has so many "ups and downs," tracking the emotional and psychosocial aspects of the disease will likely reflect physiological changes as well. Ideally, future psychological assessments will coincide with medical evaluations in order to consolidate information and continue to promote optimal treatment planning. Derogatis and colleagues (1996) suggest that a comprehensive psychological examination be conducted annually with more circumscribed, specific evaluations being conducted at intermediate visits. In this way health care personnel can monitor progress and more clearly link psychological status with medical status and treatment response.

Sources of Assessment Data

The patient is regarded as the primary fund of information. However, it is important to keep in mind that medical personnel, patients, and family members often have differing views about the patient's status and progress. For example, an elderly patient with COPD who was barely managing at home alone insisted he was "doing fine." His daughter, however, reported that his ability to care for himself had deteriorated in the last six months. She said he was not eating properly, slept a great deal, was disoriented at times, and had become more forgetful. This additional information led the treatment team to a different recommendation than if they had relied only on information from the patient. It is important to gather data from as many sources as possible in order to gain different perspectives about treatment issues and a broader understanding of the patient and his or her health status.

In another example, over the last several years we have assessed patients receiving neural implant surgery for treatment of Parkinson's disease. We have asked patients and spouses or caregivers to rate the level of disability of the patient at specific time intervals coinciding with similar ratings by examining physicians. The results of one study (McRae, Bowles, & Freed, 1994) indicated that improvement after implant surgery was rated most highly by the physicians, followed by the patients, and then the caregivers. It appears that caregivers were the least impressed with the results of surgery, perhaps because personal expectations of surgical treatment had not yet been met. Different individuals involved with a patient with chronic illness can have different perspectives that may not always agree but need to be considered in treatment planning.

Because chronic illness affects the family, and, reciprocally, the family environment impacts the patient, it is important to assess the mood and adjustment of the spouse or family. Those closest to the patient may need crisis intervention or supportive therapy in order to cope with the changing circumstances of the patient's chronic illness and their own situations.

Types of Data

There are many types of data that contribute to an understanding of the patient with chronic illness.

1. The clinical interview is vital in terms of learning what the patient and/or family consider to be important in the process of adjustment to illness: What are their fears and concerns? What information do they need? What are their expectations for the future? Do they need help considering options for treatment? What sense or meaning do they make of this disease?
2. Questionnaires, allowing for systematic collection of information, not only chart progress of the patient but also aid in clinical research and program evaluation (Belar & Deardorff, 1995).
3. Patient and/or family diaries tracking daily information can provide other assessment data points that might be helpful in treatment plan-

ning. For example, patients might be able to deduce what sorts of thoughts or interpersonal interactions lead to increased stress and thus exacerbate symptoms of their disease.

4. Direct observations of the patient can provide information not otherwise available. Watching arthritis patients as they perform a standardized series of sitting-walking-standing maneuvers provides information about pain behaviors that would be inaccessible through other forms of data collection (Keefe & Williams, 1989).

5. The clinical mental status exam or broad neuropsychological screening tool (e.g., see Strub & Black, 1993) is another area of assessment that is helpful for the counseling psychologist. It is important to include a mental status exam in the preliminary assessment of cognitive ability and psychological orientation. If there is evidence of perceptual disorientation or cognitive deterioration, follow-up assessment may be warranted and requested by the treating clinician.

Specific Assessment Domains

The referral question directs the assessment focus and limits the scope of the instruments used. Traditional assessment instruments are often used with patients with chronic medical conditions; however, results must be interpreted with caution (Nicassio & Smith, 1995). The Beck Depression Inventory (Beck, Ward, Mendelson, Mock, & Erbaugh, 1961), for example, includes a number of somatic items that represent symptoms of depression. However, the somatic items may be endorsed by medical patients because they match particular physical complaints related to their illness—in many cases these symptoms are not related to depression (Erdal, 1995). Thus, an elevation of scores on this inventory may be misinterpreted as depression in patients with chronic diseases.

In addition to the standard repertoire of psychological assessment tools, there are many instruments specifically designed to measure issues of concern in medical populations; in persons with chronic illnesses, these include social support, hope, perceived control, and coping. A listing of commonly used assessment instruments in health psychology, along with a list of suggested readings regarding assessment, may be found in Belar and Deardorff (1995). Wright, Johnston, and Weinman (1995) have developed a kit of published instruments that are often used in health assessment.

Quality of Life

Quality of life has become an important aspect of assessment in health care (Bech, 1993; Dimsdale & Baum, 1995). Instead of relying exclusively on physicians' judgments of whether the patient should be better because certain procedures have been administered, funding agencies, research institutions, and third party payers have become increasingly interested in the patient's view of how he or she is doing. Despite the lack of agreement about the definition of quality of life, assessment generally includes a number of common elements: anxiety and depression, life satisfaction, unpleasant treatment side effects, pain, and functional impairment (Taylor & Aspinwall, 1990). Also included may be intrusiveness of illness (e.g., how much the disease and/or treatment interferes with previous "normal" daily activities), perceived control or self-efficacy, social support, sexual functioning, and ability to work.

Several attempts have been made to develop comprehensive quality of life measures that can be used across diseases (Kaplan & Anderson, 1988; Ware & Sherbourne, 1992); the Medical Outcomes Study Short Form-36 is commonly used with healthy individuals as well as persons with a variety of medical conditions (Stewart, Hays, & Ware, 1988; Stewart & Ware, 1992). Other researchers have concentrated on more disease-specific measures (de Boer, Wijker, Speelman, & de Haes, 1996; Diabetes Control and Complications Trial Research Group, 1988; Jenkinson, Peto, Fitzpatrick, Greenhall, & Hyman, 1995; Morrow, Lindke & Black, 1992). The general measures offer the advantage of allowing comparison of quality of life across diseases and conditions, while the more specific measures focus on symptoms and stages of illness particular to one disease. Depending upon the situation, assessment could include both types of instruments in order to provide the most comprehensive information.

Personal Meaning of Illness

Determining the meaning of the illness or condition to the individual may be very helpful in developing specific interventions (Brenner & McRae, 1991; Elliott & Marmarosh, 1995). When assessing patients from other than the dominant culture, it is important to consider health beliefs or personal meaning in order not to miss a critical piece of information that may lead to diminished treatment adherence or explain why the patient and family are not following medical recommendations. For example, persons from other cultures may go to Western physicians because of convenience or at the advice of others in the community. However, they may remain unconvinced of the efficacy of Western medicine and seek out indigenous healers or herbalists for treatment, ignoring the prescription given by the physician.

Much can be learned from those individuals who are able to derive positive meaning from the experience of chronic illness as they may be more able to confront the adverse changes that accompany the progression of disease (Andersen, 1996; Taylor & Aspinwall, 1990). Some individuals with chronic conditions have reflected that "illness has made me value relationships more" or "I never would have stopped to think about what's important if this hadn't happened" or "each day is important now" (Brenner & McRae, 1991). These interpretations, or attempts to derive meaning from the situation, appear to enable some persons to cope more effectively with the challenges of disease.

In summary, it is important to remember that the point of assessment is to develop an understanding of

> (a) the patient and his or her physical and social environment, (b) the patient's relevant strengths and weaknesses, (c) the evidence for psychopathology, (d) the nature of the disease and treatment regimen, and (e) the coping skills being used. (Belar & Deardorff, 1995, p. 65)

In addition, psychologists should consider the prediction by Derogatis and colleagues (1996) that future developments in assessment will become more focused on specificity and standardization. As psychological assessment becomes part of the cost-utility analysis that contributes to the equation that allots health care dollars, it will become ever more important for psychologists to develop assessment packages that are brief yet comprehensive, flexible, cost-efficient, and minimally intrusive. In these ways counseling psychologists can make very meaningful contributions to the care of patients with chronic illnesses by enlarging the view of the patient and his or her environment for health care providers.

Psychological Intervention

The goals of psychological intervention include helping patients recapture, restore, or resume at least a semblance of their premorbid levels of physical and emotional functioning and life satisfaction. Not all patients or families experiencing chronic illness seek psychotherapy, nor are they referred by the health care team. In fact, many persons adjust to chronic conditions without our help (Turk, 1979). For those who are referred, intervention may come in the form of crisis counseling, or giving the patient opportunities to express anger and frustration or to mourn the perceived losses that accompany the disease process. In general, psychological interventions provide an objective, nonjudgmental environment within which patients can receive support, learn new skills, and move toward a positive adjustment to illness.

Interventions come in many forms: individual therapy with patients or family members, groups, interventions with the family, and health promotion activities designed to influence behavior. The aim of many of these interventions is to help the patient and/or family learn to manage some of the stress and anxiety that often accompany chronic illness. Whether the patient is experiencing ongoing medical complaints, frightening treatment procedures, family changes, employment problems, or the prospect of disease progression and death, stress and anxiety are often present. Many researchers have linked these emotions to the onset or exacerbation of symptoms of diabetes, coronary artery disease, pulmonary dysfunction, and rheumatoid arthritis (Gentry, 1984; Hughes, Pearson, & Reinhart, 1984; Kiecolt-Glaser & Glaser, 1988; Rahe, 1988).

Individual Therapy

Several short-term cognitive-behavioral strategies, most notably progressive muscle relaxation, guided imagery, systematic desensitization, hypnosis, and biofeedback, have been effective in countering the impact of stress and anxiety for persons with chronic illness. These strategies generally increase the sense of perceived control and enhance the individual's repertoire of available coping strategies. A meta-analysis by Hyman, Feldman, Harris, Levin, and Malloy (1989) found that stress management interventions, such as relaxation training and progressive muscle relaxation, were effective for several chronic problems, including hypertension, headaches, and insomnia. Several practitioners (Anderson, 1987; Devine, 1992; Lehrer, Carr, Sargunaraj, & Woolfolk, 1994; Ornish et al., 1990) have modified progressive muscle relaxation techniques in order to prepare patients for stressful situations like surgery, invasive treatment (injections), role reassignment in the home or office, and the emergence of social stressors related to the illness.

Systematic desensitization, biofeedback, and modeling have also been used successfully in reducing patients' physiological anxiety and anticipatory anxiety associated with chemotherapy (Redd & Andrykowski, 1982). The use of presurgery videotapes, in addition to nurses presenting information related to recovery from surgery, has elicited lower presurgery anxiety and decreased postsurgery recovery time in the hospital (Anderson, 1987).

Groups

Group psychotherapy has been effective in assisting patients with chronic illnesses gain information, receive social support, develop individual meaning for their illness, and acquire skills and adaptive behaviors with which to cope with their disease. In general, supportive group therapy provides a sense of belonging, a process of normalization and social comparison, and a place to express emotions (Forester, Kornfeld, Fleiss, & Thompson, 1993).

Groups can also provide a valuable psychoeducational component that expands a patient's knowledge and understanding of the disease. Lorig, Mazonson, and Holman (1993) reported follow-up data on the Arthritis Self-Help Course. The six-week self-efficacy enhancing program had very powerful treatment effects. Four years following the intervention, those who participated had 40 percent fewer physician visits and reported a 20 percent reduction in pain—even while physical disability increased 9 percent. Authors ascribed improvements to increases in perceived self-efficacy, which influenced motivation, perseverance, and vulnerability to stress and depression. Altruism, or the opportunity for individuals to help others in the group, was anecdotally found to be important to group members, and thus may have contributed to the patients' improvements.

Since many patients may be physically unable to attend group meetings, modern technology has provided some options. For those who have computers, internet bulletin boards, chat rooms, and video conferencing provide a vehicle through which these immobile patients can receive the benefits of group and individual contact (Troster, Paolo, Glatt, & Hubble, 1995). Indeed, a number of Parkinson's patients known to both authors use communication via the internet to both give and receive social support, exchange information about medications and the disease process, and to feel as though they are still participating in the world outside the home to which they have become confined.

Family Interventions

Depending on the needs of the family, interventions may be done with the individual couple, the nuclear or extended family, or in a group of several families. Families experiencing chronic illness are often encouraged to attend groups to share concerns, problem-solve with other families in similar circumstances, and support one another both emotionally and in tangible ways (Kerns, 1995). Sometimes information and knowledge about the changes and consequent stresses of adjustment are enough to assure families that their responses are "normal." To hear a clinician or other members of a support group say that anger and frustration in a particular situation is a healthy response can be very therapeutic. Research has shown that multifamily psychoeducational groups have been effective in reducing the emotional distress and burden associated with a family member managing cardiovascular disease (Gonzalez, Atwood, Garcia, & Meyskins, 1989). A group intervention for couples with one member diagnosed with Parkinson's disease (Brandow, 1997) was found to significantly diminish dysphoric mood in caregivers from baseline to postintervention assessment. Anecdotal observations indicated that social comparison theory may explain, at least in part, the improvement in mood reported by the spouses (Brandow, 1997).

The impact of counseling can refresh couple and family relationships and improve the patient's ability to manage the disease. The more involved families and spouses are in the medical care of the chronically ill, the less likely patients are to feel overprotected, stressed, alone, or pressured by unrealistic expectations regarding the course of their disease.

Health Promotion

An important intervention related to chronic illness is prevention, or health promotion. Many of the long-term processes that contribute to the development of chronic diseases are behavioral or psychological in nature. For example, smoking, poor diet, inadequate physical activity, alcohol consumption, and unprotected sexual intercourse are behavioral risk factors that may lead to conditions such as cardiovascular disease, hypertension, chronic obstructive pulmonary disease, emphysema, sexually transmitted diseases, and cirrhosis. Mental health professionals can use a variety of educational strategies and interventions to modify health-related attitudes and behaviors, thus affecting the risk factors that contribute to illness.

It is also important to take preventive, health promotional activities into the community in order for them to be more accessible by a larger population. For example, to enroll Hispanic participants in the Arthritis Self-Help Course, the developers of the program at Stanford University went to senior centers and churches in Hispanic areas in the San Francisco Bay area on Sunday mornings to present information about the course and to answer questions (Nacif de Bery & Gonzalez, 1997). The six-week course was then presented in the targeted neighborhoods, thus bringing education to the people who would benefit from it, but who might not have attended in a less convenient location.

Future Considerations

Among the future considerations in health care for the chronically ill are turf wars regarding many of the domains discussed in this chapter (Kaplan, 1991). The following questions are examples of issues facing our profession.

1. Will we, as counseling psychologists and mental health professionals, be able to find a niche in the fee-for-service and managed care competition? Program development, specialization in particular areas such as multiple sclerosis or movement disorders, research, and assessment are all ways to enhance our roles in the medical community.

2. Will we be able to empirically demonstrate that various psychoeducational interventions for chronically ill patients and their caregivers lead to better patient outcomes and enhance quality of life for both individuals? Research is moving in the direction of addressing health care concerns and quality of life for both the patient and the spouse or caregiver. We need to do outcome research on interventions we provide to improve treatment and to provide evidence of efficacy to insurers.

3. Will we heed the call to enlist the patient as partner in the endeavor to achieve optimal adjustment to chronic illness (Sobel, 1997)? Additional research is needed to determine the types of patients or categories of diseases that might be the most promising "partners," and to investigate the critical elements in the physician/patient relationship that promote "partnership." In summary, we need to take advantage of the training that has provided us with the skills to be both scientists and practitioners in order to be competitive in the health care marketplace.

Summary

Counseling psychologists and other mental health professionals are valuable contributors in the emerging multifaceted health care environment. Specific skills in assessment, individual, family, and group psychotherapy have enabled psychologists to assess patients' coping strategies and personality strengths, address low self-esteem, anxiety, and depressive symptomatology. The attention to developmental, cultural, and family issues has enlarged the focus of health care and placed the patient in a broader context. Chronic illness is no longer seen merely as the patient's problem; the health care environment is recognizing the importance of respecting cultural and familial variables.

Suggested Resources

There are many resources that provide information, support, and guidance in treating and living with chronic disease. Following is a very brief discussion of professional resources, reference books for patients and families, and internet resources. Readers may investigate other local and national organizations for information and support regarding specific diseases.

For an introduction and comprehensive overview of issues related to chronic illness, a primary resource is *Managing Chronic Illness: A Biopsychosocial Perspective,* edited by Nicassio and Smith (1995). A variety of broad topics are covered, including assessment, neuropsychology, ethnocultural considerations, interventions, and adherence.

Persons interested in aspects of caregiving are referred to a book by Biegel, Sales, and Schulz (1991) entitled, *Family Caregiving in Chronic Illness.* The organization of this volume is centered on specific conditions such as stroke, Alzheimer's disease, cancer, and chronic mental illness. In addition, interventions and issues common to most caregivers are discussed.

A compilation of commonly used measures in chronic illness was produced by Wright, Johnston, and Weinman (1995). *Measures in Health Psychology: A User's Portfolio* is divided into themed units containing over 40 measures with information regarding details of administration, scoring, interpretation, and normative data. Some of the units include measures on social support, coping, stress, health status and quality of life, and control beliefs.

A helpful volume for patients and families is *Living a Healthy Life with Chronic Conditions* by Lorig, Holman, Sobel, Laurent, Gonzalez, and Minor (1994). This book was designed as a general resource and includes chapters on self-managment of one's disease, exercise, communication, nutrition, and more specific information about several chronic conditions such as lung disease, heart disease, stroke, and diabetes. A similar book related specifically to arthritis is *The Arthritis Helpbook* by Lorig and Fries (1990). This book was initially designed for persons attending the Arthritis Self-Help Course offered by the Arthritis Foundation in many countries. It offers helpful information for persons with arthritis and fibromyalgia.

Several Internet Web sites have been established for patients and family members that provide up-to-date medical information. Bulletin boards where individuals can chat with others about life with a chronic illness are also available.

American Heart Association: http://www.amhrt.org

National Arthritis Foundation: http://www.arthritis.org

Society of Behavioral Medicine: http://psychweb.syr.edu/sbm/sbm.html

The following are current publications that provide a host of health-specific Internet Web sites available to the health consumer:

Ferguson, T. (1996). *Health online: How to find health information, support groups, and self-help communities in cyberspace.* Reading, MA: Addison-Wesley.

Goldstein, D., & Flory, J. (1996). *The online consumer guide to health-care and wellness.* Chicago: Irwin Professional Publishing.

Naythons, M., & Catsimatides, A. (1995). *The internet: Health, fitness, and medicine yellow pages.* New York: Osborne McGraw-Hill.

Discussion Questions

1. What developmental issues influence the process of adjustment to a chronic medical illness such as multiple sclerosis or Parkinson's disease?
2. What are the advantages and disadvantages of group counseling versus individual counseling for patients with chronic illnesses?
3. In what ways does the collaboration between psychologists and physicians positively influence patient care?
4. What are the benefits of health promotion and prevention activities?

References

Alcorn, J. D. (1991). Counseling psychology and health applications. *The Counseling Psychologist, 19,* 325–341.

Altmaier, E. M. (1991). Research and practice roles for counseling psychologists in health care settings. *The Counseling Psychologist, 19,* 342–364.

Andersen, S. (1996, October). *Disease as a challenge: A theme in the new role of the patient.* Workshop presented at the Second European Parkinson's Disease Conference, Stockholm.

Anderson, E. A. (1987). Preoperative preparation for cardiac surgery facilitates recovery, reduces psychological distress, and reduces the incidence of acute postoperative hypertension. *Journal of Consulting and Clinical Psychology, 55,* 513–520.

Bech, P. (1993). Quality of life measurement in chronic disorders. *Psychotherapy and Psychosomatics, 59,* 1–10.

Beck, A. T., Ward, C. H., Mendelson, M., Mock, J., & Erbaugh, J. K. (1961). An inventory for measuring depression. *Archives of General Psychiatry, 4,* 561–571.

Belar, C. D., & Deardorff, W. W. (1995). *Clinical health psychology in medical settings: A practitioner's guidebook.* Washington, DC: American Psychological Association.

Biegel, D. E., Sales, E., & Schulz, R. (1991). *Family caregiving in chronic illness.* Newbury Park: Sage.

Bodnar, J. C., & Kiecolt-Glaser, J. K. (1994). Caregiver depression after bereavement: Chronic stress isn't over when it's over. *Psychology and Aging, 9,* 372–380.

Brandow, R. K. (1997). *Exploring the potential for effective self-management of quality of life among Parkinson patients.* Unpublished doctoral dissertation, University of Denver.

Brenner, H. G., & McRae, C. (1991, March). *Searching for meaning: Its impact on the psychological adjustment of spinal cord injured individuals.* Poster session presented at the Society of Behavioral Medicine Twelfth Annual Scientific Sessions, Washington, DC.

Christensen, A. J., Smith, T. W., Turner, C., & Cundick, K. (1994). Patient adherence and adjustment in renal dialysis: A person X treatment interactive approach. *Journal of Behavioral Medicine, 17,* 549–566.

de Boer, A. G. E. M., Wijker, W., Speelman, J. D., & de Haes, J. C. J. M. (1996). Quality of life in patients with Parkinson's disease: Development of a questionnaire. *Journal of Neurology, Neurosurgery and Psychiatry, 61,* 70–74.

DeGood, D. E. (1983). Reducing medical patients' reluctance to participate in psychological therapies: The initial session. *Professional Psychology, 14,* 570–579.

Derogatis, L. R., Fleming, M. P., Sudler, N. C., & DellaPietra, L. (1996). Psychological assessment. In P. M. Nicassio, & T. W. Smith (Eds.), *Managing chronic illness: A biopsychosocial perspective* (pp. 59–115). Washington, DC: American Psychological Association.

Devine, E. C. (1992). Effects of psychoeducational care for adult surgical patients: A meta-analysis of 191 studies. *Patient Educational Counseling, 19,* 129–142.

Diabetes Control and Complications Trial Research Group. (1988). Reliability and validity of a diabetes quality of life measure for the diabetes control and complication trial (DCCT). *Diabetes Care, 11,* 725–732.

Dimsdale, J. E., & Baum, A. (Eds.). (1995). *Quality of life in behavioral medicine research.* Hillsdale, NJ: Lawrence Erlbaum.

Dunbar-Jacob, J., Burke, L. E., & Puczynski, S. (1996). Clinical assessment and management of adherence to medical regimens. In P. M. Nicassio, & T. W. Smith (Eds.), *Managing chronic illness: A biopsychosocial perspective* (pp. 313–349) Washington, DC: American Psychological Association.

Elliott, T. R., & Marmarosh, C. (1995). Social-cognitive processes in behavioral health: Implications for counseling. *The Counseling Psychologist, 23,* 666–681.

Erdal, K. (1995). *Depressive symptoms in Parkinson's disease.* Unpublished doctoral dissertation, Arizona State University, Tempe, AZ.

Ferguson, T. (1996). *Health online: How to find health information, support groups, and self-help communities in cyberspace.* Reading, MA: Addison-Wesley.

Forester, B., Kornfeld, D. S., Fleiss, J. C., & Thompson, S. (1993). Group psychotherapy during radiotherapy: Effects on emotional and physical distress. *American Journal of Psychiatry, 150,* 1700–1706.

Gentry, M. E. (1984). Developments in activity analysis: Recreation and group work revisited. *Social Work with Groups, 7,* 35–44.

Goldstein, D., & Flory, J. (1996). *The online consumer guide to healthcare and wellness.* Chicago: Irwin.

Gonzalez, J. J., Atwood, J., Garcia, J. A., & Meyskins, F. L. (1989). Hispanics and cancer preventive behavior: The development of a behavioral model and its policy implications. *Journal of Health and Social Policy, 12,* 55–73.

Haley, W. E., West, C. A., Wadley, V. G., & Ford, G. R. (1995). Psychological, social, and health impact of caregiving: A comparison of black and white dementia family caregivers and noncaregivers. *Psychology and Aging, 10,* 540–552.

Hughes, G. H., Pearson, M. A., & Reinhart, G. R. (1984). Stress: Sources, effects, and management. *Family and Community Health, 7,* 47–58.

Hyman, R. B., Feldman, H. R., Harris, R. B., Levin, R. F., & Malloy, G. B. (1989). The effects of relaxation training on clinical symptoms: A meta-analysis. *Nursing Research, 38,* 216–220.

Jenkinson, C., Peto, V., Fitzpatrick, R., Greenhall, R., & Hyman, N. (1995). Self-reported functioning and well-being in patients with Parkinson's disease: Comparison of the Short-form Health Survey (SF-36) and the Parkinson's Disease Questionnaire (PDQ-39). *Age and Aging, 24,* 505–509.

Kaplan, R. M. (1991). Counseling psychology in health settings: Promise and challenge. *The Counseling Psychologist, 19,* 376–381.

Kaplan, R. M., & Anderson, J. P. (1988). The quality of well-being scale: Rationale for a single quality of life index. In S. R. Walker, & R. Rosser (Eds.), *Quality of life assessment and applications* (pp. 51–77). London: MTP.

Keefe, F. J., & Williams, D. A. (1989). New directions in pain assessment and treatment. *Clinical Psychology Review, 9,* 549–568.

Kerns, R. D. (1995). Family assessment and intervention. In P. M. Nicassio, & T. W. Smith (Eds.), *Managing chronic illness: A biopsychosocial perspective* (pp. 207–244). Washington, DC: American Psychological Association.

Kiecolt-Glaser, J. K., & Glaser, R. (1988). Psychological influences on immunity: Making sense of the relationship between stressful life events and health. In G. P. Chrousos, D. L. Loriaux, & P. W. Gold (Eds.), *Mechanisms of physical and emotional stress.* (pp. 237–247). New York: Plenum.

Lehrer, P. M., Carr, R., Sargunaraj, D., & Woolfolk R. L. (1994). Stress management techniques: Are they all equivalent, or do they have specific effects? *Biofeedback and Self-Regulation, 19,* 353–401.

Levenson, J. L. (1992). Psychosocial interventions in chronic medical illness: An overview of outcome research. *General Hospital Psychiatry, 14S,* 43S–49S.

Lorig, K., & Fries, J. (1990). *The arthritis helpbook* (3rd ed.). Reading, MA: Addison-Wesley.

Lorig, K., Holman, H., Sobel, D., Laurent, D., Gonzalez, V., & Minor, M. (1994). *Living a healthy life with chronic conditions.* Palo Alto, CA: Bull.

Lorig, K., Mazonson, P. D., & Holman, H. R. (1993). Evidence suggesting that health education for self-management in patients with chronic arthritis has sustained health benefits while reducing health care costs. *Arthritis and Rheumatism, 36*, 439–446.

McRae, C., Bowles, S., & Freed, C. (1994, July). *Quality of life among persons receiving neural implant surgery for Parkinson's disease.* Paper presented at the Third International Congress of Behavioral Medicine, Amsterdam.

Morrow, G. R., Lindke, J., & Black, P. (1992). Measurement of quality of life in patients: Psychometric analyses of the Functional Living Index-Cancer (FLIC). *Quality of Life Research, 1*, 287–296.

Nacif de Bery, V., & Gonzalez, V. M. (1997). Recruiting for arthritis studies in hard to reach populations: A comparison of methods used in an urban Spanish-speaking community. *Arthritis Care and Research, 10*, 64–71.

Naythons, M., & Catsimatides, A. (1995). *The internet: Health, fitness, and medicine yellow pages.* New York: Osborne McGraw-Hill.

National Center for Health Statistics. (1992). *Vital statistics of the United States, 1992* (DHHS Publication No. HE 20.6210). Washington, DC: U.S. Government Printing Office.

Nicassio, P. M., & Smith, T. W. (Eds.). (1995). *Managing chronic illness: A biopsychosocial perspective.* Washington, DC: American Psychological Association.

Olbrisch, M. E., & Levenson, J. L. (1995). Psychosocial assessment of organ transplant candidates: Current status of methodological and philosophical issues. *Psychosomatics, 36*, 236–243.

Ornish, D., Brown, S. E., Scherwitz, L. W., Billings, J. H., Armstrong, W. T., Ports, T., McLanahan, S. M., Kirkeeide, R. L., Brand, R. J., & Gould, K. L. (1990). Can lifestyle changes reverse coronary heart disease? The Lifestyle Heart Trial. *Lancet, 336*, 129–133.

Pope, A. M., & Tarlov, A. R. (1991). *Disability in America: Toward a national agenda for prevention.* Washington, DC: National Academy.

Rahe, R. H. (1988). Anxiety and physical illness symposia: Consequences of anxiety. *Journal of Clinical Psychiatry, 49*, 26–29.

Redd, W. H., & Andrykowski, M. A. (1982). Behavioral intervention in cancer treatment: Controlling aversion reactions to chemotherapy. *Journal of Consulting and Clinical Psychology, 50*, 1018–1029.

Reitan, R. M., & Davidson, L. A. (1974). *Clinical neuropsychology: Current status and applications.* Washington, DC: V. H. Winston.

Sobel, D. (1997, April). *Mind matters, money matters: Improving health and cost outcomes with clinical behavioral medicine.* Paper presented at the Eighteenth Annual Scientific Sessions of the Society of Behavioral Medicine, San Francisco.

Stewart, A. L., Hays, R. D., & Ware, J. E., Jr. (1988). The MDS Short-form General Health Survey: Reliability and validity in a patient population. *Medical Care, 26*, 724–735.

Stewart, A. L., & Ware, J. E., Jr. (Eds.). (1992). *Measuring functioning and well-being. The Medical Outcomes Study approach.* Durham, NC: Duke University.

Strub, R. L., & Black, F. W. (1993). *The mental status examination in neurology* (3rd ed.). Philadelphia: F. A. Davis.

Taylor, S. E., & Aspinwall, L. G. (1990). Psychological aspects of chronic illness. In P. T. Costa, Jr., & G. R. VandenBos (Eds.), *Psychological aspects of serious illness: Chronic conditions, fatal diseases, and clinical care* (pp. 3–60). Washington, DC: American Psychological Association.

Thoresen, C. E., & Eagleston, J. R. (1985). Counseling for health. *The Counseling Psychologist, 13*, 15–87.

Troster, A. I., Paolo, A. M., Glatt, S. L., & Hubble, J. P. (1995). "Interactive video conferencing" in the provision of neuropsychological services to rural areas. *Journal of Community Psychology, 23,* 85–88.

Tucker, C. M. (1991). Counseling psychology and health psychology: A response. *The Counseling Psychologist, 19,* 387–391.

Turk, D. C. (1979). Factors influencing the adaptive process with chronic illness. In I. G. Sarason, & C. D. Spielberger (Eds.), *Stress and anxiety (Vol. 6)* (pp. 291–308). Washington, DC: Hemisphere.

Ware, J. E., Jr., & Sherbourne, C. D. (1992). The MOS 36-item Short Form Health Survey (SF-36): I. Conceptual framework and item selection. *Medical Care, 30,* 473–483.

Wright, S., Johnston, M., & Weinman, J. (1995). *Measures in health psychology: A user's portfolio.* Windsor, England: NFER-Nelson.

Young, K., & Zane, N. (1995). Ethnocultural influences in evaluation and management. In P. M. Nicassio, & T. W. Smith (Eds.), *Managing chronic illness: A biopsychosocial perspective* (pp. 163–206). Washington, DC: American Psychological Association.

Zarit, S. H., Reever, K. E., & Bach-Peterson, J. (1980). Relatives of impaired elderly: Correlates of feeling of burden. *The Gerontologist, 20,* 649–655.

7
Psychological Perspectives on Life-Threatening Illness: Cancer and AIDS

Thomas V. Merluzzi
Mary Ann Martinez Sanchez

It is not uncommon to hear about someone living with an illness that years ago would have been considered in most instances imminently fatal. For many people, heart disease, renal disease, diabetes, childhood leukemia, and a host of other conditions are now treatable or at least manageable. The transformation of these once-terminal conditions to the status of life threatening or chronic is due to early detection and aggressive treatment. However, mortality rates for many of these diseases are still very high because early detection presumes that individuals are educated with respect to screening procedures or warning signs. Also, unfortunately, some cancers are not detected early and other diseases such as amyotrophic lateral sclerosis (ALS or Lou Gehrig's disease) and acquired immune deficiency syndrome (AIDS) are associated with limited life expectancy in spite of treatments. Each of these conditions has a critical psychological component that may affect the person's adjustment to the illness and the course of the illness. In this chapter we have chosen to focus on cancer and AIDS as examples of illnesses that are life threatening and that also have a substantive psychological component.

For many people, a diagnosis of cancer or AIDS is tantamount to dying. For those in the most advanced stages of these diseases, dying is an inevitable outcome in most instances. However, recent advances in early diagnosis and aggressive treatment of certain types of cancer and the advent of certain compounds such as AZT and protease inhibitors (Adams & Merluzzi, 1993) for treating AIDS raise hopes for increasing longevity after diagnosis. In fact, while the incidence of both diseases has increased, so too have the long-term survival rates. The focus on both short- and long-term survival has brought attention to the psychosocial aspects of cancer and AIDS. At all stages of these diseases, even the most advanced, with few exceptions, one has time to cope, to worry, to plan, to hope, to be sad, to be joyful, to escape, to love. The work of Antoni (Antoni, Baggett, et al., 1991), Fawzy (Fawzy et al., 1993), Ironson (Ironson, Antoni, & Lutgendorf, 1995), and Spiegel (Spiegel, Bloom, Kraemer, & Gottheil, 1989) are examples of how mental health professionals might help people with these life-threatening illnesses make advantageous use of that time, whether it be weeks, months, years, or a lifetime.

Overview of AIDS and Cancer

AIDS

AIDS is a viral infection that is transmitted by exposure to fluid that contains human immunodeficiency virus (HIV). It can be sexually transmitted, acquired by using a needle that is tainted with AIDS-infected blood, or by exposure to AIDS-infected blood (e.g., through an open wound). However, it is a weak virus that is not easily transmitted and is easily killed by a number of ordinary substances (e.g., bleach). AIDS is a retrovirus that enters certain cells in the immune system (helper T cells), replicates itself, and may remain undetected for some time. It is usually diagnosed by a blood test that detects HIV, however, the presence of opportunistic infections (e.g., shingles) may signal the onset of AIDS. Normally the immune system would be able to cope with these infections, but the compromised nature of the immune system makes it difficult to mount resources needed to combat the virus.

A four-step classification system (McCutchan, 1990) has been proposed to describe the progression of HIV infection:

1. At acute infection most people will experience flu-like symptoms that dissipate in 3–10 days.
2. The asymptomatic stage may last a long time, during which the immune system gradually declines.

3. The symptomatic stage represents a time in the disease course when serious and, at times, life-threatening illnesses may occur. It is evident from the symptoms or combination of symptoms that the immune system is seriously compromised.
4. Finally, within a year after the onset of the symptomatic stage, full-blown AIDS may be diagnosed, characterized by opportunistic infections (e.g., a fungal type of pneumonia called PCP), cancer (e.g., skin lesions such as Kaposi's sarcoma), and a helper T cell count less than 200 (1000 is normal).

The medical management of AIDS includes the treatment of symptoms that arise out of the compromised immune system as well as two types of drugs that are designed to inhibit the replication of HIV: Reverse transcriptase (RT) inhibitors such as azidothymidine (AZT) and dideoxyinosine (DDI) have been used for a number of years and appear to be somewhat successful in the maintenance of T cell counts. Protease inhibitors such as nevirapine are new additions to the medical management of HIV/AIDS. Clinically, the protease inhibitors have been quite successful in arresting or slowing the progression of the virus and promoting a reversal of the wasting syndrome which is characterized by loss of weight and energy. Many persons with AIDS are on a combination of RT and protease inhibitors, as well as a number of other compounds to combat side effects and other illnesses. While AIDS is fatal, there has been some optimism that the new combination therapies will prolong the lives of those with AIDS and particularly those who begin these regimes early in the asymptomatic stage. Risk reduction is critical in controlling the spread of HIV/AIDS; however, treatment of that subject is beyond the scope of this chapter.

Cancer

Cancer is another pervasive disease in our society. However, cancer is not really one disease, as there are many types of cancer. Moreover, the incidence of some types of cancer varies considerably by ethnicity. For example, African-American men have higher rates of prostate cancer than Caucasian men. Also, mortality rates are higher among African Americans compared to Caucasians; however, that may be due to later detection and less access to the medical system.

Cancers generally take a long time to develop. For example, a lung tumor may take 15 years to develop to the point where it may be detected.

Exposure to risk factors may not lead to cancer. For example, if we were to follow prospectively people who have smoked a pack of cigarettes a day for 20 years, not all would develop lung cancer. Thus, the dysfunction in DNA that disrupts growth and reproduction is not a uniform response to risk.

For most cancers there is a staging process that occurs at diagnosis. Generally, four stages are used and represent increasing seriousness of the disease:

- Stage I represents disease that is localized and has not infiltrated surrounding tissue.
- Stage II signifies that the cancer has spread minimally to surrounding tissue but has not migrated far beyond the initial site.
- Stages III and IV indicate disease that has spread beyond the original site. The prognosis for long-term survival is poor when a stage IV is given at diagnosis.

Medical treatment of cancer may include surgery, chemotherapy (delivered both intravenously and orally), and/or radiation. Usually, cancer patients who have operable tumors will have surgery and chemotherapy. In some instances, the site of the tumor is radiated after surgery. Chemotherapy consists of a combination of drugs that is designed to interfere with the reproduction of all cells. However, given that cancer cells proliferate at a much higher rate than normal cells, they are particularly vulnerable to the necrotic (cell-killing) effects of chemotherapy. Because the stomach lining regenerates rapidly, it is also very vulnerable to the effects of chemotherapy, which often cause nausea. However, recent advances in treating nausea and protecting white blood cell counts (a component of the immune system) have improved the quality of life of patients on chemotherapy.

Radiation is used for curative and palliative treatment. Patients usually will receive daily radiation treatment for two to four weeks. Some may receive it in combination with chemotherapy; however, these combination regimens are intense and may compromise quality of life. Palliative radiation therapy may be used to relieve some symptoms (e.g., pain) or improve functioning (e.g., improve walking).

Other than lung cancer, the cure rates for cancer have increased, but not improved dramatically, over the past 20 years. The marginal improvements may be due to early detection and changes in lifestyle rather than the effectiveness of chemotherapy. Therefore, reduction of risk and early detection are the keys to survival. Based on that premise, a great deal of attention has been given to the importance of screening for breast cancer, prostate cancer, and colon cancer. Now that the gene that causes cancer (BRCA-1) has been isolated, persons with an extensive history of cancer in their family may choose to be tested to determine if they are at risk.

In sum, the diagnosis of any life-threatening illness represents a serious challenge to the health of the individual and involves a complex series of medical decisions. With the possible exception of some stage I tumors, most people who are diagnosed with cancer or AIDS will receive treatments that are debilitating, may cause severe side effects (e.g., nausea, vomiting, hair loss, depression), and may be very disruptive of the patient's daily life. In the remaining sections of the chapter we will discuss how people cope with these life-threatening diseases and treatments.

Chronology of Events in the Coping Process

Cancer and AIDS involve stress-inducing events that require a patient to call upon coping resources to meet each challenge. Initially the diagnosis of cancer or AIDS may cause distress (Hughes, 1993; Levy et al., 1992). Most people will recover from that initial shock; others, however, may experience a continuation of stress or depression because their coping styles may prolong or increase distress (Stanton & Snider, 1993). For example, after being diagnosed with cancer, many people have surgery or surgery plus radiation. Chemotherapy may follow, with the attendant nausea and other side effects. For some people, pain may become an intermittent or persistent problem. Even if treatment is successful, there is still the worry of recurrence. At each point in this process, the demands of the situation may exceed coping resources and some patients may become overwhelmed. Others will manage the demands and recover functioning to a great extent. Each milestone in the chronology of the disease should be understood in order to treat the patient effectively.

Diagnosis

Cancer

For someone diagnosed with a life-threatening illness there is the immediate task of coming to terms with the diagnosis. In a study of women who were about to receive results of a breast biopsy, Stanton and Snider (1993) found that emotions varied at various points from prebiopsy to postsurgery. Both the benign group and the cancer group were comparable prior to the biopsy. However, after the biopsy but before surgery the cancer group was more tense, depressed, angry, fatigued, and confused than the benign group. At postsurgery, the cancer group was more fatigued and had less vigor than the benign group but did not differ on other mood states. Thus, with respect to their emotional reactions, the women with cancer did seem to recover rapidly. Younger patients, those who were less optimistic, and those who engaged in cognitive avoidance were more distressed than those who were older, optimistic, and had a positive focus. In light of these findings, care providers should encourage patients to seek social support and discourage avoidance in order to maximize the protective factors of a social network and, at the same time, optimize the processing of medical information and problem solving.

After a diagnosis of breast cancer, women often have the option of having a mastectomy or a lumpectomy. A recent study comparing these two treatments (Hughes, 1993) found no differences in distress at diagnosis or quality of life during the initial course of treatment for stage I and II patients. One prominent study, however, does not entirely confirm these findings. Levy, Heberman, Lee, Lippman, and d'Angelo (1989) assessed the mood and functional status of lumpectomy and mastectomy patients shortly after surgery. About half of the patients were given a choice of treatment and the other half were randomly assigned to receive a lumpectomy or masectomy. Although there were no differences between groups that were randomly assigned, months after surgery lumpectomy patients in the choice condition were more distressed than the mastectomy patients. At a 15-month follow-up (Levy et al., 1992), the lumpectomy patients were rated by others as more functional than the mastectomy patients; however, they viewed themselves as having less energy and less support than those who had mastectomies. Finally, the acute distress of the lumpectomy patients did dissipate over time. Although we might expect lumpectomy patients to recover more quickly than the mastectomy patients, that may not be the case. In fact, they may require more attention and support.

Because cancer is many diseases, the generalization of results from one type of cancer to another may not be possible. For a sample of lymphoma patients, Devlen, Maguire, Phillips, and Crowther (1987) found that depression and anxiety were greatest before treatment but also affected some patients after treatment and during follow-up. While it may be safe to assume that the period after diagnosis and before treatment is difficult and fraught with uncertainty, there actually may be some emotional relief once treatment decisions have been made and implemented. However, during that time between diagnosis and treatment it is important to focus on the problem-solving style and capabilities of the patient. Nezu and colleagues (1994) found that newly diagnosed cancer patients who exhibited problem-solving styles that were negative, avoidant, and impulsive also reported high levels of depressive and anxiety symptoms and a higher number of cancer-related problems.

AIDS

For persons with AIDS, the diagnosis may be a stepwise process. First, the decision to be tested is usually associated with identifying oneself as at risk for a disease that is socially stigmatizing, and knowing that even with assurances of confidentiality there is a risk of disclosure. Then there is the waiting period between testing and finding out serostatus (whether one is positive or negative for the virus). Finally, there is the process of dealing with the HIV+ diagnosis, including its personal and social implications. Thus, it is not surprising that between 9 and 28 percent of those tested in different samples did not return for the results of the testing (Folkman & Chesney, 1995).

When informed of their HIV+ status, most individuals experience an increase in anxiety, depression, and general psychological distress (Ostrow et al., 1989). In a very well-controlled prospective study by Antoni, Baggett, and others (1991), men learned of their serostatus after having been in a stress management group or in a control group for five weeks. Those who had the benefit of treatment showed significantly less increase in depression and no increase in anxiety. In another study, in which counseling was provided prior to notification of serostatus, Perry and colleagues (1990) reported no increase in psychological distress following notification of an HIV+ status.

Following the HIV testing there may be an asymptomatic period that can last for many years. Several studies have shown that anxiety and depression during this time may not be out of the normal range (Folkman & Chesney, 1995; Krikorian, Kay, & Liang, 1995). However, when significant symptomatology is present, anxiety and depression levels dip.

In the vocational, domestic, sexual, and social domains of psychosocial adjustment, men with AIDS are more poorly adjusted than asymptomatic seropositive men and uninfected men. Moreover, there is some evidence that men who are depressed when they are asymptomatic seropositive may have overall greater T cell decrement over time (six years) than those who were not depressed (Burack et al., 1993). Because depression is treatable and therapy may alter the course of the disease, the early diagnosis of depression might be important for the subsequent well-being of the person who is HIV+. However, currently there is no evidence that survival rates are any different for depressed versus nondepressed persons who are asymptomatic and seropositive (Lyketsos et al., 1993).

Perhaps what characterizes the asymptomatic stage of HIV infection most is uncertainty. There are a host of dilemmas that might be faced at that point: disclosure of HIV status, modification of health and sexual behaviors, maintenance of emotional balance, and so on. Weitz (1989) has suggested that uncertainty may provoke attempts to assert control. This process is similar to what Taylor and Brown (1988) have termed "positive illusions," described in the following section. Finally, for men who are HIV+, satisfaction with their social support network and participation in the AIDS community appear to be related to more healthy coping strategies (Leserman, Perkins, & Evans, 1992).

Psychological and Physical Reactions to Treatments

Following diagnosis and after treatment decisions have been made, many patients must confront the prospect of surgery, radiation, chemotherapy, or a combination of those treatments. For those with cancer or AIDS there may be many months or years of drug treatment with concomitant side effects. Accompanying the treatments is concern about maintaining physical functioning and uncertainty about the success of treatments.

Depression is more common among cancer patients than in the general population (which is about 6 percent). In their review of the studies on the psychosocial adjustment of breast cancer patients, Irvine, Brown, Crooks, Roberts, and Browne (1991) noted that about 20–30 percent of women experience some emotional problems, such as depression. In a sample of men with mixed cancer diagnoses who had been diagnosed within six weeks of testing, Gooding, McAnulty, Wittrock, Britt, and Khansur (1995) noted that about 39 percent reported symptoms of moderate to severe depression. Based on a select review of research, Massie and Holland (1990) concluded that about 25 percent of hospitalized cancer patients are likely to experience depression. Those at highest risk for depression had a prior history of affective disorder or alcoholism, advanced stages of cancer, poorly controlled pain, or treatment with medications that may produce depressive symptoms.

Finally, Maunsell, Brisson, and Deschênes (1992) found that "the number of stressful life events and a history of depression before breast cancer diagnosis are strong indicators of the risk of high psychological distress in the 18-month period after initial treatment for breast cancer" (p. 123). Depression also increases the risk of suicide. Although suicide attempts are close to the same level as the general population, persons with cancer have increased suicide mortality (Allebeck & Bolund, 1991).

Treatments for both cancer and AIDS have a substantial impact on psychological functioning. For cancer, cytoxic treatment causes side effects that are related to the necrotic effects of aggressive chemotherapies. The case of Melanie, a 42-year-old married cancer patient with three children, provides a clear example of how medical treatment can interfere with mood. When Melanie came for a psychological evaluation she complained of crying all the time, not caring about anything anymore, and just wanting it "all to end." She blamed herself for being "weak" and for being a "bad mother" because she did not have the energy to spend time with her children. Melanie was being treated with interferon injections and had been on this treatment regimen for several months. She finally inquired if her depressive symptoms could be a side effect of her treatment, since her mood had begun to change only after the treatment had begun. Melanie was extremely relieved to discover that there was a medical explanation for what she was feeling, and that there were possible psychological and psychopharmacologic treatments for it.

In addition to the side effects caused by the drugs, there may also be a conditioned response to the chemotherapy. A conditioned response may be acquired when the patient pairs the medical setting and the medical staff with the nausea and vomiting caused by the injected drugs. The conditioned stimuli may include nurses who administer the drugs, the smell of the hospital or clinic, or the building itself. Thus, sometime prior to the actual administration of chemotherapy, conditioned symptoms such as nausea, vomiting, anxiety, dread, or depression may emerge. These conditioned symptoms may also occur either during the administration of the drugs before their toxicity has begun or afterward as the person recalls the experience. Bovbjerg and colleagues (1990) have also established that the conditioning process extends to the immune system. That is, immunosupression occurred in women who were waiting in the doctor's office for chemotherapy, but it did not when they were at home several days prior to treatment. Finally, there may be some relationship between the conditioned response pattern and traditional notions of stress when stress is predictable. For example, Morrow and colleagues

(1992) found that the anticipation of chemotherapy was directly related to arousal prior to the treatments.

Physicians often encounter the situation in which patients drop out of the chemotherapy regimen. Gilbar (1991) found that dropouts experienced poorer quality of life than those who completed chemotherapy. This difference was particularly salient in the domains of vocational and social adjustment; however, the largest difference occurred in psychological distress and in adjusting to medical care. The implications from this study are that dropouts may be people who do not adjust well to the medical setting, are not satisfied with their quality of life, and/or are emotionally upset.

The process of coping with treatments for cancer and AIDS may include the emergence of depression, medically caused emotional responses, stress reactions that may resemble classical conditioning, and poor quality of life that may affect compliance with treatment regimens. Early recognition of these problems by medical staff may promote referrals for psychological treatment to prevent disruption in medical care.

Coping Processes

The term *coping* is often used with cancer and AIDS patients. The implication is that these diseases are perceived as a threat or challenge that may tax the resources of the individual. Thus, cognitive, emotional, and behavioral responses are needed to render the threat more manageable. According to Rowland (1989), there are at least three domains that may determine the coping response that is needed:

1. disease-related determinants, for example, site, stage, type of treatment
2. individual determinants, such as developmental stage, personality, values and beliefs, and perceived support
3. sociocultural factors, for example, community attitudes, availability of social resources

Obviously, advanced stage at diagnosis of full-blown AIDS and aggressive or disfiguring treatments for cancer will be more difficult to cope with. The timing of the disease is also a critical factor in the coping process. For example, contracting breast cancer at age 25 is not construed as age-normative and, therefore, will be more threatening than the same disease in a woman who is 80. In addition to the age-normative occurrence of cancer at age 80, the older person also has had a lifetime of experiences to bring to bear upon the coping process. As for AIDS, it is for the most part a disease that affects young people and, therefore, is almost always "off timing" developmentally.

Cancer

Research on coping with cancer indicates that active coping styles and perceptions of control are associated with a more positive adjustment to the disease than are coping styles characterized by avoidance (Dunkel-Schetter, Feinstein, Taylor, & Falke, 1992; Stanton, & Snider, 1993). Consistent with those findings, Carver and colleagues (1993) reported that the coping strategies of acceptance, the use of humor, and positive framing were associated with low distress following treatments for breast cancer. Additionally in that study, overt denial and behavioral disengagement were associated with higher levels of distress. Carver and colleagues also found evidence for some reciprocal causation that resulted in a cascade of negative coping and distress. For example, low acceptance of cancer before initial surgery predicted denial and disengagement at a three-month follow-up, which, in turn, predicted higher levels of distress at a six-month follow-up. Moreover, they found that dispositional optimism was related to greater acceptance and less denial and behavioral disengagement.

Taylor's (1983) theory of cognitive adaptation to illness includes three coping processes that seem to bode well for positive adjustment to cancer. She found that women with metastatic breast cancer adapted better if they perceived that they had control over some aspect of their life, if they attached meaning to their disease (e.g., how they acquired the disease), and if they made downward social comparisons (e.g., "someone else has it worse"). In terms of control, women might change their diet, engage in some form of complementary medicine, or change some other manageable aspect of their daily life. The meaning or explanation attached to the acquisition of the disease did not have to be medically correct to be functional. Finally, the social comparisons did not have to be made relative to an actual person. For example, someone who had a mastectomy might claim that she was much better off than someone who had both breasts removed. In all three processes, the person may be creating illusions of control, meaning, and social comparison, which Taylor (1983) describes as "positive illusions." These illusions are distortions that enhance positive self-evaluations, maintain perceptions of control, and promote an optimistic perspective (Taylor & Brown, 1988).

AIDS

The data on coping with AIDS have some parallels with the literature on coping with cancer. Namir, Wolcott, Fawzy, and Alumbaugh (1990) found that men with AIDS who used avoidant coping experienced more psychological distress than those who used social support or active-behavioral approaches to problem solving. Moreover, avoidant coping was associated with higher levels of depression, more health concerns, lower levels of social support, and lower self-esteem when compared to active-behavioral coping. Interestingly, sole reliance on changing thoughts (i.e., thinking positively) was associated with obsessional and ruminative strategies that were not successful in reducing distress. The authors concluded that mastery over AIDS involves increasing self-efficacy and the sense that one is in control of one's behavior.

The notion that control strategies may be related to positive adjustment to AIDS was also studied by Reed, Taylor, and Kemeny (1993). These authors distinguished personal control beliefs from vicarious control beliefs. The former refers to personal actions that might be taken to alter the situation or lead to a desired outcome; the latter refers to control that is vested in powerful others to provide positive outcomes. Obviously, in the medical setting the "powerful others" are the health care staff, including physicians. Reed and colleagues found that personal control beliefs that relate to day-to-day symptoms and the overall course of the illness were associated with positive adjustment to AIDS. Whereas, vicarious control "over the course of the illness and over medical care and treatment were negatively associated with adjustment to AIDS" (p. 813). The authors concluded that men who adjust well to AIDS view themselves not as passive victims of the disease but as having control over certain daily aspects of the disease and the overall course of the disease. As with cancer patients, there may be few benefits to reinforcing realism. Instead, there may be some adaptive benefit to holding positive illusions that may foster hope and positive states of mind.

The few recent studies of long-term survivors of AIDS reinforce the beneficial effects of active, positive coping. The descriptive research on long-term survival of AIDS seems to indicate that survivors (i.e., those who are alive three years after diagnosis) have active coping styles and are relatively free of mood disorders and other psychological distress. In addition, most long-term survivors have had bouts with life-threatening illness and seemed to bounce back after each setback. Moreover, they tended to believe that they would experience good times and felt strongly that their lives were important (Rabkin, Remien, Katoff, & Williams, 1993). They were also more likely to believe that chance or personal control are associated with health outcomes rather than the actions of powerful others. That is, they tended to believe that medical interventions can help but are not a panacea. There is very little, if any, use of denial among long-term survivors. Moreover, there is flexible use of many different types of active coping strategies (Remien, Rabkin, Williams, & Katoff, 1992).

In general, the diagnosis of cancer or AIDS constitutes a major life event that evokes the need for adjustments. Active, problem-oriented coping styles that foster control or perceived control produce better adjustment than coping styles characterized by denial, avoidance, or passivity. For many people this process may result in some personal adjustments that are manageable. Once the initial crisis of the diagnosis has passed and the treatment decisions have been made, these people may recover functioning. For others, the coping process may be more difficult and result in an adjustment disorder with depressed mood or a major depressive disorder. Those who are more active copers with no premorbid history will probably weather the crisis. However, coping with cancer and AIDS is a process that requires a degree of resilience; that is, the ability to persistently recover as much as possible from a number of setbacks over an extended period of time.

A Model for Adjustment to Cancer and AIDS

There has been little theory guiding research on coping with cancer and AIDS. However, one of the most promising theoretical perspectives for research in this area is self-regulation (Bandura, 1991) and, in particular, self-efficacy. Self-efficacy refers to confidence judgments one makes about one's ability to perform particular behaviors. Thus, from the perspective of self-efficacy (Bandura, 1986), coping with cancer and AIDS refers to confidence judgments one makes about one's ability to perform particular adaptive behaviors related to those illnesses.

Theoretically, self-efficacy operates as a mediating variable because it transforms or changes the relationship between two other variables (Baron & Kenny, 1986). As such, efficacy judgments are made after compiling, sorting, and integrating information from the external environment and from inside the person. With respect to life-threatening illness, that information might include the degree to which the disease and its treatments affect the functioning of the person, the availability of social support, coping style, personality characteristics, developmental stage, attitudes toward the disease, and a number of other variables. Outcomes, such as psychological adjustment, quality of life, and longevity, are projected from these efficacy judgments. Research on coping with acute pain, abortion, and cancer (Litt, 1988; Major et al., 1990; Merluzzi & Martinez Sanchez, 1994) supports the mediating role of efficacy expectations.

For a woman with breast cancer, one of the self-efficacy judgments concerns her confidence that she can cope with treatment-related side effects, such as nausea or hair loss. In order to make that judgment, she may survey the demands of the situation (i.e., enduring those physical changes) and assess her coping resources (e.g., support from spouse, previous coping patterns under stress). If she feels that her coping resources are sufficient given her perceptions of the demands of the situation, she may be confident that she can manage nausea and hair loss. Another person may not be as confident if she feels that she does not possess or have access to the resources she needs to manage the side effects. Thus, according to self-efficacy theory, these women survey their own internal resources as well as resources in their environment (e.g., the social support of others, information from doctors, tumor marker values) and then make subjective judgments about their coping capacity. The more confident (more efficacious) a person is, the better she will cope with the disease and treatment side effects (Cunningham, Lockwood, & Cunningham, 1991; Telch & Telch, 1986).

The proposed model for coping with cancer and AIDS starts with variables that may have a direct impact on self-efficacy expectations that, in turn, affect outcomes such as adjustment, quality of life, and longevity (figure 7.1). In the paragraphs below, several of these variables are reviewed and recommendations for assessment are offered. With respect to the overall model, special attention is given to social support, disease impact, and quality of life because they play a prominent role in the literature on cancer and AIDS. Finally, while the model proposes that a number of variables affect outcome through the mediation of self-efficacy, many of these variables may also affect the outcome variables directly. The assumption of the model is that self-efficacy may mediate wholly or partially the effects of those predictor variables on outcomes.

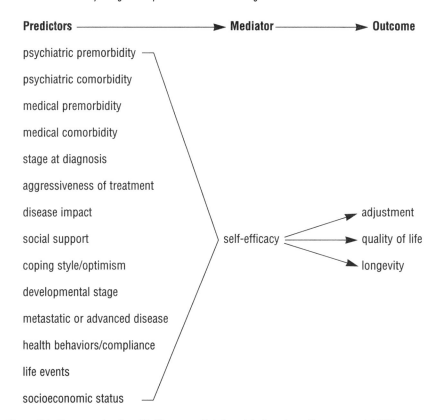

Figure 7.1. Components of a self-efficacy mediated model of coping with cancer and AIDS.

Components of the Model and Assessment Strategies

Social Support

No other aspect of coping with cancer and AIDS has received as much attention as social support. This area of research is driven by the belief that social relationships and social support provide a basic human need that has an influence on our health and well-being. The distinctions between types of support (Helgeson & Cohen, 1996) have included such categories as:

- emotional support, which involves the communication of caring and concern,
- informational support, which includes the provision of guidance and advice, and
- instrumental or tangible support, which involves providing material goods such as money, transportation, or direct physical assistance.

For the most part, emotional support has been well studied and appears to be related to adjustment to cancer. Also, in most studies the most unhelpful type of support was actually the absence or withdrawal of emotional support; that is, avoiding the patient, minimizing the patient's problems, and forced cheerfulness (Helgeson & Cohen, 1996). These behaviors prevent the patient from openly discussing the illness.

Similarly, Zich and Temoshok (1990) found that persons with AIDS preferred emotional support over informational (problem-solving) support. They suggested that emotional support can be offered by a variety of people, but that informational support may be better accepted from an expert. Perhaps persons with AIDS and cancer have received both helpful and unhelpful informational support and perceive problem-solving support from an "unqualified" person as annoying and unhelpful (Zich & Temoshok, 1990). Finally, Zich and Temoshok found that higher levels of social support were associated with low levels of hopelessness and depression, but the latter two constructs were not correlated with physical symptoms. This finding may suggest that thoughts of suicide may be related more to the loss of support rather than to the disease. Thus, social support may be a modifiable variable that may change the course of adjustment to the disease.

There may be some optimal matching between the source of support and the type of support desired. Rose (1990) asked newly diagnosed cancer patients about the type of support they wanted from family, friends, and health professionals. They preferred tangible aid from family members, modeling from friends who had cancer, and open communication and clarification from their health professionals. Tangible aid includes food, clothing, money, transportation, help with insurance, and so on. The desire that family members would provide this type of support is based on the social obligations that we have for family compared to others in our social network. The need for modeling from other cancer patients illustrates the desire to learn from others who are not a part of the family. A support group or some informal support system provides this type of support. The desire for open communication and clarification from health professionals may stress the importance of the health professional–patient relationship. While patients expected intimacy and tolerance of their need to vent from both family and friends, they hoped for reassurance, esteem, guidance, and advocacy from all three sources (i.e., family, friends, and health professionals).

There is also a distinction between perceived and actual support. Construed as the belief that support (of a variety of types) is available from those with whom we have interpersonal relationships, perceived support has been described as a cognitive personality variable that affects our perception and recall of interpersonal relationships (Lakey & Cassady, 1990). Actual support is similar to tangible or instrumental support. In our research on actual social support, self-efficacy, and adjustment to cancer (Martinez Sanchez & Merluzzi, 1997), we found that when functional impairment was minimal, high levels of actual support detracted from efficacy and adjustment. Conversely, at high levels of physical impairment, high levels of actual support enhanced efficacy and adjustment to cancer. Thus, when supplied to someone who is not very debilitated by cancer, actual support may be detrimental, either promoting or reinforcing helplessness or sick role behavior.

Assessment of Social Support

1. *The Interpersonal Support Evaluation List* (Cohen, Mermelstein, Kamarack, & Hoberman, 1985) is one of the most used measures of social support. It is designed to assess perceived support in four areas: tangible support, such as "instrumental aid"; appraisal support, such as the "availability of someone to talk to about one's problems"; self-esteem support, such as "the availability of a positive comparison when comparing oneself with others"; and belonging support, such as "the availability of people one can do things with" (Cohen et al., 1985, pp. 74–75).
2. *The Inventory of Socially Supportive Behaviors* (Barrera, Sandler, & Ramsey, 1981) is a useful measure of actual support. This 40-item scale is based on three criteria: behavioral specificity so that items can be easily interpreted, broad wording so that items would be applicable to many populations, and omission of references to psychological adjustment so that the scale would not overlap with scales designed to assess that construct.
3. *The Interview Schedule for Social Interaction* (Bergeman, Plomin, Pedersen, McClearn, & Nesselroade, 1990) is another measure of social support. This measure contains 24 items that distinguish support from family members and relatives versus support received from friends.

Disease Impact

Rowland (1989) suggested that the "medical context" (p. 25) of the patient is an important consideration in the patient's psychological adjustment to cancer. Defining medical context as stage of disease, type of treatment the patient is receiving, and sites affected, she suggested that all of these components contribute to the level of physiological functioning of the patient and his or her ability to engage in the tasks of daily living. Further, Holland (1989) stated, "a patient's quality of life and adaptation at a given point in illness represents the balance between the medical facts and the mitigating effects of psychological state and social supports" (p. 75). Thus, adaptation, quality of life, and adjustment to cancer are related to the physiological and functional impact of the disease.

In our research on the self-efficacy mediated model (Merluzzi & Martinez Sanchez, 1994), the disease impact of the patient had both a modest direct effect on adjustment as well as a substantial effect mediated by self-efficacy. Stage of cancer, which is usually determined at the time of diagnosis, is also a critical piece of information because advanced stage at diagnosis is associated with much poorer prognosis than early stage detection.

Assessment of Disease Impact

1. *The Sickness Impact Profile* (SIP) is the most widely used measure of disease impact and functional ability. It is a general measure that assesses the impact of any disease or disability (Karoly, 1985), and was designed for use with a variety of demographic groups, cultural groups, and severity levels of illness (Bergner, Bobbitt, Carter, & Gilson, 1981).

2. *The Karnofsky Performance Status* (KPS), widely used in cancer research (Greico & Long, 1984; Karoly, 1985), relates the disease to daily functioning. Performance status criteria are divided into percentage scores ranging from "0," dead, to "100," normal with no complaints. The physician, technologist, nurse, or other observer assigns a single percentage score, which falls on that continuum of functioning.

It is important to take medical premorbidity and comorbidity into account (Andersen, 1994). The presence of other diseases, particularly chronic diseases, will exacerbate decrements in functional capacity and promote deterioration of efficacy and adjustment. A review of the patient's medical history will provide this information.

The assessment of pain is also a critical aspect of determining the impact of disease and medical treatments on the functioning of the patient. There are three instruments that may be useful: the *Melzack-McGill Pain*

Questionnaire (MMPQ; Melzack, 1975), the *Wisconsin Brief Pain Inventory* (BPI; Daut, Cleeland, & Flannery, 1983), and the *West Haven-Yale Multidimensional Pain Inventory* (WHYMPI; Kerns, Turk, & Rudy, 1985). The MMPQ and WHYMPI are well-respected inventories that are used for a variety of pain etiologies. The BPI was developed specifically for cancer pain. It is also important to note that a high degree of pain is usually associated with elevations in depression and anxiety. Therefore, if there are significant pain symptoms, it would be advisable to also assess depression. Illustrating comorbidity, Spiegel and Sands (1988) found that 28 percent of patients with significant self-reported pain also met the criteria for major depressive disorder; whereas none in a "low pain" group met those criteria.

Assessing Coping Style, Optimism, and Psychological Functioning
Because the role of coping has been discussed in earlier sections of this chapter we will focus on the assessment of coping. The *COPE Scale* (Carver, Scheier, & Weintraub, 1989) assesses coping styles and strategies an individual is presently using in response to stress. The COPE contains three primary areas of coping: problem-focused, emotion-focused and "coping responses that arguably are less useful" (p. 1). These areas are represented by 13 subscales. The specificity of the 13 subscales makes this instrument valuable in assessing ineffective coping styles.

Dispositional optimism has been associated with positive adaptation to illness as well as psychological and physical well-being (Scheier & Carver, 1992). *The Life Orientation Test* (LOT; Scheier, Carver, & Bridges, 1994) is a 10-item self-report measure that assesses expectancies for positive versus negative outcomes. The LOT was developed to assess optimism as a stable personality characteristic; therefore, it assesses generalized expectancies for outcomes.

In addition to coping style and optimism, it is important to assess the patient's premorbid and comorbid psychological problems. For example, a history of depression places the patient at much higher risk for depression after AIDS or cancer is diagnosed (Andersen, 1994). Also, depression and other psychiatric problems have an additive effect in terms of the impact on the person's functional capacity, efficacy, and adjustment.

Assessing Self-Efficacy
The Cancer Behavior Inventory (CBI; Merluzzi & Martinez Sanchez, 1997a, 1997b) is a comprehensive measure of self-efficacy for behaviors related to

coping with cancer. For each item in the CBI, persons with cancer rate how confident they are that they can perform or accomplish the behavior. It is important to note that patients rate each behavior even if they have not yet had to perform it. Thus, efficacy judgments are not based necessarily on past performance alone but also on some estimation of the confidence that, in the near or distant future, one could perform the task. The CBI contains six scales: (1) maintaining activity and independence, (2) coping with treatment related side effects, (3) seeking and understanding medical information, (4) accepting cancer/maintaining positive attitude, (5) affective regulation, and (6) seeking social support.

To date, no comparable measure for AIDS is available. However, the CBI could be readily adapted for AIDS by rewording the items. This alteration of the original instrument may affect its psychometric properties; therefore, the use of such a revised measure in a clinical setting should be done cautiously.

Quality of Life

Concern about the impact of disease and treatment on the patient and his or her family has led to the concept of quality of life (QOL). Whereas survival deals with the quantity of life, the subjective well-being of the patient in a number of areas (e.g., psychological, social, vocational, physical) is the domain of QOL (Aaronson & Beckman, 1987; Ware, 1984). Moreover, Cella (1995) has noted that treatments that improve QOL but not survival may be considered effective.

In one of the more well developed research programs on QOL, Cella and colleagues (1993) have identified four dimensions of QOL: physical well-being, functional well-being, emotional well-being, and social well-being. Physical well-being refers to the perceptions of bodily functions and includes nausea, pain, hair loss, fatigue, and so on. The concept of physical well-being is a combination of the effects of the disease and treatments. Functional well-being deals with the ability to carry on normal self-care and social and vocational roles. So, physical well-being may affect functional well-being, but not necessarily. For example, a person with AIDS may be able to work in spite of some of the side effects of treatment. Functional well-being may not be severely hampered, although physical well-being is compromised. Emotional well-being taps both positive states of mind as well as negative affect or distress. Finally, social well-being concerns the maintenance of social relationships with family, friends, and intimates. It is different from functional well-being in that social well-being taps the quality of those relationships.

In an interesting study on the relative importance of QOL and other variables in determining treatment preference (standard or aggressive), persons with cancer were asked to consider the relative importance of a number of factors such as age, having a partner, having children, inability to work due to side effects, the nature of side effects, life expectancy, and QOL (Kiebert et al., 1994). It appears that if there is a good chance of a cure, patients are willing to accept negative QOL. On the other hand, when the prognosis is poor, patients appear to opt for high QOL in spite of the limits on longevity. After probability of cure, patients' baseline QOL seemed to be a critical factor. That is, persons with already compromised health may not wish to endure any further decrement in QOL and therefore refuse treatments that someone with a higher threshold of QOL might be willing to endure. Having a partner and children may also affect the decision to endure more treatments that compromise QOL. Also, being younger contributes to the decision to endure treatments that greatly affect QOL. Interestingly, the nature of side effects and the possibility that work might be missed were the least of concerns.

Persons with AIDS spend a great deal of the day on health-related activities. It has been estimated that up to about seven hours each day may be spent on personal medical care, paperwork, getting extra rest needed to sustain activity, and so on. It is clear from this rather simple statistic that QOL plays a large role in the life of a person with AIDS. In addition, there is the added stigma, which can result in job discrimination and social isolation. The stigma once attached to cancer has changed somewhat over the years as more information is available about the disease. However, the stigma attached to AIDS is related to attitudes toward homosexuality and IV drug abuse. Generally, there is the attribution of blame with AIDS that is not as prevalent with most cancers. Thus, AIDS carries with it the burden of personal health issues that are very time consuming and the social burden of being stigmatized. Thus, QOL may be affected by both the disease and the social stigma attached to it.

Assessment of Quality of Life

1. *The Functional Assessment of Cancer Therapy* (FACT; Cella et al., 1993) is one of the most commonly used measures of QOL. It has a

general 28-item scale (FACT-G) and a number of disease-specific sub-scales for different types of cancer (e.g., breast, lung, prostate) and cancer treatments (e.g., bone marrow transplant). The FACT yields a total QOL score as well as scale scores for physical well-being, social/family well-being, emotional well-being, functional well-being, and disease-specific information. The FACT is a well-established measure of QOL with excellent psychometric properties. Cella and colleagues (1996) also have developed a measure of QOL for persons with HIV. That measure consists of the basic items from the FACT-G with an additional 20 items that are tailored to HIV.

2. *The Cancer Rehabilitation Evaluation System* (CARES-SF; Schag & Heinrich, 1988) is another well developed measure of QOL. It is a 59-item self-report inventory of the problems that cancer patients encounter (e.g., fatigue, pain, in ability to work). This measure yields a general score that reflects global QOL as well as scores of subscales that include physical, medical interaction, psychosocial, sexual, marital, and several miscellaneous scales.

3. *The Psychosocial Adjustment to Illness Scale* (PAIS-SR; Derogatis & Derogatis, 1990) was constructed to assess the psychosocial adjustment to disease ranging from mild disorders to life-threatening diseases. The 46-item scale measures seven areas of adjustment: health care orientation, vocational environment, domestic environment, sexual relationship, extended family relationships, social environment, and psychological distress. The PAIS-SR has been factor analyzed using data from a sample of 502 cancer patients with varying diagnoses (Merluzzi & Martinez Sanchez, 1997c). In general, the factors derived from that analysis appear to confirm the original conceptually derived scales. For a review of other measures of quality of life see Cella, 1995.

Psychosocial Treatments for Cancer and AIDS

Recently, there has been a great deal of interest in the impact of psychological treatments on the quality of life of persons with cancer and AIDS. Moreover, several well-controlled studies have also explored the longevity of persons who receive these treatments. This area of research is still emerging and large-scale replication studies are in progress. However, the results are very promising; participation in group intervention appears to benefit both quality of life and longevity.

Interventions for Anticipatory Nausea and Stress

Treatments for conditioned symptoms such as anticipatory nausea and anxiety have included relaxation training with imagery to enhance relaxation as well as "general coping preparation" (Burish, Snyder, & Jenkins, 1991). Generally, the treatments based on relaxation and imagery do reduce the conditioned side effects. In addition, Burish and colleagues (1991) found that a preparatory coping program that consisted of a tour of the treatment facility, a videotaped presentation of patients receiving chemotherapy, question-and-answer sessions with oncology nurses, and written materials was as effective in reducing conditioned side effects as the relaxation-imagery training.

Other approaches to treating these symptoms include cognitive restructuring aimed at modifying attitudes, beliefs, and thoughts that may cause or exacerbate stress. Also, stress inoculation training is recommended for anticipating stressful situations that might occur on a regular basis in the life of someone with cancer or AIDS (Golden, Gersh, & Robbins, 1992).

Interventions for Pain

Pain is one of the most common complaints from cancer patients (Syrjala & Roth-Roemer, 1996). The most comprehensive approach to cancer- and AIDS-related pain from a psychological perspective is the cognitive-behavioral approach (Golden et al., 1992). The first step is a reconceptualization of the pain as a well-specified problem rather than a vague concern or experience. The main focus of this reconceptualization is to reduce the purely sensory perspective of pain and to present a more multicomponent view that takes into account cognitive, affective, and sociocultural influences. This reframing of the pain process also helps reduce resistance to the treatment. The next step focuses on cognitive restructuring in which the patients' thoughts and beliefs are probed in order to enhance control-oriented thoughts and abandon irrational beliefs that may exacerbate the pain (e.g., catastrophic or bipolar and polarized thinking). The intention of this portion of the treatment is to enhance the inhibition of pain by controlling mechanisms that block pain messages to the brain or inhibit pain intensity (see Melzack & Wall, 1965). Patients are then taught a variety of skills, such as problem solving, relaxation and controlled breathing, and attention-diversion. In order to generalize and maintain treatment gains, patients are encouraged to use the skills each day and report on their effectiveness. Finally, follow-up sessions are scheduled to boost the effects of the treatment.

Perhaps the strongest controlled clinical trial data in this area points to the efficacy of support combined with imagery or hypnosis (Spiegel & Bloom, 1983; Syrjala & Chapko, 1995; Syrjala, Cummings, & Dondaldson, 1992). In a meta-analysis of cognitive-behavioral interventions for pain that was not limited to cancer pain, Fernandez and Turk (1989) found that all the cognitive-behavioral strategies were effective, but that imagery consistently showed the greatest effect. In addition, current research clearly indicates that long-term treatment is not necessary, and that brief, focused interventions can be effective (Fawzy, Fawzy, Arndt, & Pasau, 1995; Syrjala & Chapko, 1995; Syrjala & Roth-Roemer, 1996).

The use of cognitive-behavioral strategies to control cancer pain is illustrated with the case of Dennis. Dennis, a 36-year-old multiple myeloma patient, complained of severe mouth and throat pain following bone marrow transplantation. Dennis was taught the imagery technique of sensory transformation. After a brief induction, consisting of deep breathing followed by progressive muscle relaxation, Dennis was asked to imagine holding an ice cube in his mouth. The suggestion was made for Dennis to hold the ice cube on his tongue and to "feel the soothing icy numbness spreading through the tissues of [his] mouth, layer by layer." As the ice melted he was told he could feel that same "soothing icy numbness running down the back of [his] throat." He was told he could hold that icy numbness there, in his mouth and throat, for as long as he needed to, and that he could let it recede whenever he wished. It was also suggested that he could bring back this feeling of soothing numbness whenever he needed to, simply by "closing [his] eyes, focusing on [his] breathing, and bringing back the image of holding an ice cube or some ice-cold liquid in [his] mouth." By using this technique, Dennis was able to have control over his own comfort at a time when so little else was under his control.

Psychosocial Interventions to Promote Adjustment, Quality of Life, and Longevity

We are at the point in the treatment of cancer and AIDS that the beneficial effects of psychosocial interventions on adjustment, quality of life, and longevity are no longer in question. Three recent reviews of the literature on the effects of psychosocial interventions conclude that the results of those interventions include improvements in coping, affect, QOL, immune functioning, and survival (Fawzy et al.,1995; Ironson et al., 1995; Meyer & Mark, 1995). For example, in their meta-analysis of psychosocial interventions, Meyer and Mark (1995) concluded that these interventions have "positive effects on emotional adjustment, functional adjustment, and treatment- and disease-related symptoms" (p. 104). Furthermore, the effect sizes were in a range that is considered typical for psychological interventions.

In a critical review of some of the same literature, Fawzy and colleagues (1995) concluded that persons with cancer benefit from a wide variety of psychological interventions, including individual and group counseling. They recommend a structured intervention for newly diagnosed patients that consists of health education, stress management, coping and problem-solving skills, and group support. They contend that using a structured intervention for newly diagnosed patients is important because it helps to reduce distress and anxiety and provides patients with skills to mobilize their coping responses. These conclusions were primarily based on the Fawzy and colleagues' (1993) six-year follow-up study of patients newly diagnosed with malignant melanoma who had participated in the short-term structured intervention. At six years posttreatment, of the 34 patients in the control group 13 had recurrences and 10 of the 34 died, compared to 7 having recurrence and 3 of 34 dying in the experimental group.

For persons whose diagnosis is beyond the initial stages of a disease, a weekly group meeting over an extended period of time seems to be more appropriate than the short-term structured interventions. The extended time frame of this type of group fosters processes such as self-disclosure, interpersonal feedback, and mutual support, which lead to group cohesion. In addition, the group encourages its members to talk about feelings, be creative, determine what is important, develop a life project (accomplish something important), realign social networks, enhance family support, and work on doctor-patient communication. Group members can also be trained in self-hypnosis and relaxation for pain control (Spiegel, 1991).

In an initial study (Spiegel et al., 1989), women with late-stage breast cancer in a year-long therapy group lived on average three years compared to one and a half years for women in the control group. Moreover, there was a dose-related effect; the more time spent in the group, the greater the benefit. This result gives more credence to the notion that there was something about the group that contributed to survival time. It is also important to note that the divergence in survival did not occur until 20 months into the study; that is, about 8 months after the termination of the intervention.

For persons with AIDS, research on psychosocial interventions to enhance quality of life have begun to appear. These interventions are even more timely given the introduction of protease inhibitors, which appear to be effective in arresting or slowing the progression of the disease (Adams & Merluzzi, 1993). However, survival studies like those conducted with cancer patients have not yet been conducted.

The most well-developed approach to psychosocial interventions for persons with HIV was offered by Antoni (1991), who suggested that interventions aimed at increasing adaptive coping, social support, and self-efficacy would decrease distress and depression and enhance a sense of well-being. These, in turn, would positively impact neuroendocrine and immunologic functioning. The intervention and improved physiological functioning would also positively impact social and role functioning, resulting in decreases in risk behavior and substance abuse. The outcomes in this model are decreased disease progression and increased functional abilities.

In a study designed to test some of those assumptions, Antoni, Baggett, and others (1991) randomly assigned gay men to either a cognitive-behavioral stress management intervention or a control group. Five weeks into the intervention, the men were informed of their serostatus and then continued in the treatments for another five weeks. The cognitive-behavioral stress management treatment included work on recognizing the signs of stress and negative automatic thoughts, relaxation training, as well as information on AIDS and the immune system, sexual risk behaviors, and social support. The stress management and information sessions alternated with relaxation sessions. Men in the control group who were notified that they were seropositive showed significant increases in anxiety and depression while those in the cognitive-behavioral stress management group evidenced no changes in anxiety and just a slight increase depression. The buffer effect of the intervention seemed to be related to the amount of relaxation homework in which the men engaged during the five-week prenotification period. In addition to the differences in psychological responses, the control group had decrements in immunological responses after serostatus notification.

At a one-year follow-up, coping strategies such as denial and disengagement were associated with increased depression (Antoni, Goldstein, Gookin, Fletcher, & Schneiderman, 1991). On the other hand, coping skills such as active coping, planning, and positive reappraisal were associated with decreased depression. At a two-year follow-up (Antoni, Goldstein, et al., 1991), predictors of disease progression included degree of distress at time of diagnosis, denial, poor attendance in the group, and failure to comply with relaxation homework. Thus, the functional status of men who did not use denial and who participated fully in the intervention was better than in those who used denial and did not adhere to the treatment protocol.

Psychological interventions for persons with cancer and HIV have beneficial effects on psychosocial functioning and QOL, and, in the case of cancer, survival. The common threads that seem to be woven through these interventions are group support, fear reduction, problem solving, and stress management. Perhaps these groups increase the self-efficacy and the perception of control, which is crucial to positive adaptation in patients with cancer or AIDS. The patients may feel that they have more control over their lives and the disease. The results of the longevity studies would suggest that this positive illusion of control may have some impact on the course of the disease.

Summary and Future Directions

In this chapter we have presented an overview of some of the major issues in coping with cancer and AIDS. We have not attempted to be comprehensive in our approach; for example, areas that were not touched upon at all include prevention, caregiving, and death and dying. This chapter focused on aspects of cancer and AIDS that might occur after diagnosis and during the process of coping with those diseases. We encourage those in the helping profession to conceptualize the process of coping with life-threatening disease as having different challenges at different points in the course of the disease. The self-efficacy mediated model of coping might provide a conceptual framework for assessment and treatment. Finally, outcome studies seem to indicate that quality of life and longevity may be positively affected by psychological interventions.

Perhaps the most critical area for future research, with direct implications for practice, is the study of the impact of psychosocial interventions and psychological variables (e.g., self-efficacy) on the quality of life and longevity of persons with cancer or AIDS. There is no question that the biological aspects of these diseases will be the most effective predictors of medical outcomes and longevity. However, there may be some effect that certain behaviors and states of mind have on the response to medical interventions (e.g., chemotherapy, protease inhibitors) that may promote a more (or less) favorable response to treatment. That response, in turn, may affect longevity. The obvious focus of that mediating or moderating mechanism is the immune system. Some attempts to link behavior (or states of mind), the immune system, and quality of life and longevity have begun to appear (Fawzy et al., 1993) and others are in process. The results of these research efforts over the next decade will have a substantial effect on the clinical practice of psychologists who work with patients who have cancer or AIDS.

Suggested Resources

On the subject of cancer, *Everyone's Guide to Cancer Therapy* (Dollinger & Rosenbaum, 1998) is an excellent resource that is accessible to both psychologists and patients. A more specialized resource is *Breast Cancer: The Complete Guide* (Hirshaut & Pressman, 1997)

For AIDS, numerous resources are available that describe the disease and its treatments. One that describes the discovery of the disease is *And the Band Played On* (Shilts, 1995). Two recent books on AIDS are very accessible and useful for patients: *The Guide to Living with HIV Infection* (Bartlett & Finkbeiner, 1996) and *Living with HIV and AIDS* (Gifford, Lorig, Laurent, & Gonzalez, 1996) Psychologists interested in working with patients who have cancer or AIDS might want to consult *Psychological Treatment of Cancer Patients: A Cognitive-Behavioral Approach* (Golden, Gersh, & Robbins, 1992). In addition, the October 1991 issue of the *Counseling Psychologist* (19[4]), was devoted to counseling persons with HIV/AIDS.

Journals that would be of interest to counseling psychologists are *Health Psychology, Psycho-Oncology, Journal of Psychosocial Oncology,* and the *Annals of Behavioral Medicine.*

Discussion Questions

1. There are many ways in which persons with the same disease (e.g., prostate cancer, early-stage AIDS), whose medical treatments are identi-

cal, may vary in terms of their coping with the disease. What are some of the psychological aspects of cancer and AIDS that may contribute to those individual differences?

2. How does the developmental perspective of counseling psychology contribute to the survivor perspective that was taken in this chapter?

3. How might group interventions for persons with cancer or AIDS affect the quality of outcomes for persons in those groups?

4. How might you tailor the assessment of coping resources of a person with cancer or AIDS to take into account the unique characteristics of that individual client?

5. How might you use the concept of quality of life in the course of treating patient who is having difficulty coping with advanced disease?

References

Aaronson, N. K., & Beckman, J. (1987). *The quality of life of cancer patients.* Monograph Series of the European Organization for Research on Treatment of Cancer (Vol. 17). New York: Raven Press.

Adams, J., & Merluzzi, V. J. (1993). Discovery of nevirapine, a nonnucleoside inhibitor of HIV-1 reverse transcriptase. In J. Adams, & V. J. Merluzzi (Eds.), *The search for antiviral drugs* (pp. 45–70). Boston: Birkhäuser.

Allebeck, P., & Bolund, C. (1991). Suicides and suicide attempts in cancer patients. *Psychological Medicine, 21,* 979–984.

Andersen, B. L. (1994). Surviving cancer. *Cancer, 74,* 1484–1495.

Antoni, M. (1991). Psychosocial stressors and behavioral interventions in gay men with HIV infection. *International Review of Psychiatry, 3,* 383–399.

Antoni, M., Baggett, H. L., Ironson, G., LaPerriere, A., August, S., Klimas, N., Schneiderman, N., & Fletcher, M. (1991). Cognitive-behavioral stress management intervention buffers distress responses and immunologic changes following notification of HIV-1 seropositivity. *Journal of Consulting and Clinical Psychology, 59,* 906–915.

Antoni, M., Goldstein, D., Gookin, K., Fletcher, M. A., & Schneiderman, N. (1991). Coping responses to HIV-1 serostatus notification predict short and long-term affective distress. *Psychosomatic Medicine, 53,* 227.

Bandura, A. (1986). *Social foundations of thought and action: A social cognitive theory.* New Jersey: Prentice Hall.

Bandura, A. (1991). Social cognitive theory of self-regulation. *Organizational Behavior and Human Decision Processes, 50,* 248–287.

Baron, R. M., & Kenny, D. A. (1986). The moderator-mediator variable distinction in social psychological research: Conceptual, strategic, and statistical considerations. *Journal of Personality and Social Psychology, 55,* 1173–1181.

Barrera, M., Sandler, I. N., & Ramsey, T. B. (1981). Preliminary development of a scale of social support: Studies on college students. *American Journal of Community Psychology, 9,* 435–447.

Bartlett, J. G., & Finkbeiner, A. K. (1996). *The guide to living with HIV infection.* Baltimore: Johns Hopkins.

Bergeman, C. S., Plomin, R., Pedersen, N. L., McClearn, G. E., & Nesselroade, J. R. (1990). Genetic and environmental influences on social support: The Swedish adoption/twin study of aging. Journal of Gerontology: *Psychological Sciences, 45,* 101–106.

Bergner, M., Bobbit, R. A., Carter, W. B., & Gilson, B. S. (1981). The Sickness Impact Profile: Development and final revision of a health status measure. *Medical Care, 19,* 787–805.

Bovbjerg, D. H., Redd, W. H., Maier, L. A., Holland, J. C., Lesko, L. M., Niedzwiecki, D., Rubin, S. C., & Hakes, T. B. (1990). Anticipatory immune suppression and nausea in women receiving cyclic chemotherapy for ovarian cancer. *Journal of Consulting and Clinical Psychology, 58,* 153–157.

Burack, J. H., Barrett, D. C., Stall, R. D., Chesney, M. A., Ekstrand, M. L., & Coates, T. J. (1993). *Journal of the American Medical Association, 270,* 2568–2573.

Burish, T. C., Snyder, S. L., & Jenkins, R. A. (1991). Preparing patients for cancer chemotherapy: Effects of coping preparation and relaxation interventions. *Journal of consulting and Clinical Psychology, 59,* 518–525.

Carver, C. S., Pozo, C., Harris, S. D., Noriega, V., Scheier, M. F., Robinson, D. S., Ketchem, A. S., Moffat, F. L., & Clark, K. C. (1993). How coping mediates the effect of optimism on distress: A study of women with early stage breast cancer. *Journal of Personality and Social Psychology, 65,* 375–390.

Carver, C. S., Scheier, M. F., & Weintraub, J. K. (1989). Assessing coping strategies: A theoretically based approach. *Journal of Personality and Social Psychology, 56,* 267–283.

Cella, D. F. (1995). Methods and problems in measuring quality of life. *Supportive Care in Cancer, 3,* 11–22.

Cella, D. F., McCain, N. L., Peterman, A. H., Mo, F., & Wolen, D. (1996). Development and validation of the Functional Assessment of Human Immunodeficiency virus infection (FAHI) quality of life instrument. *Quality of Life Research, 5,* 450–463.

Cella, D. F., Tulsky, D. S., Gray, G., Sarafin, B., Linn, E., Bonomi, A., Silberman, M., Yellen, S. B., Winicor, P., Brannon, J., Eckberg, K., Lloyd, S., Purl, S., Blendowski, C., Goodman, M., Barnicle, M., Stewart, I., McHale, M., Bonomi, P., Kaplan, E., Taylor, S., Thomas, C., & Harris, J. (1993). The Functional Assessment of Cancer Therapy Scale: Development and validation of the general measure. *Journal of Clinical Oncology, 11,* 570–579.

Cohen, S., Mermelstein, R., Kamarck, T., & Hoberman, H. M. (1985). Measuring the functional components of social support. In I. G. Sarason, & B. R. Sarason (Eds.), *Social support: Theory, research and applications* (pp. 73–94). New York: Martin Nijhoff

Cunningham, A. J., Lockwood, G. A., & Cunningham, J. A. (1991). A relationship between perceived self-efficacy and quality of life in cancer patients. *Patient Education and Counseling, 17,* 71–78.

Daut, R. L., Cleeland, C. S., & Flannery, R. C. (1983). Development of the Wisconsin Brief Pain Questionnaire to assess pain in cancer and other diseases. *Pain, 17,* 197–210.

Derogatis, L. R., & Derogatis, M. F. (1990).*The Psychosocial Adjustment to Illness Scale: Administration, scoring, and procedures manual—II.* Towson, MD: Clinical Psychometric Research.

Devlen, J., Maguire, P., Phillips, P., & Crowther, D. (1987). Prospective study (II). *British Medical Journal, 295,* 955–965.

Dollinger, M., & Rosenbaum, E. H. (1998). *Everyone's guide to cancer therapy.* New York: Andrews & McMeel.

Dunkel-Schetter, C., Feinstein, L. G., Taylor, S. E., & Falke, R. L. (1992). Patterns of coping with cancer. *Health Psychology, 11,* 79–87.

Fawzy, F. I., Fawzy, N. W., Arndt, L. A., & Pasau, R. O. (1995). Critical review of psychosocial interventions in cancer care. *Archives of General Psychiatry, 52,* 100–113.

Fawzy, F. I., Fawzy, N. W., Hyun, C. S., Elashoff, R., Guthrie, D., Fahey, J. L., & Morton, D. (1993). Malignant melanoma: Effects of an early structured psychiatric intervention, coping and affective state on recurrence and survival 6 years later. *Archives of General Psychiatry, 50,* 681–689.

Fernandez, E., & Turk, D. D. (1989). The utility of cognitive coping stratgies for altering perception of pain: A meta-analysis. *Pain, 38,* 123–135.

Folkman, S., & Chesney, M. (1995). Coping with HIV infection. In M. Stein, & A. Baum (Eds.), *Chronic diseases* (pp. 115–133). Mahwah, NJ: Erlbaum.

Gifford, A. L., Loring, K., Laurent, D., & Gonzalez, V. (1996). *Living well with HIV and AIDS.* New York: Bell.

Gilbar, O. (1991). The quality of life of cancer patients who refuse chemotherapy. *Social Science and Medicine, 32,* 1337–1340.

Golden, W. L., Gersh, W. D., & Robbins, D. M. (1992). *Psychological treatment of cancer patients: A Cognitive-behavioral approach.* Needam Heights, MA: Allyn & Bacon.

Gooding, P. R., McAnulty, R. D., Wittrock, D. A., Britt, D. M., & Khansur, T. (1995). Predictors of depression among male cancer patients. *The Journal of Nervous and Mental Disease, 183,* 95–98.

Greico, A., & Long, C. J. (1984). Investigation of the Karnofsky Performance Status as a measure of quality of life. *Health Psychology, 3,* 129–142

Helgeson, V. S., & Cohen, S. (1996). Social support and adjustment to cancer: Reconciling descriptive, correlational, and intervention research. *Health Psychology, 15,* 135–148.

Hirshaut, Y., & Pressman, P. I. (1997). *Breast cancer: The complete guide.* New York: Bantam.

Holland, J. C. (1989). Clinical course of cancer. In J. C. Holland, & J. H. Rowland (Eds.), *The handbook of psychooncology* (pp. 75–100). New York: Oxford University.

Hughes, K. K. (1993). Psychosocial and functional status of breast cancer patients: The influence of diagnosis and treatment choice. *Cancer Nursing, 16,* 222–229.

Ironson, G., Antoni, M., & Lutgendorf, S. (1995). Can psychological interventions affect immunity and survival? Present findings and suggested targets with a focus on cancer and human immunodeficiency virus. *Mind Body Medicine, 1,* 85–110.

Irvine, D., Brown, B., Crooks, D., Roberts, J., & Browne, G. (1991). Psychosocial adjustment in women with breast cancer. *Cancer, 67,* 1117–1991.

Karoly, P. (1985). Measurement strategies in health psychology. New York: Wiley.

Kerns, R., Turk, D. C., & Rudy, T. E. (1985). The West Haven-Yale Multidimensional Pain Inventory (WHYMPI). *Pain, 23,* 345–356.

Kiebert, G. M., Stiggelbout, A. M., Kievit, J., Leer, J.-W. H., van de Veide, & De Haes, H. J. C. J. M. (1994). Choices in oncology: Factors that influence patient's treatment preference. *Quality of Life Research, 3,* 175–182.

Krikorian, R., Kay, J., & Liang, W. M. (1995). Emotional distress, coping, and adjustment in human immunodeficiency virus infection and acquired immune deficiency syndrome. *The Journal of Nervous and Mental Diseases, 183,* 293–298.

Lakey, B., & Cassady, P. B. (1990). Cognitive processes in perceived social support. *Journal of Personality and Social Psychology, 59,* 337–343.

Leserman, J., Perkins, D. O., & Evans, D. L. (1992). Coping with the threat of AIDS: The role of social support. *American Journal of Psychiatry, 149,* 1514–1520.

Levy, S. M., Hayes, L. T., Herberman, R. B., Lee, J., McFeeley, S., & Kirkwood, J. (1992). Mastectomy versus breast conservation surgery: Mental health effects at long-term follow-up. *Health Psychology, 11,* 349–354.

Levy, S. M., Heberman, R. B., Lee, J. K., Lippman, M. E., & d'Angelo, T. (1989). Breast conservation versus mastectomy: Distress sequelae as a function of choice. *Journal of Clinical Oncology, 7,* 367–375.

Litt, M. D. (1988). Self-efficacy and perceived control: Cognitive mediators of pain tolerance. *Journal of Personality and Social Psychology, 54,* 149–160.

Lyketsos, C. G., Hoover, D., Guccione, M., Senterfitt, W., Dew, M. A., Wesch, J., VanRaden, M., Treisman, G., & Morgenstern, H. (1993). Depressive symptoms as predictors of medical outcomes in HIV infection. *Journal of the American Medical Association, 270,* 2563–2567.

Major, B., Cozzarelli, C., Schiacchitano, A. M., Cooper, M. L., Testa, M., & Mueller, P. M. (1990). Perceived social support, self-efficacy, and adjustment to abortion. *Journal of Personality and Social Psychology, 59,* 452–463.

Martinez Sanchez, M. A., & Merluzzi, T. V. (1997). *Perceived and actual support and the mediational role of self-efficacy in adjusting to cancer.* Unpublished manuscript, University of Notre Dame.

Massie, M. J., & Holland, J. C. (1990). Depression and the cancer patient. *Journal of Clinical Psychiatry, 51,* 12–19.

Maunsell, E., Brisson, J., & Deschênes, L. (1992). Psychological distress after initial treatment for breast cancer: A comparison of partial and total mastectomy. *Journal of Clinical Epidemiology, 42,* 765–771.

McCutchan, J. A. (1990). Virology, immunology, and clinical course of HIV infection. *Journal of Consulting and Clinical Psychology, 58,* 5–12.

Melzack, R. (1975). The McGill Pain Questionnaire: Major properties and scoring methods. *Pain, 1,* 277–299.

Melzack, R., & Wall, P. D. (1965). Pain mechanisms: A new theory. *Science, 50,* 971–979.

Merluzzi, T. V., & Martinez Sanchez, M. A. (1994). The mediating effects of self-efficacy on adjustment to cancer. Boston: Society of Behavioral Medicine.

Merluzzi, T. V., & Martinez Sanchez, M. (1997a). Assessment of self-efficacy and coping with cancer: Development and validation of the Cancer Behavior Inventory. *Health Psychology, 16,* 145–155.

Merluzzi, T. V., & Martinez Sanchez, M. (1997b). Perceptions of coping behaviors by persons with cancer and health care providers. *Psycho-Oncology, 6,* 114–121.

Merluzzi, T. V., & Martinez Sanchez, M. A. (1997c). Factor structure of the Psychosocial Adjustment to Illness Scale (Self-Report) for persons with cancer. *Psychological Assessment, 9,* 269–276.

Meyer, T. J., & Mark, M. M. (1995). Effects of psychosocial interventions with adult cancer patients: A meta-analysis of randomized experiments. *Health Psychology, 14,* 101–108.

Morrow, G. R., Asbury, R., Hammon, S., Dobkin, P., Caruso, L., Pandya, K., & Rosenthal, S. (1992). Comparing the effectiveness of behavioral treatment for chemotherapy-induced nausea and vomiting when administered by oncologists, oncology nurses, and clinical psychologists. *Health Psychology, 11,* 250–256.

Namir, S., Wolcott, D. L., Fawzy, F. I., & Alumbaugh, M. J. (1990). Implications of different strategies for coping with AIDS. In L. Temoshok, & A. Baum (Eds.), *Psychosocial perspectives on AIDS* (pp. 173–190). Hillsdale, NJ: Erlbaum.

Nezu, A. M., Nezu, C. M., Faddis, S., Houts, P. S., DelliCarpini, L. A., Pfeiffer, E. J., & Rothenberg, J. L. (1994). *Problem solving and distress among recently diagnosed cancer patients.* San Diego: Association for the Advancement of Behavior Therapy.

Ostrow, D. G., Monjan, A., Joseph, J., VanRaden, M., Fox, R., Kingsley, L., Dudley, J., & Phair, J. P. (1989). HIV-related symptoms and psychological functioning in a cohort of homosexual men. *American Journal of Psychiatry, 146,* 737–742.

Perry, S., Jacobsberg, L. B., Fishman, B., Weiler, P. H., Gold, J. W. M., & Frances, A. J. (1990). Psychological responses to serological testing for HIV. *AIDS, 4,* 145–152.

Reed, G. M., Taylor, S. E., & Kemeny, M. E. (1993). Perceived control and psychologica l adjustment in gay men with AIDS. *Journal of Applied Social Psychology, 23,* 791–824.

Remien, R. H., Rabkin, J. G., Williams, J. B., & Katoff, L. (1992). Coping strategies and health beliefs of AIDS long-term survivors. *Psychology and Health, 6,* 335–345.

Rabkin, J. G., Remien, R., Katoff, L., & Williams, J. B. (1993). Resilience in adversity among long-term survivors of AIDS. *Hospital and Community Psychiatry, 44,* 162–167.

Rose, J. H. (1990). Social support and cancer: Adult patients' desire for support from family, friends, and health professionals. *Journal of Community Psychology, 18,* 439–464.

Rowland, J. H. (1989). Intrapersonal resources: Coping. In J. C. Holland, & J. H. Rowland (Eds.), *The handbook of psychooncology* (pp. 44–57). New York: Oxford University.

Schag, C. A., & Heinrich, R. L. (1988). *Cancer Rehabilitation Evaluation System: Manual.* Los Angeles: CARES Consultants.

Scheier, M. F., & Carver, C. S. (1992). Effects of optimism on psychological and physical well-being: Theoretical overview and empirical update. *Cognitive Therapy and Research, 16,* 201–228.

Scheier, M. F., Carver, C. S., & Bridges, M. W. (1994). Distinguishing optimism from neuroticism (and trait anxiety, self-mastery, and self-esteem): A reevaluation of the life orientation test. *Journal of Personality and Social Psychology, 67,* 1063–1078.

Shilts, R. (1995). *And the band played on.* New York: Penguin.

Spiegel, D. (1991). A psychosocial intervention and survival time of patients with metastatic breast cancer. *Advances, 7,* 10–19.

Spiegel, D., & Bloom, J. R. (1983). Group therapy and hypnosis reduce metastatic breast carcinoma pain. *Psychosomatic Medicine, 45,* 333–339.

Spiegel, D., Bloom, J. R., Kraemer, H. C., & Gottheil, E. (1989). Effect of psychosocial treatment on survival of patients with metastatic breast cancer. *Lancet, 2,* 888–891.

Spiegel, D., & Sands, S. H. (1988). Pain management in the cancer patient. *Journal of Psychosocial Oncology, 6,* 205–216.

Stanton, A. L., & Snider, P. R. (1993). Coping with a breast cancer diagnosis: A prospective study. *Health Psychology, 12,* 16–23.

Syrjala, K. L., & Chapko, M. E. (1995). Evidence for a biopsychosocial model of cancer treatment-related pain. *Pain, 61,* 69–79.

Syrjala, K. L., Cummings, C., & Donaldson, G. (1992). Hypnosis or cognitive behavioral training for the reduction of pain and nausea during cancer treatment: A controlled clinical trial. *Pain, 48,* 137–146.

Syrjala, K. L., & Roth-Roemer, S. (1996). Cancer pain. In J. Barber (Ed.), Hypnosis and suggestion in the treatment of pain: A clinical guide (pp. 121–157). New York: Norton.

Taylor, S. E. (1983). Adjustment to threatening events: A theory of cognitive adaptation. *American Psychologist, 41,* 1161–1173.

Taylor, S. E., & Brown, J. D. (1988). Illusion and well-being: A social psychological perspective on mental health. *Psychological Bulletin, 103,* 193–210.

Telch, C. F., & Telch, M. J. (1986). Group skills instruction and supportive group therapy for cancer patients: A comparison of strategies. *Journal of Consulting and Clinical Psychology, 54,* 802–808.

Ware, J. E. (1984). Conceptualizing disease impact and treatment outcomes. *Cancer, 53,* 2316–2326.

Weitz, R. (1989). Uncertainty and the lives of persons with AIDS. *Journal of Health and Social Behavior, 30,* 270–281.

Zich, J., & Temoshok, L. (1990). Perceptions of social support, distress, and hopelessness in men with AIDS and ARC: Clinical implications. In L. Temoshok, & A. Baum (Eds.), *Psychosocial perspectives on AIDS* (pp. 201–227). Hillsdale, NJ: Erlbaum.

8

Pain Management

Jeffrey L. Okey

Pain is fundamentally a subjective experience and, as such, difficult to objectify and define. Perhaps the best known, most comprehensive, and most widely accepted definition of pain is provided by the International Association for the Study of Pain (IASP), which defines pain as "an unpleasant sensory and emotional experience, associated with actual or potential tissue damage, or described in terms of such damage" (Merskey & Bogduk, 1994). The implications of this definition are vitally important for the mental health professional working in a health care setting. More specifically, the hallmark of this definition is that it implies the importance of both sensory experiences (i.e., medical or physical problems) and emotional experiences (i.e., subjective responses and feelings) in understanding pain. It also allows for the fact that a given experience of pain may be related either to physical damage already done ("actual" damage) or to the fear and/or anticipation of damage that may occur ("potential" damage). It also suggests that while a given experience of pain may be described in terms of tissue damage, such objective, physical damage may not exist. In short, this conceptualization of pain as a subjective experience with both sensory and emotional components suggests that any appropriate assessment and treatment for pain will carefully consider both factors.

Inherent in this definition is both a calling and a warning for the mental health professional practicing in the health care setting. The calling is this: Because pain is a subjective experience with significant emotional components, it is incumbent upon mental health professionals to assert their perspective and skills in understanding and treating patients with pain. The warning is this: Because pain will always have a significant physical or sensory component, or at least reports of such a component, even in what may ultimately turn out to be primarily a psychiatric disorder, close coordination with appropriate medical personnel is vital. The successful mental health professional in the health care setting will be the one who is best able to educate both professionals and patients alike regarding the influence of emotional and psychological factors on pain, while also allowing themselves to learn from and defer to both medical professionals and patients regarding the medical and sensory aspects of pain.

The Problem

The significance of pain as a primary concern and focus of intervention in the health care setting can hardly be overstated. Recent estimates suggest that approximately 30 percent of the population of economically developed countries suffer from chronic pain (Bonica, 1987). Of the 70 million Americans who report chronic pain, more than 50 million are partially or totally disabled for periods ranging from a few days to weeks or months (Fordyce, 1995). Pain as a presenting problem accounts for 80 percent of all physician visits (Gatchel & Turk, 1996), and back pain alone is the second leading symptomatic reason for physician office visits in the United States (Fordyce, 1995). Pain, of course, is not limited to patients with low back problems and is, in fact, often an associated symptom—if not the primary one—with a number of chronic medical problems, including arthritis, cancer, fibromyalgia, headache, mandibular disorders, and myofascial pain syndromes.

Perhaps the most insidious aspect of pain is its ability to precipitate a downward spiral of interconnecting symptoms and problems that may ultimately lead to a fully entrenched "chronic pain syndrome," characterized by sleep disturbance, interpersonal difficulties, symptoms of stress, anxiety, and depression, and functional and/or occupational disability (Sternbach, 1987). The case of Ms. S, a licensed practical nurse, provides an example of this phenomenon. Ms. S, a 37-year-old, single parent of three small children, herniated a spinal disc while moving a patient as a routine part of her duties one year ago. Since that time she has undergone lumbar surgery, which stabilized her spinal condition and alleviated the severe pain radiating into her lower extremity. She now presents with chronic, diffuse pain in the lumbar region, which is exacerbated by any physical activity. She also reports significant sleep disturbance, a number of symptoms of depression and anxiety, and considerable fear that she will continue to deteriorate physically and emotionally and not be able either to care for her children or to return to work. She once again presents to her physician seeking a cure for her pain, which she believes is necessary for her to move forward with her life.

Theories of Pain

Theories of pain have evolved over the years to increasingly consider and incorporate the role of psychological and social factors in the individual's experience and reporting of pain. The biomedical theory of pain, a lasting but fading legacy of Western medicine's assumption of the split between mind and body, asserts that an individual's complaints should result from a specific biological problem or disease state (Turk, 1996). The failure or limitation of this theory, however, is clear in a case such as Ms. S's: Given that her "biological problem" or "disease" has already been "fixed" or "cured," how can one best account for and treat her pain problem?

The first generally accepted attempt to integrate the role of both biological and psychological factors in the understanding of pain was provided by the gate control theory (Melzack & Wall, 1965). This theory of pain states that an individual's experience of pain is dependent upon the amount of pain signal that ultimately makes its way through a series of "gates" in the peripheral and central nervous systems. It further states that there are a number of factors that determine how open or closed these gates are, including psychological factors such as emotional state and cognitive processes. While the gate control theory represented a true paradigm shift in the understanding and treatment of pain, the next evolution is found in the more recent and generally accepted biopsychosocial theory of pain (Turk, 1996).

The biopsychosocial theory holds that the individual's experience and reporting of pain are the result of the complex interplay between biological, psychological, and social factors (Turk, 1996). For example, in the case of Ms. S, the biopsychosocial theory would hold that her pain is best accounted for by the interaction of biological factors (such as her postsurgical lumbar condition, her sleep disturbance, and compromised biochemistry) with psychological factors (such as her beliefs and emotions) and with social factors (such as interpersonal relations, social support, and interaction with a disability/compensation system). The biopsychosocial theory is obviously more comprehensive than either the biomedical or gate control theory alone, is consistent with the IASP definition of pain, and is certainly the generally accepted umbrella under which psychological approaches have emerged and gained favor as an integral, essential part of effective pain management.

As an expert in the psychological understanding and treatment of patients, the mental health practitioner in the pain management setting has the significant opportunity and responsibility to assess and treat the psychosocial components of the biopsychosocial equation. The successful practitioner will variously assume the roles of psychiatric diagnostician, student in medical matters, teacher in psychological matters, patient advocate, consultant, psychotherapist, and team member. The following diagnostic and intervention considerations comprise a basic primer for the mental health practitioner attempting to integrate the biopsychosocial theory into his or her practice.

Diagnosis and Assessment

In order to effectively and ethically diagnose and assess a given patient's pain problem, the mental health clinician will need to operate from a multi-disciplinary perspective and consider physical, psychological, social, and developmental factors. More simply put, the clinician will need to assess the whole person in the greater context of life, not simply his or her pain. In order to accomplish this, the clinician must carefully consider and address the following factors:

1. the nature of the referral
2. medical assessment and diagnosis
3. the individual's developmental history
4. psychiatric diagnosis
5. the patient's subjective experience and treatment goals
6. integrated assessment and treatment planning

Referral Information

The first telling piece of diagnostic information is the nature of the referral itself. For example, if a potential patient has self-referred to a mental health professional for assistance in managing headache or neuromuscular pain because he or she sees it as perhaps stress-related, this may imply good motivation and "buy in" on the patient's part regarding the impact of psychological and emotional factors in the management of pain. It may also imply, however, that the patient has prematurely self-referred and has not yet sought sufficient medical evaluation. Another example may be the patient who is referred either by an attorney or a worker's compensation system for pain management related to low back pain and resulting disability. Such a referral raises the possibility of potential secondary gain factors to be evaluated or at least suggests the clear impact of the social context for the person in pain. Referrals will also often come directly from medical personnel and may greatly vary in terms of their specificity. A physician, for example, may refer a patient for "ten sessions of biofeedback therapy targeting the frontalis musculature for assistance with tension headache pain management" or perhaps, much more generally, for "psychological evaluation and treatment recommendations."

The important factor here is to carefully consider the nature of the referral itself when formulating impressions and recommendations. For example, in reference to the sample referral scenarios noted above: If a patient has not yet sought adequate medical evaluation for his or her pain problem, such a referral must be made. If an attorney or workers' compensation system has made the initial referral, one may wish to conclude (at least until data indicate otherwise) that secondary gain factors are a significant factor in the etiology or maintenance of the pain problem. If a physician has made a referral—general or specific—the mental health clinician will do well to consider any implicit information that can be inferred based upon previous work with that physician (for example, a given physician may only specifically refer patients seen as having potential substance dependence problems). In short, the astute mental health practitioner may begin forming tentative clinical impressions by simply noting the source of the referral itself.

Medical Assessment and Diagnosis

It cannot be stressed strongly enough that any patient being evaluated by a mental health clinician for a pain problem should first have had a complete and comprehensive medical evaluation. Once the clinician is reasonably assured that adequate medical evaluations and procedures have been completed, it is incumbent upon the clinician to review, understand, and appropriately apply the information contained in these medical reports. Herein lies perhaps the biggest challenge for the mental health clinician working in the health care setting—learning medical diagnoses, terminology, procedures, and prognoses at a level sufficient to enable empathy with the patient, communication with medical personnel, and accurate completion of the psychosocial diagnosis and assessment. Here are two specific examples:

1. In order to assess the degree to which a patient's emotional state is contributing to his experience of pain, one must first understand the extent to which his sensory experience is contributing to his experience of pain, that is, just how severe are the objective medical findings in the particular case?
2. In order to assess a patient's educational or informational deficit as regards a given medical diagnosis or procedure, the clinician must be educated in these diagnoses or procedures.

Though some mental health clinicians may have the good fortune of a personal medical background or the benefit of formal medical or behavioral medicine training, the majority of clinicians will need to educate themselves in "real time" in the clinical setting. The best immediate or short-term resource in this regard is to avail oneself of the medical expertise available in the multidisciplinary health care setting. More specifically, the mental health practitioner should identify a respected physician or nurse on the team, ask specific medical questions, or ask more general questions regarding suggested readings or learning opportunities. Not only will the medical personnel involved likely appreciate the interest and offer their expertise, but such questioning may also model and enourage their querying the mental health practitioner regarding psychosocial matters. A longer term, more comprehensive approach to gaining the necessary medical knowledge is to begin an individualized course of study based upon a recognized, standard knowledge base, such as is found in the *Core Curriculum for Professional Education in Pain,* published by the IASP (Fields, 1995). The *Core Curriculum* outlines the basic parameters of medical and psychosocial knowledge regarding pain (including anatomy and physiology, pharmacology, and the role of the various medical specialties in pain treatment) and also cites the seminal references for the information outlined. The curriculum provides an ideal framework for either self-study or for more formalized classroom education or pain management team staff development training.

Developmental History

It is important to take a standard psychological and developmental history so as to understand the patient's current pain in the context of his or her overall life. When taking the history, the clinician will have to answer for him- or herself such questions as:

- What did this patient learn about the meaning of pain, suffering, or disability from his or her family?
- Has the patient experienced any significant traumas or losses—either in childhood or more recently—that may impact upon the current experience of pain?
- Is the current medical problem and/or pain significant either in that it is the patient's first experience of difficulty and loss, or is it the "last straw" in an endless litany of personal medical and family problems?

While practitioners will, of course, develop a clinical interview style or protocol consistent with their individual orientation and personal style, the following questions must somehow be integrated into any comprehensive developmental history:

1. What was your basic family structure during your childhood? Who were your parents or guardians? Natural parents? Any parental divorce or remarriage? Who did you live with? Did you have brothers or sisters? Were you oldest? Youngest?
2. Did you experience any traumas or losses as a child? Were you physically, sexually, and/or emotionally abused? If so, what was the nature and extent of the abuse?
3. Did you or any of your family have any significant health or pain problems? If so, please elaborate.
4. When did you leave home? For what reason? What is your educational and vocational history?
5. What is your adult relationship history? Do you have children? What ages?
6. What is your adult health history?
7. Have you experienced any recent traumas or losses?
8. What is your current living situation? Relationship status? Vocational status?

Psychiatric Diagnosis

As with medical evaluations and reports, it is important to gather and consider available information from previous psychological or psychiatric evaluations or treatments. It is not unusual for patients being referred in the context of the health care setting, however, to have had no prior experiences with mental health practitioners. This may be simply because the patient has not previously perceived the need for such assistance or help, or because he or she is more likely to present with medical rather than emotional difficulties, a fact that is, of course, important in diagnosis and assessment in and of itself.

In most health care settings the mental health clinician will be called upon to form diagnostic impressions in accord with the *Diagnostic and Statistical Manual of Mental Disorders, Fourth Edition* (*DSM-IV*; American Psychiatric Association, 1994). The clinician will, over time, potentially see patients representing the full range of *DSM-IV* disorders. It will be especially important for the clinician to be intimately familiar with the mood, anxiety, somatoform, and adjustment disorders. Pain, particularly when it is in the context of chronic disabling or life-threatening illness, is often a precipitant to episodes of major depression or adjustment disorders, as well as the precipitant to an exacerbation of other mood and anxiety disorders. When physical symptoms are present that suggest a general medical condition (pain being but one symptom example) and yet are not fully explained by a general medical condition present in the patient, then a clinician will need to consider and diagnose one or more of the somatoform disorders.

While a complete review of the somatoform disorders and considerations in differential diagnosis are beyond the scope of this chapter, it is important to note that the *DSM-IV* includes a specific diagnosis called "Pain Disorder," which is considered an Axis I disorder (see table 8.1). This diagnostic classification has two subcategories:

1. pain disorder associated with psychological factors, which is diagnosed when psychological factors are judged to have the major role in the onset, severity, exacerbation, or maintenance of the pain
2. pain disorder associated with both psychological factors and a general medical condition, diagnosed when both psychological factors and a general medical condition are judged to have important roles in the onset, severity, exacerbation, or maintenance of the pain

---

Table 8.1
***DSM-IV* Diagnostic Criteria for Pain Disorder**

A. Pain in one or more anatomical sites is the predominant focus of the clinical presentation and is of sufficient severity to warrant clinical attention.

B. The pain causes clinically significant distress or impairment in social, occupational, or other important areas of functioning.

C. Psychological factors are judged to have an important role in the onset, severity, exacerbation, or maintenance of the pain.

D. The symptom or deficit is not intentionally produced or feigned (as in Factitious Disorder or Malingering).

E. The pain is not better accounted for by a Mood, Anxiety, or Psychotic Disorder and does not meet criteria for Dyspareunia.

From APA, 1994, p. 461.

The importance of these or any other specific diagnoses ultimately depends upon the extent to which they inform prognoses and treatment recommendations, as well as the extent to which they serve the needs within the social context, whether that be for insurance reimbursement or understanding and acceptance within the referring medical community. What is always important, however, is being well versed in the differential diagnoses of the noted disorders and obtaining appropriate training and credentialing prior to making such diagnoses.

Patient's Subjective Experience and Treatment Goals

When a patient is referred for psychological evaluation regarding a pain complaint or for pain management, it is essential to understand the patient's experience of pain as comprehensively as possible. This is difficult because, by definition, pain is fundamentally a subjective experience with no direct, objective measurement possible. It is possible, however, to help the patient express this subjective experience in somewhat objective terms by means of various instruments and/or questions. The simplest gross measure of pain intensity is the Visual Analogue Scale (VAS), wherein the patient is asked to mark the pain level on a 10-point scale, ranging from "no pain" to "worst pain ever" (Melzack & Katz, 1994). While this is useful as a gross screen, it does not describe the specific sensory qualities of the pain, the affective qualities associated with these sensations, or the overall evaluation of the pain experience.

The McGill Pain Questionnaire (MPQ) is designed to elicit this further level of specificity and is a reliable instrument often used as a standard in the health care setting (Melzack & Katz, 1994). The MPQ is a pencil-and-paper instrument that asks the patient to make a total of 20 fine discriminations among descriptions of pain sensations such as among "pulsing" or "throbbing" or "pounding," or among "miserable" or "intense" or "unbearable." The finished protocol provides both a rich qualitative description of the patient's subjective experience and an overall numerical "pain rating index," which allows for quantitative comparison with other patients, as well as with the patient him- or herself over time.

Beyond the MPQ or any other standardized protocol used, however, it is important in one way or another to answer the following questions:

1. Where is the pain located? How is the actual sensation of the pain described? What is the severity, intensity, or duration of the pain?
2. What does the pain mean for the patient, that is, what does it signify or stand for?
3. Is there a relationship between the patient's emotions and his or her pain, that is, do emotions either precipitate or result from the pain?
4. What does the patient currently do to manage the pain?
5. Are there any behavioral contingencies modifying the pain, for example, family responses, workers' compensation system contingencies, etc.?
6. What are the patient's goals regarding management of the pain, for example, to eliminate it completely or just to reduce the most severe pain episodes?

In short, the mental health clinician will want to ask a full range of questions designed to illicit the overall significance of the pain for the patient, both in terms of its role as a cause and as an effect.

Integrated Assessment and Treatment Planning

The final step in the diagnosis and assessment process will be integrating all of the above information and material into a written report, note, or treatment plan that will form the basis of effective communication with both the patient and what is likely to be a multidisciplinary group of health care professionals. Form and content of written reports will obviously depend on the needs and context of the particular setting in which the clinician works, though documentation should at minimum delineate a clear conceptualization of the psychosocial factors perceived as contributing to the patient's pain problem, psychosocial interventions recommended to address these problems, and an anticipated course of treatment and prognosis. All reports and treatment plans should take into consideration the patient's goals and wishes, and delineate specifically where these goals and wishes coincide with the treatment recommendations and where they do not. A final step is for the mental health clinician to take these recommendations and actively, assertively communicate them to all the relevant parties, including the patient, family members, other health care professionals, and any other social agency or institution involved in the patient's care.

A standard, comprehensive consultation report by the mental health practitioner should ideally include appropriately detailed elaboration under the following headings: referral/identifying information; *DSM-IV* diagnoses; developmental/social history; description of pain and patient goals; mental status/psychometric testing; overall clinical impressions; and treatment recommendations. The formality of written documentation will help educate the medical personnel about the relevant psychosocial issues, enable better continuity of care for the patient, and further help the mental health practitioner to plan and prepare the interpersonal clinical interventions he or she will implement directly with the multidisciplinary team and patient.

Intervention

To maximize effectiveness, recommended interventions in pain management should be based as specifically as possible on the results of diagnosis and assessment and should use as wide a range of modalities as possible given the available resources and patient's wishes. The following is a brief review of the therapeutic modalities typically used by mental health clinicians in the health care setting with comments regarding their application.

Individual Counseling and/or Psychotherapy

If a specific psychiatric diagnosis is made during the assessment phase, the mental health professional will certainly want to recommend and offer the standard course of therapy typically associated with the diagnosis. For example, if a patient is experiencing a major depressive disorder in conjunction with the pain problem, depending on the clinician's theoretical frame of reference and the patient's stated desire, the clinician may wish to recommend weekly individual psychotherapy for a period of three to six months concurrent with the appropriate evaluation regarding medical management of the more severe symptoms of depression. Even in cases where no specific psychiatric disorders are present, most patients with significant pain problems or complaints are likely to benefit from a time-limited course of cognitive-behavioral psychological intervention (10 to 15 sessions over a two- to four-month period of time) designed to enhance the patient's coping strategies through a process of education, support, and training in pain coping strategies.

There are a number of cognitive-behavioral protocols or models available designed to address specific pain problems or diagnoses, such as rheumatoid arthritis (Bradley, 1996), cancer (Syrjala & Roth-Roemer, 1997), and low back pain (Hanson & Gerber, 1990). While such protocols vary in the specifics, they all address the four essential components of cognitive-behavioral interventions: education, skills training, cognitive and behavioral rehearsal, and generalization and maintenance (Bradley, 1996). Mental health practitioners in the pain management setting will do well to obtain and implement a relevant protocol and, if necessary, to gradually modify its contents to meet the needs of their patient population.

Relaxation Training and/or Biofeedback Therapy

Relaxation training, a broad concept that incorporates a number of techniques and modalities such as progressive relaxation, hypnosis, imagery, and biofeedback, is well documented as an effective, essential component of any comprehensive approach to pain management (Arena & Blanchard, 1996; Syrjala & Abrams, 1996). Which selected techniques are most effective for a given patient or population is an empirical question, though one for which there are clearly emerging answers. To cite just one example, hypnosis is proving to be an extremely effective tool in cancer pain management (Syrjala & Roth-Roemer, 1996). Biofeedback therapy, which uses physiological instrumentation to provide patients with "real-time" feedback on their state of arousal or relaxation, is also empirically supported as an effective modality for providing relaxation training across a number of techniques and patient populations (Arena & Blanchard, 1996).

Given the established effectiveness of relaxation approaches to pain management, is it incumbent upon mental health practitioners to learn and implement a range of techniques appropriate for their setting. Such relaxation training could be provided in the context of individual or group counseling or could be recommended and provided as a separate treatment modality. As with individual psychotherapy recommendations, the particular course of therapy will depend upon diagnosis, patient motivation, and availability of resources. A time-limited course of relaxation or biofeedback therapy (10 to 12 sessions over a two- to three-month period of time), however, will provide most patients with a solid base of relaxation training and pain management ability.

Couples and/or Family Counseling

Not only does the patient's pain exist in the context of his or her whole life, but it also exists in the context of his or her significant relationships. Whenever and wherever possible, the patient's significant other and extended family or social group should be brought into the treatment plan. Unless familial distress is identified as an independent problem, an extended course of couple or family therapy is not indicated for pain management. It is almost always helpful, however, to include significant others in two or three sessions to provide them with education related to the patient's diagnosis and pain program, support during this difficult time, and strategies whereby they can best help their loved one in pain. For example, the family of a patient with chronic low back pain might benefit from education and counsel regarding the reciprocal nature and effects of their behaviors and responses, that is, the manner in which pain behavior elicits typical family responses, and how these responses may in turn affect the patient's experience and expression of pain (Kerns & Payne, 1996).

Group Support, Education, and/or Counseling

A particularly important and helpful modality for patients with pain, particularly pain related to chronic disease and disability, is group support or counseling (Spiegel & Bloom, 1983). An ideal group would consist of patients with similar diagnoses, thus providing patients with an opportunity to receive education related to the specific medical problem, to benefit from the sense that they are not alone in experiencing this difficulty, and to provide an overall consistent frame of reference, thus enabling a quick establishment of trust and rapport.

Education

Inherent in all of the above modalities is the importance of education: education of patients regarding pain, any underlying disease or disorder, and the available treatment or coping strategies; education of the patient's family regarding these same issues; and education of the other multidisciplinary health care professionals regarding the impact of emotional and social factors on the patient's experience of pain. In short, it is important for mental health professionals to remember that they are likely the most important—if not the only—advocate of the patient in recognizing the importance of these psychosocial factors in regard to pain. In addition, they should see it as their mission to educate all relevant parties in regard to these issues. Specific educational interventions for patients include providing them with relevant literature, implementing specific cognitive-behavioral protocols, and offering detailed information on an individual basis regarding diagnostic and treatment issues. Educational interventions for interdisciplinary staff members may include sharing relevant professional literature and offering to conduct staff development seminars regarding the psychosocial aspects of pain and pain management.

Strategic, Comprehensive Intervention

Finally, when developing and implementing a treatment plan, the clinician must strive to make it as comprehensive, multimodal, and strategic as possible. While any of the noted interventions may be significantly valuable in and of themselves, their value multiplies exponentially when provided in combination by a coordinated, multidisciplinary treatment team. For example, if the patient has the motivation and available resources to participate in a comprehensive multidisciplinary pain management program, he or she may simultaneously be provided with individual psychotherapy, individual relaxation and/or biofeedback training, psychoeducational and psychotherapeutic groups, as well as family conferencing and meetings. All of these occur in the context of a medical environment with appropriate physician management and physical and occupational therapy modalities. While the ability to offer such a comprehensive treatment program obviously depends on a number of personal and social factors, approaching pain management from such a multimodal perspective can significantly enhance treatment efficacy (Feuerstein & Zastowny, 1996).

Controversies

The importance of emotional and psychological factors in pain management has become increasingly accepted in both professional and lay circles. Perhaps most symbolically evidencing the public's acceptance of the mind-body connection was Bill Moyers's 1993 Public Television series and companion book, *Healing and the Mind,* wherein portraits were drawn of a number of mental health professionals working in the health care setting, particularly in the field of pain management. Still, there remains some controversy regarding the extent to which the role of emotions and psychological factors in precipitating and managing pain should be considered. As Spiegel (1995) points out in *Living Beyond Limits,* there is a danger in attributing too much significance to the role of psychological factors. He notes that this idea—that if one could be perfectly in tune with his or her emotions and properly meditate upon the correct images, that one could either prevent pain or cure even the most significant diseases such as cancer—is pure fallacy. Calling this fallacy the "prison of positive thinking," he warns that such an extreme view may well be just as inaccurate and potentially damaging as the earlier view that emotions and psychological factors had no significant role in disease or pain processes. To what extent psychological intervention can ultimately improve one's management of pain remains an experiential and empirical question.

Other controversies in the field of pain management reflect the controversies in psychology as a whole. Issues relating to philosophical and theoretical orientation of the practitioner are always controversial and certainly affect every aspect of the clinician's professional identity and role. For example, is there a place for a psychodynamically informed or trained practitioner in the pain management setting (Grzesiak, Ury, & Dworkin, 1996)? If so, how does one integrate such a longer-term, depth-oriented psychotherapeutic approach with the pain management setting's proclivity for shorter-term interventions and techniques? Every controversy that exists in the greater field of psychology exists for the mental health practitioner in the pain management setting, but is further complicated by the social context and demands of that setting.

An additional controversial issue in the field of pain management regards what constitutes adequate training to claim expertise in this field. As a result of the relatively recent acceptance and proliferation of mental health practitioners in the arena of pain management, many current clinicians have garnered their expertise through "on the job training," attending relevant workshops, and/or personal reading of the professional and popular literature. As the field becomes more formalized, more training programs and postgraduate training fellowships in pain management are being offered and such training will likely become the standard of training necessary for legal credentialing and ethical functioning. During this growth phase in the field of pain management, it will be especially important for mental health practitioners to reflect upon their level of expertise and confidence and to restrict their practice within this realm in accord with the relevant ethical and legal guidelines.

A final crucial controversy for the clinician working as a pain management specialist in the health care setting is how to maintain appropriate patient confidentiality while also giving other members of the multidisciplinary professional team—as well as insurance providers, for that matter—the information necessary to provide appropriate treatment. There are no easy answers here, and an in-depth exploration of the issues involved would constitute a book in its own right. Suffice it to say that perhaps more often than in other settings there is a conflict between the patient's right to confidentiality and the needs of others to know pertinent information. Clinicians need to become intimately aware of the relevant ethical and legal guidelines related to their profession and jurisdiction, to reflect upon their personal stance on these matters, and to proactively formulate a method or protocol by which they will handle difficult decisions in this area.

Summary

As the significance of psychological and social factors in the experience and reporting of pain has become more accepted, the mental health clinician has become an integral part of the multidisciplinary professional team in the pain management setting. By nature of their training and orientation, mental health practitioners are in a unique position to be an integrative voice on such multidisciplinary teams and to take on an important role as patient advocates. There are a wide range of psychological interventions available that have proven effective in helping many patients manage their pain and improve their function. While mental health practitioners from a wide range of philosophical and theoretical orientations can successfully work in the field of pain management, it is important that clinicians garner the necessary training, education, and experience in terms of medical understanding, relaxation training, and multidisciplinary team functioning so as to work effectively in the pain management setting.

Suggested Resources

Gatchel and Turk (1996) provide a comprehensive overview of both pain management theory and practice; *Psychological Approaches to Pain Management* is likely the single best resource available. This volume reviews in detail the theories of pain highlighted in this chapter and all of the major treatment approaches. It also addresses issues applicable to special populations, such as children, the elderly, and injured workers.

Books targeted most specifically for patients with pain are also excellent resources for the clinician just entering the field, both in terms of providing basic familiarity with pain management approaches and in providing clinically useful techniques or exercises. Two particularly excellent examples are *The Chronic Pain Control Workbook* (Catalano & Hardin, 1996) and *Mastering Pain* (Sternbach, 1987).

Core Curriculum for Professional Education in Pain (Fields, 1995) provides an excellent outline and reference list for the clinician invested in pursuing an expert level of study in the field of pain management.

Pain management clinicians should also continue to study, practice, and integrate a range of relaxation techniques. *Relaxation Dynamics* (Smith, 1985) offers a good overview of a wide range of techniques, including progressive relaxation, hypnosis, imagery, and meditation. *Full Catastrophe Living* (Kabat-Zinn, 1990) is a popular, modern "classic" on incorporating meditative approaches to pain management in the medical setting.

In addition, the serious student of pain management would do well to contact and consider membership in the International Association for the Study of Pain (IASP), a dynamic, multidisciplinary, professional organization that emphasizes advocacy for and education in pain management. The address for the IASP is: 909 NE 43rd Street, Suite 306, Seattle, WA, 98105.

Discussion Questions

1. Why is pain considered a subjective experience? Why is it difficult to objectify and define?
2. Why is the role of the mental health clinician so integral to effective pain management treatment?
3. What additional training should the mental health clinician seek in order to work in the area of pain management?
4. Why are multidisciplinary, multimodal treatment approaches particularly important in pain management?

References

American Psychiatric Association (1994). *Diagnostic and statistical manual of mental disorders* (4th ed.). Washington, DC: Author.

Arena, J. G., & Blanchard, E. B. (1996). Biofeedback and relaxation therapy for chronic pain disorders. In R. J. Gatchell, & D. C. Turk (Eds.), *Psychological approaches to pain management* (pp. 179–230). New York: Guilford.

Bonica, J. J. (1987). Importance of the problem. In S. Andersson, M. Bond, M. Mehta, & M. Swerdlow (Eds.), *Chronic non-cancer pain* (p. 13). Lancaster, UK: MTP.

Bradley, L. A. (1996). Cognitive-behavioral therapy for chronic pain. In R. J. Gatchell, & D. C. Turk (Eds.), *Psychological approaches to pain management* (pp. 131–147). New York: Guilford.

Catalano, E. M., & Hardin, K. N. (1996). *The chronic pain control workbook* (2nd ed.). Oakland, CA: New Harbinger.

Feuerstein, M., & Zastowny, T. R. (1996). Occupational rehabilitation: Multidisciplinary management of work-related musculoskeletal pain and disability. In R. J. Gatchell, & D. C. Turk (Eds.), *Psychological approaches to pain management* (pp. 458–485). New York: Guilford.

Fields, H. L. (Ed.). (1995). *Core curriculum for professional education in pain* (2nd ed.). Seattle, WA: IASP.

Fordyce, W. E. (Ed.). (1995). *Back pain in the workplace: Management of disability in nonspecific conditions.* Seattle, WA: IASP.

Gatchel, R. J., & Turk, D. C. (Eds.). (1996). *Psychological approaches to pain management.* New York: Guilford.

Grzesiak, R. C., Ury, G. M., & Dworkin, R. H. (1996). Psychodynamic psychotherapy with chronic pain patients. In R. J. Gatchell, & D. C. Turk (Eds.), *Psychological approaches to pain management* (pp. 148–178). New York: Guilford.

Hanson, R. W., & Gerber, K. E. (1990). *Coping with chronic pain: A guide to patient self-management.* New York: Guilford.

Kabat-Zinn, J. (1990). *Full catastrophe living.* New York: Delta.

Kerns, R. D., & Payne, A. (1996). Treating families of chronic pain patients. In R. J. Gatchell, & D. C. Turk (Eds.), *Psychological approaches to pain management* (pp. 283–304). New York: Guilford.

Melzack, R., & Katz, J. (1994). Pain measurement in persons in pain. In P. D. Wall, & R. Melzack (Eds.), *Textbook of pain* (3rd ed.) (pp. 337–351). London: Churchill Livingstone.

Melzack, R., & Wall P. D. (1965). Pain mechanisms: A new theory. *Science, 50,* 971–979.

Merskey, H., & Bogduk, N. (Eds.). (1994). *Classification of chronic pain* (2nd ed.). Seattle, WA: IASP.

Moyers, B. (1993). *Healing and the mind.* New York: Doubleday.

Smith, J. C. (1985). *Relaxation dynamics.* Champaign, IL: Research.

Spiegel, D. (1995). *Living beyond limits.* New York: Times Books.

Spiegel, D., & Bloom, J. R. (1983). Group therapy and hypnosis reduce metastatic breast carcinoma pain. *Psychosomatic Medicine, 45,* 333–339.

Sternbach, R. A. (1987). *Mastering pain.* New York: Ballantine.

Syrjala, K. L., & Abrams, J. R. (1996). Hypnosis and imagery in the treatment of pain. In R. J. Gatchell, & D. C. Turk (Eds.), *Psychological approaches to pain management* (pp. 231–258). New York: Guilford.

Syrjala, K. L., & Roth-Roemer, S. L. (1996). Hypnosis and suggestion for managing cancer pain. In J. Barber (Ed.), *Hypnosis and suggestion in the treatment of pain* (pp. 121–157). New York: Norton.

Syrjala, K. L., & Roth-Roemer, S. L. (1997). Non-pharmacologic approaches to pain. In A. Berger, R. K. Portenoy, & D. E. Weissman (Eds.), *Principles and practice of supportive oncology.* Philadelphia: Lippincott.

Turk, D. C. (1996). Biopsychosocial perspective on chronic pain. In R. J. Gatchell & D. C. Turk (Eds.), *Psychological approaches to pain management* (pp. 3–32). New York: Guilford.

9
Rehabilitation Medicine

Kathleen Chwalisz

Rehabilitation medicine is one of the fastest growing health care areas, and it appears to be an area in which psychologists can achieve parity with physicians, while meeting a unique and specific need (Frank, Gluck, & Buckelew, 1990). Although 21 percent of psychologists working in certified rehabilitation settings are counseling psychologists (Parker & Chan, 1990), this area has received relatively little attention in the counseling psychology literature. In contrast, 60 percent are clinical psychologists, who primarily identify themselves as neuropsychologists, so they appear to be engaged in very different activities from what one might expect from a counseling psychologist. There is a significant niche for counseling psychologists in rehabilitation settings that has not been fully realized.

Rehabilitation Psychology

Rehabilitation psychology is a discipline that "applies psychological knowledge and behavioral science to any and all aspects of physical disability at the individual, group, and systems level" (Grzesiak, 1981, p. 413). This chapter focuses on physical medical rehabilitation, although there are a wide variety of other rehabilitation settings and activities (e.g., substance abuse rehabilitation, psychiatric rehabilitation, rehabilitation of learning disabilities). Rehabilitation in a medical setting is prototypical of traditional philosophies and techniques used by mental health professionals in rehabilitation.

The Rehabilitation Setting

One of the distinguishing aspects of the rehabilitation setting is the patient population. Patients in rehabilitation

- have suffered "dramatic and catastrophic violation of their physical integrity" (Gold, Meltzer, & Sherr, 1987, p. 279),
- enter the rehabilitation setting hoping for a full recovery,
- view the primary problem to be a physical one,
- are active agents in their treatment, and
- may experience dramatic physical improvements during the initial stages of rehabilitation (Stutts, 1991).

Therefore, the counseling psychologist may have a more peripheral role in the early stages of rehabilitation.

A recent Uniform Data System report on 108 hospitals (Granger & Hamilton, 1992) showed that the largest proportion of inpatient rehabilitation patients have suffered strokes (33 percent) and patients have primarily been diagnosed with orthopedic disorders (29 percent), brain injuries (8 percent), spinal cord injuries (5 percent), and neurological disorders (5 percent). The average age of inpatient rehabilitation patients is 67 years, but ages range from late adolescence through the very elderly.

A given patient's presentation depends on such factors as:

- the nature of the illness or injury
- the circumstances surrounding the disability
- the developmental life stage in which the loss occurred
- the personal and social resources available to the patient

Common to all patients, however, is the task of adjusting to losses of a nature and degree not previously experienced. Psychotherapy helps patients to assimilate those losses (Stutts, 1991).

Several other features distinguish the rehabilitation setting.

1. Given that the ultimate goal is to return the patient to his or her home or community, the family unit is actually the "patient" in a rehabilitation situation (Stutts, 1991).
2. Rehabilitation intervention is typically conducted by multidisciplinary teams, which include a physiatrist (i.e., a physician specializing in rehabilitation medicine), a psychologist or other mental health professional, a social worker specializing in case management, a physical

therapist, an occupational therapist, a speech pathologist, and one or more rehabilitation nurses.

3. The Americans with Disabilities Act (ADA) has begun to shape the very nature of practice in this area, shifting the focus of rehabilitation efforts from changing the person with the disability to match the perceived demands of the workplace to changing the workplace to meet the person's needs (Bell, 1993).

Diagnosis and Assessment

The predominant psychological issues among rehabilitation patients are feelings of depression, isolation, and loneliness. These problems are typically related to situational or environmental factors (e.g., loss of independent status, lack of mobility, inaccessible living conditions), rather than preexisting psychological problems (Gold et al., 1987). Therefore, a more pressing need in rehabilitation is for the psychologist to reach a functional understanding of the patient's impairments, rather than consider a diagnosis of mental illness. Any diagnosis should lead directly to rehabilitation goals, with problems analyzed from a competence perspective. Competencies may be linked to psychological consequences, such that symptoms disappear when competence is gained (McFall, 1993). Assessment, including neuropsychological assessment, should include an assessment of everyday functioning (Faust, 1993). In writing assessment reports, it is desirable to use functional descriptions rather than categorizing or stigmatizing the individual with a diagnosis (Sachs & Redd, 1993).

Vocational concerns are a frequent presenting problem, and rehabilitation mental health professionals are often called upon to conduct vocational assessment, provide vocational counseling, and assist patients in being integrated into the workplace (e.g., Bond & Dietzen, 1993; Sachs & Redd, 1993).

In rehabilitation settings, not only do psychologists assess individual patients, but they also assess rehabilitators, training, services, outcomes, environments, and patient preferences (Sechrest, 1993). Although a variety of approaches are used to accomplish these various assessment goals, the most frequently used assessment tools are geared toward individual assessment.

Assessment Instruments

Bolton and Brookings (1993) summarized and critiqued eight categories of commonly used assessment tools (see table 9.1).*

Table 9.1
Categories of Assessment Instruments Used in Rehabilitation

Category of Instruments	Examples
1. Vocational assessment instruments	Functional Assessment Inventory Preliminary Diagnostic Questionnaire Minnesota Importance Questionnaire United States Employment Service Interest Inventory
2. Work behavior rating scales	Becker Work Adjustment Profile Work Personality Profile Work Adjustment Rating Form

3. Independent living scales	Rehabilitation Indicators
	Social and Prevocational
	  Information Battery
	National Independent Living Skills
	  Assessment Instruments

4. Psychosocial assessment instruments	MMPI-2 16PF (Form E) Acceptance of Disability Scale
5. Tests of intellectual abilities	Hiskey-Nebraska Test of Learning Ability WAIS-R GATB
6. Rehabilitation outcome measures	Minnesota Satisfactoriness Scales Levels of Cognitive Function Scale Service Outcome Measurement Form
7. Attitude toward disability scales	Disability Factor Scales–General Attitudes Toward Disabled Persons Scale
8. Work sample systems	Valpar Work Sample Series TOWER System

---

*For a more extensive review of rehabilitation assessment instruments, there are a number of detailed volumes available, for example, Bolton, 1988; Fuhrer, 1987; Halpern & Fuhrer, 1984.

1. *Vocational assessment instruments* measure work-relevant attitudes, behaviors, values, and preferences and appear to serve two purposes in rehabilitation. The first is employability; that is, to what extent can the individual return to the workforce? The Functional Assessment Inventory (Crewe & Athelstan, 1984) focuses on vocationally relevant behaviors and capabilities, and is particularly useful with elderly persons. The Preliminary Diagnostic Questionnaire (PDQ; Moriarty, 1981), a more broadly useful employability measure, taps four functional domains: cognitive, motivation or disposition to work, physical, and emotional.

The second purpose is to help patients make vocational choices in the event that a disability results in a change of job or career. The Minnesota Importance Questionnaire (Gay, Weiss, Hendel, Dawis, & Lofquist, 1971), used to assess work-related values, and the United States Employment Service Interest Inventory (USES-II; U.S. Department of Labor, 1982a), used to assess vocational interests, are commonly used and well-validated in rehabilitation. The USES-II was designed to be used with the General Aptitude Test Battery (U.S. Department of Labor, 1982b), the most thoroughly occupationally validated multiaptitude test available (Bolton & Brookings, 1993).

2. *Work behavior rating scales* are used to observe patients in a real or simulated work setting. The Becker Work Adjustment Profile (BWAP; Becker, 1989) assesses work habits/attitudes, interpersonal relations, cognitive skills, and work performance skills to identify deficits in a patient's work behavior that may become goals for vocational training. The Work Personality Profile (WPP; Bolton & Roessler, 1986) has well-established reliability and validity with rehabilitation populations and has been widely used, particularly in psychiatric rehabilitation. Work behavior rating scales are used for the primary purpose of identifying work-related deficits that may be remediated. These measures differ somewhat in terms of the types of behaviors and skills they tap, so psychologists may choose a particular measure based on previous information or hypotheses about a particular patient's skills.

3. *Independent living scales* assess functioning in activities of daily living (e.g., self-help, mobility, communication). The Rehabilitation Indicators (Brown, Diller, Fordyce, Jacobs, & Gordon, 1980) include status indicators (i.e., statuses or roles crucial to the client's functioning), activity pattern indicators (i.e., daily living activities described in terms of frequency, duration, social interaction, and assistance need), and skill indicators (i.e., behav-

ioral tools needed by the client to attain rehabilitation goals). The Social and Prevocational Information Battery (SPIB; Halpern, Irwin, & Mundres, 1986), the independent living scale most extensively investigated, was designed to assess the social and prevocational knowledge of persons with developmental disabilities.

4. *Psychosocial assessment instruments* measure traits, needs, motives, and adjustment to disability. Standard clinical personality assessment instruments, such as the MMPI-2 (Hathaway & McKinley, 1989), may be used in some cases. It is important to remember, however, that rehabilitation assessment is not conducted solely for the purpose of diagnosis; it must lead to rehabilitation goals. A more commonly used personality instrument in rehabilitation is the Sixteen Personality Factor Questionnaire-Form E (16PF-E; Institute for Personality and Ability Testing, 1985). Bolton and Brookings (1993) noted that the 16PF has been used in at least 20 studies of personality traits associated with disability, and psychometric studies of the 16PF-E have established reliability and validity for use with rehabilitation clients.

Psychosocial assessment has focused primarily on acceptance of disability. The Acceptance of Disability Scale (ADS; Linkowski, 1987) has been widely used in studies of persons with a range of disabilities. For example, greater pain severity was reported by persons with spinal cord injuries who were less accepting of their disability (Summers, Rapoff, Varghese, Porter, & Palmer, 1991).

5. *Tests of intellectual abilities* include those developed for use with persons with disabilities as well as more commonly used intelligence tests. The Hiskey-Nebraska Test of Learning Ability (Hiskey, 1966) was developed for use with individuals with severe hearing impairment. The Wechsler Adult Intelligence Scale-Revised (WAIS-R; Wechsler, 1981) and the General Aptitude Test Battery (GATB; U.S. Department of Labor, 1982b) can be used with the more general rehabilitation population, and the GATB is linked to other U.S. Department of Labor occupational exploration materials.

6. *Rehabilitation outcome measures* evaluate patient outcomes as a result of participating in rehabilitation services. The Minnesota Satisfactoriness Scale (MSS; Gibson, Weiss, Dawis, & Lofquist, 1970) can be completed in about five minutes and yields scores on four subscales—performance, conformance, personal adjustment, and dependability. The Service Outcome Measurement Form (SOMF; Westerheide, Lenhart, & Miller, 1975) assesses case difficulty, economic/vocational issues, physical functioning, adjust-

ment to disability, and social competency. As with other functional measures, outcome measures are available to tap different domains, and the psychologist will need to be aware of which instruments best tap the domains of interest for a particular rehabilitation client.

7. *Attitudes toward people with disability scales* measure attitudes toward others and how individuals might be expected to react to their own disability. Antonak and Livneh (1988) reviewed 22 of these scales; the most widely used are the Disability Factor Scales-General (DFS-G; Siller, 1969) and the Attitudes Toward Disabled Persons Scale (ATDPS; Yuker, Block, & Young, 1970). The DFS-G is designed to assess seven components of attitudes toward people with physical disabilities with items that express reactions, describe assumed attributes, and advocate policies toward people with nine types of disabling conditions such as facial scars, paralysis, cancer, and deafness (Bolton & Brookings, 1993). Attitude instruments are generally used for research purposes; clinical applications of such scales appear to be focused on item content (Bolton & Brookings, 1993). For example, responses to particular items might be used to make clinical decisions.

8. *Work sample systems* are standardized procedures for assessing vocational aptitudes and skills via work samples. Botterbusch (1987) reviewed and evaluated 21 commercial work sample systems. The Valpar Work Sample Series (Valpar Corporation, 1986) is the most extensively studied work sample system. The series consists of 19 standardized work samples, representing worker characteristics from the Dictionary of Occupational Titles (DOT; e.g., clerical comprehension and aptitude, simulated assembly work, whole body range of motion). Work samples are used to assess patients for particular functional limitations which might prohibit them from performing all aspects of a job, and most systems provide references that link results in some way to specific job-related information (e.g., DOT).

Rehabilitation assessment has been criticized as having limited validity and clinical utility. McFall (1993) questioned the constructs on which many rehabilitation assessment instruments are based. Although predictive validity has been suggested as the criterion for evaluating these instruments, commonly used vocational assessment approaches have been questioned with respect to their ability to sufficiently predict outcomes for persons with disabilities (Bond & Dietzen, 1993). Rehabilitation assessment instruments have also been criticized for not meeting the scientific standards for utility in clinical practice, which require that instruments: (a) provide an adequate description of target behaviors, (b) propose an explanation of factors that influence or control the behaviors of interest, (c) correlate with external criteria relevant to the behaviors of interest, and (d) lead to a specific treatment plan (Glueckauf, 1993).

Assessment and the Americans with Disabilities Act

The ADA has significant implications for rehabilitation assessment, as it prohibits the use of selection assessment criteria that screen out persons with disabilities unless these criteria are shown to be job-related and consistent with business necessity. Current testing practices with persons with disabilities for employment and postsecondary school admission do not fully comply with antidiscrimination regulations (Nester, 1993). Validity issues are related to the nonstandard procedures that are often used (e.g., changes to test medium, time limits, test content). Further, mental health professionals in rehabilitation settings are also cautioned about labeling test results as involving nonstandard procedures, because this may alert employers regarding an applicant's disability status (Nester, 1993).

Interventions

The "rehabilitation psychologist's prime concern is to ensure that proper psychosocial conditions exist for positive interaction among all persons involved in the continuing rehabilitation effort" with the goal of enhancing individual development (Eisenberg & Jansen, 1983, p. 5). This broad statement illustrates the wide variety of interventions and "clients" the mental health professional encounters in a rehabilitation setting. The rehabilitation psychologist works with individual patients, family members, rehabilitation team members, programs, administrators, third-party payers, and employers.

Patients

There are more than 130 different therapeutic approaches available to mental health professionals (Eisenberg & Jansen, 1983). Two additional therapeutic approaches in rehabilitation are group therapy for persons with similar disabilities and role playing, which allows patients to practice behaviors in a controlled setting. Biofeedback is most often used for muscle retraining, eliminating tension and migraine headaches, lowering blood pressure, reducing seizure activity, and treating stress-related difficulties. Hypnosis has been applied to pain management, psychosomatic illness, major neurotic disturbances, psychophysiologic correlates of neurological diseases, and addictive processes involved in obesity, smoking, and drug and alcohol dependency (Eisenberg & Jansen, 1983). Other common therapeutic interventions include role modeling, behavioral rehearsal, assertiveness training, and systematic desensitization (Ince, 1981).

Whereas intervention strategies are universal, the model from which rehabilitation psychologists operate is unique. Hershenson (1990) distinguished rehabilitation activities in terms of primary, secondary, and tertiary prevention. Rehabilitation professionals operate in the realm of tertiary prevention, which involves "preventing long-term residual conditions from having any greater disabling effects than necessary, once the secondary prevention fields have done all they can to cure or limit the disease/disabling process" (Hershenson, 1990, p. 170).

At the primary prevention level (i.e., preventing the onset), Jarvikoski and Lahelma (1981) designed a workplace intervention for early identification and intervention with persons likely to be disabled from work. Clients were either self-referred or identified by numbers of sick days taken. A network of contact people in different work units provided support and information about the program, a rehabilitation team provided assessment and interventions (e.g., counseling and instructions, group rehabilitation training, medical treatment, ergonomic changes), and a labor protection committee oversaw the progress of the program. Although this is a promising area for rehabilitation, evaluation data were not presented, and not much literature in this area has appeared since. It appears that primary prevention is still not accepted as the realm of rehabilitation.

Therapeutic activities depend on the area affected by the disability. For example, if the patient's assets and skills are affected, the psychologist's role is to coordinate programs designed to restore or replace these, such as physical therapy to restore muscle tone after an injury. Rehabilitation psychologists provide counseling if the goal is to reintegrate self-image or reformulate goals, and they would be involved in consultation if there is a need to restructure the individual's work or home environment (Hershenson, 1990).

Much of the literature on intervention has focused on helping patients adapt to their disability. In fact, a plethora of stage models of adaptation exist (see Livneh, 1986, for a review). Livneh and Sherwood (1991) attempted to identify specific intervention strategies and criteria for change as they applied to different stages of adaptation from eight common psychotherapy theories (e.g., person-centered, gestalt, behavioral).

An example of an intervention occurring after an individual has completely adapted to his or her disability is Thompson and Hutto's (1992) employment counseling model for college students with disabilities. This program addresses problems of higher unemployment rates and longer job search time for college graduates with disabilities; it includes individual counseling, role-played mock interviews, training in disability reduction techniques for impression management, preparation of resumes and cover letters focusing on skills and abilities, and student work-related activities. Programs addressing issues that go beyond the traditional rehabilitation setting are an exciting new direction for rehabilitation intervention.

Family Members

Most patients hope to return home upon completion of the rehabilitation program; therefore, a patient's physical impairment or disability becomes a family affair. Family members experience a wide variety of emotional reactions to the disability and often have unrealistic expectations regarding the patient's recovery during the early stages of the rehabilitation process (Lezak, 1986). They often lack information regarding the patient's illness or injury and may not understand the process in which they find themselves, making them reluctant to completely trust the rehabilitation staff (Barry & O'Leary, 1989). While all family members may experience some role changes, spouses, who most often become the primary caregiver, are likely to experience the most stress. Finally, family interactions may be negatively altered as a result of a member's disability, or premorbid unhealthy interactions may interfere with the patient's rehabilitation. The rehabilitation psychologist may act as an intermediary between the team and the family, provide psychotherapy for individual family members, provide family therapy, or provide support groups for family caregivers of persons with similar disabilities. Therefore, rehabilitation psychologists must have an understanding of family systems and systems theory.

Seventy-three-year-old Mr. P suffered a stroke that left him paralyzed on the right side, wheelchair-bound, and no longer able to run his business. His wife was not present much of the time during his hospitalization, and the rehabilitation team did not have much information about her. As the team psychologist, I was working individually with Mr. P regarding his adjustment to the changes in his life and plans for when he returned home. I began receiving calls from the couple's three adult children, who were living in different parts of the state, expressing concerns regarding their father's care.

It turned out that Mr. and Mrs. P had been "living separate lives" in the same home for a number of years before the stroke. Mrs. P, upon interview, had no intention of being caregiver for her husband, and we spent a few sessions discussing her feelings of guilt and resentment regarding this ascribed role. The children expressed resentment toward both parents, and none was interested in caregiving. A family session was held so that members could voice the feelings and concerns that each had discussed with me individually, and the family mutually made decisions regarding Mr. P's care.

The family dynamics were a critical aspect of this case and significantly influenced the functioning of the rehabilitation team. First, most team members had assumed that Mrs. P would be an active caregiver. The knowledge I provided about the family dynamics resulted in several treatment plan changes. For example, the social worker arranged for more in-home health care services than usual. Mrs. P also experienced some negative reactions and comments from the physiatry resident on the team (whose own mother was a caregiver). I found it necessary to intervene with him on several occasions when he was making disparaging comments to her or about her in the team meetings. Clearly, working with the family and understanding their dynamics was key to the successful rehabilitation plan for this patient.

The Rehabilitation Team

The rehabilitation process appears to be more effective when it occurs in the context of an interdisciplinary team, involving a problem- or function-focused interactive process among professionals of different disciplines (Barry & O'Leary, 1989). A multidisciplinary team, in which team members of different disciplines contribute to the care of the patient individually but maintain professional boundaries, appears to be somewhat less effective. These two team approaches can be contrasted with the transdisciplinary approach, characterized by "role release," in which all team members share disciplinary responsibilities (Woodruff & McGonigel, 1988).

Sensitivity to the rehabilitation team's dynamics and skill in facilitating interactions among team members are important aspects of the psychologist's role on the rehabilitation team. In addition, the psychologist might follow the research literature on team effectiveness and suggest new approaches to the team. The psychologist on a rehabilitation team may also find him- or herself attending to issues of patient confidentiality among team members, helping team members determine which aspects of the information shared with them are relevant to treatment outcomes.

Programs

Psychologists' research training generally puts them in a unique position among rehabilitation team members to develop and implement program evaluation research (Barry & O'Leary, 1989). Accountability and cost containment are forces behind increased program evaluation efforts in both inpatient and outpatient rehabilitation programs. Psychologists in rehabilitation may be asked to identify program goals, identify or create measures to assess the extent to which goals are attained, collect and manage data, and communicate program evaluation results. Glueckauf (1993) suggested that evaluation research should be developed with the assistance of a consultation network of well-informed consumers and key staff. The psychologist engaged in a program evaluation task may find it useful to think of this different team role as that of a consultant, clarifying expectations, questions of confidentiality, and who the "client" is when the evaluation is initiated by parties external to the team.

Administrators and Third-Party Payers

Rehabilitation and other health care programs are increasingly being run by people with business backgrounds rather than clinical backgrounds (Leri, 1995). When a patient is admitted to an inpatient program, the rehabilitation team needs to be able to accurately estimate the expected length of stay, total charges for the program, and expected functional independence to be achieved. After the patient's completion of the program, the program needs to document to what extent goals were met and how efficiently program resources were used (Carey, 1990).

Rehabilitation staff are now more actively involved in gathering marketing and accountability data for administrators, accrediting bodies, and third-party payers. At the same time, business-oriented administrators may not have any significant understanding of patient needs, the treatment processes, or the stresses associated with clinical work. Thus, the experiences of health-care professionals with managed care have often been unpleasant and frustrating (Leri, 1995). Rehabilitation professionals must be prepared to deal with changes due to administrative or third-party payer initiatives such as cost-cutting measures that limit services or issues of confidentiality or professional autonomy in communicating with payers' case managers.

Employers

The ADA has created a number of opportunities for psychologists in rehabilitation. Rehabilitation psychologists are in an excellent position to educate employees and employers in developing ADA-mandated accommodation solutions (Sachs & Redd, 1993). In fact, a new practice area, ADA consultation, has grown out of this important legislation. An ADA consultant will (Pape & Tarvydas, 1993):

- analyze the suitability of an individual with a disability for a particular job;
- determine both the worker's traits and his or her needs for job accommodations;
- determine whether the needed accommodations would result in undue hardship for the potential employer;
- assess the needs of the other participants in the work setting (e.g., coworkers, supervisors) if the person with a disability were placed in the job;
- may also work with employers and other relevant persons to facilitate job acquisition and entry transitions for the employee with the disability; and
- may assist the worker with a disability in adjusting to other workers' reactions to him or her.

These new roles and activities may require rehabilitation mental health professionals to acquire additional training. Pape and Tarvydas (1993) provide training recommendations and a comprehensive list of principles, knowledge, and functions in the areas of disability, rehabilitation, and the ADA that should be present for effective functioning as an ADA consultant.

Issues and Controversies

Managed care is one of the most controversial forces in rehabilitation today. Whereas managed care in theory is designed for both cost containment and increased quality of care, in reality cost containment has been the focus (Leri, 1995). Insurance carriers have been known to drop insured people when they suffer an illness or injury resulting in severe physical disability or to reduce costs by cutting coverage to various service delivery providers such as inpatient rehabilitation programs. Rehabilitation professionals need to find ways to determine and justify the costs of their services. They will also need to find ways to manage the negative emotional reactions associated with the changing economic realities in rehabilitation, which could potentially damage the rehabilitation program environment and limit treatment effectiveness (Leri, 1995). Rehabilitation psychologists may also seek additional credentials such as the American Board of Rehabilitation Psychologists (ABRP) certification, although some third-party payers may mistakenly perceive such credentials as adding unnecessarily to service costs.

ADA consultation places rehabilitation professionals in roles not previously explored. For example, employers may request consultation to determine site accessibility, establish job descriptions, and determine the essential and marginal functions of a job for purposes of selection or accommodation development. Not many rehabilitation professionals have been trained in these activities, and ADA consultants might quickly find themselves functioning outside their areas of expertise (Pape & Tarvydas, 1993). New roles associated with the ADA may also create new liabilities for rehabilitation professionals (Bell, 1993). For example, "What can a counselor tell an employer about a client's disability without violating ADA?" (Bell, 1993, p.113). The ADA consultant might also be held liable if an employer refused to hire an individual after learning about a disability from the consultant.

Counseling Psychology and Rehabilitation

For a number of reasons, counseling psychology programs may be a new arena for rehabilitation professionals in the future. Clearly, specific knowledge related to rehabilitation is needed, but counseling psychology programs provide a configuration of training activities that both complement and supplement traditional training in rehabilitation. Counseling psychology identity and philosophy, with a focus on "normal" populations, is particularly suited to working with persons who were premorbidly high functioning. Counseling psychologists should have a "particular stake" in rehabilitation because of the "inherent emphases on assessing and utilizing assets and on reintroducing an individual into the community" (Berg, Pepinsky, & Shoben, 1980, p. 112). Furthermore, there are areas unique to counseling psychology training that make counseling psychologists particularly suited to working with rehabilitation populations.

1. *Vocational psychology training.* Counseling psychology's focus on training in vocational psychology and counseling can be very beneficial to rehabilitation settings. Persons who have a disability are most often considered by society to be disabled from work or school, rather than from other areas of life. Hershenson (1990) noted that "a principal premise is that rehabilitation counseling is ultimately concerned with the vocational sphere of functioning and with other areas of life functioning as they impinge on vocational functioning" (p. 272). Practitioners in rehabilitation settings often find that vocational concerns are quite salient for clients and for the discipline of rehabilitation.

Twenty-three percent of working-age persons with disabilities are working full-time, and at least 66 percent would like to be (National Council on the Handicapped, 1988). Many people with disabilities have not had access to vocational counseling to assist them in making vocational or educational choices or changes that they needed. Furthermore, opportunities are often limited by the types or degrees of accommodations employers are willing or able to make. More vocational psychologists who are broadly knowledgeable and very creative are needed in rehabilitation settings to assist persons with disabilities in maximizing their options.

2. *Multicultural psychology training.* Persons with disabilities are the most disadvantaged minority group in America (DeLoach, 1992), yet relatively little attention has been directed toward understanding the experiences of this group. Rehabilitation professionals not only need to understand the cultural factors associated with being an individual with a disability, but they must also be aware of how persons of diverse cultures view and react to disability. In a survey of vocational rehabilitation evaluators, 72 percent of the respondents indicated a need for training in cultural issues (Eldredge, Fried, & Grissom, 1991).

Counseling psychology's focus on multicultural issues and multicultural counseling training is very beneficial in working with rehabilitation populations. For example, different cultures have different reactions to disability, and professionals working with clients adjusting to disability need to understand how these different reactions affect adjustment. For another example, suffering an illness or injury that results in disability suddenly makes a person a member of a minority group. For some clients, this event requires adjustment to moving from the majority culture to being a member of a minority group. For other clients, this event results in a "multiple oppression," as a person becomes a member of more than one minority group, or it may compound a previous multiple oppression. Cultural issues can result in a wide variety of reactions to disability, and cultural sensitivity is an invaluable asset. Counseling psychologists might draw from knowledge of ethnic minority identity development models (e.g., Atkinson, Morten, & Sue, 1979) to formulate models of identity development for persons with disabilities.

3. *Training in developmental theory.* Counseling psychology philosophy emphasizes viewing client difficulties within a growth-oriented developmental model, which is consistent with rehabilitation philosophy and techniques. Most counseling psychology training programs provide extensive training in developmental theory, which will likely be a significant asset in practice. An example might be the case of a 50-year-old man who is no longer able to work after suffering a spinal cord injury in an automobile accident. From a developmental perspective, his adjustment to the physical disability may be complicated by a life stage characterized by the need to establish one's generativity versus stagnation (Erikson, 1950). In this case, specific knowledge of developmental issues provides for a much richer (and perhaps more effective) approach to counseling the rehabilitation client.

Counseling psychologists have also applied developmental theory to the rehabilitation process itself. For example, Gannon and Gold (1988) suggested that traumatic loss often reactivates early developmental issues. Their model applies developmental theory from an object relations perspective to the rehabilitation process itself, suggesting that the rehabilitation patient may actually go through a process of psychological "rebirth" in rehabilitation. This model suggests that the rehabilitation team is the "mother" and the patient is the "infant," and that they go through stages of symbiosis, practicing, rapprochement, and object constancy. Developmental applications such as this can provide a more complex understanding of the rehabilitation process.

4. *Research.* Within the scientist-practitioner training model, counseling psychologists get solid training in research methodology in addition to their practice-related skills. At the same time, a number of writers have suggest-

ed that the quality of rehabilitation research needs to be increased (e.g., Parker, 1986; Rubin & Rice, 1986). It has been suggested that an effective point of entry into the health care system for counseling psychologists is to involve themselves in health-related research (Tucker, 1991). A number of authors have called for greater attention to the validity of assessment tools in rehabilitation (e.g., Bond & Dietzen, 1993; McFall, 1993), and the measurement training offered by most programs makes counseling psychologists well-equipped to judge and establish reliability and validity of relevant assessment instruments.

Suggested Resources

For an introduction to disability and issues related to disability, *Perspectives on Disability* (Nagler, 1993) is an excellent resource. This volume covers such wide-ranging topics as what it means to be disabled, societal reactions to disability, medical and psychological issues, family issues, legal and ethical issues, and more. This information might be quite useful to educate rehabilitation patients as they adjust to a newly acquired disability.

A counseling psychologist interested in working in rehabilitation should also be familiar with rehabilitation theory and research. Elliott and Byrd (1986) identified frequently cited authors, works, and sources of research cited in *Rehabilitation Psychology.* These sources represent a good orientation to rehabilitation psychology theory and research. More current issues of *Rehabilitation Psychology,* the American Psychology Association Division 22 publication, presents state-of-the-art theory and interventions in rehabilitation. Other sources regarding interventions are the *Rehabilitation Counseling Bulletin* and the *Journal of Applied Rehabilitation Counseling.*

The Handbook of Health and Rehabilitation Psychology, edited by Goreczny (1995), summarizes health psychology and rehabilitation psychology interventions related to a wide variety of physical disorders and disabilities. The *Advances in Clinical Rehabilitation* series, edited by Eisenberg and Grzesiak (1987, 1988, 1990), presents state-of-the-art interventions and research more specific to rehabilitation populations. *Physical Medicine and Rehabilitation* (Washburn, 1981) provides a nice illustration of common physical rehabilitation techniques.

For information on assessment, one might consult *Psychological Assessment in Medical Rehabilitation* (Cushman & Sherer, 1995), which summarizes and critiques measures and instruments in various areas of rehabilitation assessment (e.g., coping and reaction to disability, functional assessment, assessment of vocational interests and aptitudes, neuropsychological assessment). *Improving Assessment in Rehabilitation and Health* (Glueckauf, Sechrest, Bond, & McDonel, 1993) presents more specific issues regarding rehabilitation assessment.

Rehabilitation psychologists should also educate themselves about the ADA. In addition to learning the contents of the law itself, there have been a number of published discussions of the implications of the ADA. A 1993 special section of *Rehabilitation Psychology* (38[2]) includes discussions of ADA implications for assessment, consultation, rehabilitation of persons with neurological impairments, and injured workers.

Discussion Questions

1. How does the patient population in a rehabilitation setting differ from other inpatient physical or mental health care settings?
2. What does counseling psychology training provide that respresents a particularly unique contribution to work in rehabilitation settings?
3. What additional training should a counseling psychologist seek in order to work in a rehabilitation setting?
4. What are some of the ethical issues surrounding practice in the new field of ADA consultation?

References

Antonak, R. F., & Livneh, H. (1988). *The measurement of attitudes toward people with disabilities: Methods, psychometrics, and scales.* Springfield, IL: Charles C. Thomas.

Atkinson, D. R., Morten, G., & Sue, D. W. (1979). *Counseling American minorities: A cross-cultural perspective.* Dubuque, IA: W. C. Brown.

Barry, P., & O'Leary, J. (1989). Roles of the psychologist on a traumatic brain injury rehabilitation team. *Journal of Applied Rehabilitation Counseling, 22*(3), 28–46.

Becker, R. L. (1989). *Becker Work Adjustment Profile: Evaluator's manual.* Columbus, OH: Elbern.

Bell, C. G. (1993). The Americans with Disabilities Act and injured workers: Implications for rehabilitation professionals and the worker's compensation system. *Rehabilitation Psychology, 38*(2), 103–115.

Berg, I., Pepinsky, H. B., & Shoben, E. J. (1980). The status of counseling psychology: 1960. In J. M. Whitely (Ed.), *The history of counseling psychology* (pp. 105–124). Monterey, CA: Brooks/Cole.

Bolton, B. (1988). *Vocational assessment and rehabilitation testing: Current practices and test reviews.* Austin, TX: Pro-Ed.

Bolton, B., & Brookings, J. B. (1993). Appraising the psychometric adequacy of rehabilitation instruments. In R. L. Glueckauf, L. B. Sechrest, G. L. Bond, & E. C. McDonel (Eds.), *Improving assessment in rehabilitation and health* (pp. 109–134). Newbury Park, CA: Sage.

Bolton, B., & Roessler, R. (1986). *Manual for the Work Personality Profile.* Fayetteville, AR: Arkansas Research and Training Center for Vocational Rehabilitation.

Bond, G. R., & Dietzen, L. L. (1993). Predictive validity and vocational assessment: Reframing the question. In R. L. Glueckauf, L. B. Sechrest, G. L. Bond, & E. C. McDonel (Eds.), *Improving assessment in rehabilitation and health* (pp. 61–86). Newbury Park, CA: Sage.

Botterbusch, K. (1987). *Vocational assessment and evaluation systems: A comparison.* Menomonie, WI: University of Wisconsin—Stout, Materials Development Center.

Brown, M., Diller, L., Fordyce, W., Jacobs, D., & Gordon, W. (1980). Rehabilitation indicators: Their nature and uses for assessment. In B. Bolton, & D. Cook (Eds.), *Rehabilitation client assessment* (pp. 102–117). Baltimore: University Park.

Carey, R. (1990). Integrating Case Management, program evaluation, and marketing for inpatient and outpatient rehabilitation programs. *Advances in Clinical Rehabilitation, 3,* 219–249.

Crewe, N. W., & Athelstan, G. T. (1984). *Functional Assessment Inventory manual.* Menomonie, WI: University of Wisconsin—Stout, Materials Development Center.

Cushman, L. A., & Sherer, M. J. (1995). *Psychological assessment in medical rehabilitation.* Washington, DC: American Psychological Association.

DeLoach, C. (1992). Disabling attitudes: When image begets impairment. In N. Hablutzel, & B. T. McMahon (Eds.), *The Americans with Disabilities Act: Access and accommodations* (pp. 9–33). Orlando, FL: Paul M. Deutsch.

Eisenberg, M. G., & Grzesiak, R. C. (Eds.). (1987). *Advances in clinical rehabilitation* (Vol. 1). New York: Springer.

Eisenberg, M. G., & Grzesiak, R. C. (Eds.). (1988). *Advances in clinical rehabilitation* (Vol. 2). New York: Springer.

Eisenberg, M. G., & Grzesiak, R. C. (Eds.). (1990). *Advances in clinical rehabilitation* (Vol. 3). New York: Springer.

Eisenberg, M. G., Jansen, M. A. (1983). Rehabilitation psychology: State of the art. *Annual Review of Rehabilitation, 3,* 1–31.

Eldredge, G. M., Fried, J. H., & Grissom, J. K. (1991). *Vocational evaluator training needs: Food for thought. Vocational Evaluation and Work Adjustment Bulletin, 24,* 11–13.

Elliott, T. R., & Byrd, E. K. (1986). Frequently cited authors, works, and sources of research in Rehabilitation Psychology. *Rehabilitation Psychology, 31*(2), 111–115.

Erikson, E. H. (1950). *Childhood and society.* New York: W. W. Norton.

Faust, D. (1993). The use of traditional neuropsychological tests to describe and prescribe: Why polishing the crystal ball won't help. In R. L. Glueckauf, L. B. Sechrest, G. L. Bond, & E. C. McDonel (Eds.), *Improving assessment in rehabilitation and health* (pp. 87–108). Newbury Park, CA: Sage.

Frank, R. G., Gluck, J. P., & Buckelew, S. P. (1990). Rehabilitation: Psychology's greatest opportunity? *American Psychologist, 45*(6), 757–761.

Fuhrer, M. J. (Ed.). (1987). *Rehabilitation outcomes: Analysis and measurement.* Baltimore: Paul H. Brookes.

Gannon, S., & Gold, J. R. (1988). Rebirth: The rehabilitation process. *Professional Psychology: Research and Practice, 19*(6), 632–636.

Gay, E. G., Weiss, D., Hendel, D. D., Dawis, R. V., & Lofquist, L. H. (1971). *Manual for the Minnesota Importance Questionnaire.* Minneapolis: University of Minnesota, Vocational Psychology Research.

Gibson, D. L., Weiss, D. J., Dawis, R. V., & Lofquist, L. H. (1970). *Manual for the Minnesota Satisfactoriness Scales.* Minneapolis: Minnesota Studies in Vocational Rehabilitation.

Glueckauf, R. L. (1993). Use and misuse of assessment in rehabilitation: Getting back to basics. In R. L. Glueckauf, L. B. Sechrest, G. L. Bond, & E. C. McDonel (Eds.), *Improving assessment in rehabilitation and health* (pp. 135–155). Newbury Park, CA: Sage.

Glueckauf, R. L., Sechrest, L. B., Bond, G. L., & McDonel, E. C. (Eds.). (1993). *Improving assessment in rehabilitation and health.* Newbury Park, CA: Sage.

Gold, J. R., Meltzer, R. H., & Sherr, R. L. (1987). Professional transition: Psychology internships in rehabilitation settings. In R. H. Dana, & W. T. May. (Eds.). *Internship training in professional psychology* (pp. 278–284). Washington: Hemisphere.

Goreczny, A. J. (1995). (Ed.). *Handbook of health and rehabilitation psychology.* New York: Plenum.

Granger, C. V., & Hamilton, B. B. (1992). UDS report. The Uniform Data System for Medical Rehabilitation report of first admissions for 1990. *American Journal of Physical Medical Rehabilitation, 71*(2), 108–113.

Grzesiak, R. C. (1981). Rehabilitation psychology, medical psychology, health psychology, and behavioral medicine. *Professional Psychology, 12*(4), 411–413.

Halpern, A. S., & Fuhrer, M. J. (Eds.). (1984). *Functional assessment in rehabilitation.* Baltimore: Paul H. Brookes.

Halpern, A. S., Irwin, L. K., & Mundres, A. W. (1986). *Social and Prevocational Information Battery-Revised: Examiner's manual.* Monterey, CA: CTB/McGraw-Hill.

Hathaway, S. R., & McKinley, J. C. (1989). *MMPI-2: Manual for administration and scoring.* Minneapolis: University of Minnesota.

Hershenson, D. B. (1990). A theoretical model for rehabilitation counseling. *Rehabilitation Counseling Bulletin, 33*(4), 268–278.

Hiskey, M. (1966). *Manual for the Hiskey-Nebraska Test of Learning Aptitude.* Lincoln, NE: Union College.

Ince, L. P. (1981). *Behavorial psychology in rehabilitation medicine.* Baltimore: Williams & Wilkins.

Institute for Personality and Ability Testing. (1985). *Manual for Form E of the 16PF.* Champaign, IL: Author.

Jarvikoski, A., & Lahelma, E., (1981). Early rehabilitation and its implementation at the work place. *Internation Journal of Rehabilitation Research, 4*(4), 519–530.

Leri, J. E. (1995). The psychological, political, and economic realities of brain injury rehabilitation in the 1990s. *Brain Injury, 9*(5), 533–542.

Lezak, M. D. (1986). Psychological implications of traumatic brain damage for the patient's family. *Rehabilitation Psychology, 31*(4), 241–150.

Linkowski, D. C. (1987). *The Acceptance of Disability Scale.* Washington, DC: George Washington University, Rehabilitation Research and Training Center.

Livneh, H. (1986). A unified approach to existing models of adaptation to disability: Part I, A model adaptation. *Journal of Applied Rehabilitation Counseling, 17*(1), 5–16.

Livneh, H., & Sherwood, A. (1991). Application of personality theories and counseling strategies to clients with physical disabilties. *Journal of Counseling and Development, 69,* 525–538

McFall, R. M. (1993). The essential role of theory in psychological assessment. In R. L. Glueckauf, L. B. Sechrest, G. L. Bond, & E. C. McDonel (Eds.), *Improving assessment in rehabilitation and health* (pp. 11–32). Newbury Park, CA: Sage.

Moriarty, J. B. (1981). *Preliminary Diagnostic Questionnaire.* Dunbar, WV: West Virginia Rehabilitation Research and Training Center.

Nagler, M. (1993). *Perspectives on disability.* Palo Alto, CA: Health Markets Research.

National Council on the Handicapped. (1988). *On the threshold of independence. A report to the President and Congress.* Washington, DC: Author.

Nester, M. A. (1993). Psychometric testing and reasonable accommodation for persons with disabilities. *Rehabilitation Psychology, 38*(2), 75–85.

Pape, D. A., & Tarvydas, V. M. (1993) Responsible and responsive rehabilitation consultation on the ADA: The importance of training for psychologists. *Rehabilitation Psychology, 38*(2), 117–131.

Parker, H. J., & Chan, F. (1990). Psychologists in rehabilitation: Preparation and experience. *Rehabilitation Psychology, 35*(4), 239–248.

Parker, R. M. (1986). Vicissitudes of rehabilitation research. *Rehabilitation Counseling Bulletin, 30*(1), 48–52.

Rubin, S., & Rice, J. (1986). Quality and relevance of rehabilitation research: A critique and recommendations. *Rehabilitation Counseling Bulletin, 30,* 33–42.

Sachs, P. R., & Redd, C. A. (1993). The Americans with Disabilities Act and individuals with neurological impairments. *Rehabilitation Psychology, 38*(2), 87–101.

Sechrest, L. B. (1993). Measurement in rehabilitation: From beginning to what end? In R. L. Glueckauf, L. B. Sechrest, G. L. Bond, & E. C. McDonel (Eds.), *Improving assessment in rehabilitation and health* (pp. 253–273). Newbury Park, CA: Sage.

Siller, J. (1969). *The general form of the Disability Factor Scales series (DFS-G).* New York: New York University, Department of Educational Psychology.

Stutts, M. L. (1991). Supervision in comprehensive rehabilitation settings: The terrain and the traveler. *Clinical Supervisor, 9*(1), 33–57.

Summers, J. D., Rapoff, M. A., Varghese, G., Porter, K., & Palmer, R. E. (1991). Psychosocial factors in chronic spinal cord injury pain. *Pain, 47*(2), 183–189.

Thompson, A. R., & Hutto, M. D. (1992). An employment counseling model for college graduates with severe disabilities: A timely intervention. *Journal of Applied Rehabilitation Counseling, 23*(3), 15–17.

Tucker, C. M. (1991). Counseling psychology and health psychology: Is this a relationship whose time has come? *The Counseling Psychologist, 19*(3), 387–391.

U.S. Department of Labor (1982a). *Manual for the USES Interest Inventory.* Minneapolis: Intran.

U.S. Department of Labor. (1982b). *Manual for the General Aptitude Test Battery, section I: Administration and scoring.* Minneapolis: Intran.

Valpar Corporation. (1986). *VALPAR Component Work Sample Series Manuals.* Tucson, AZ: Author.

Washburn, K. B. (1981). *Physical medicine and rehabilitation* (2nd Ed.). Garden City, NY: Medical Examination Publishing Co., Inc.

Wechsler, D. (1981). *WAIS-R manual: Wechsler Adult Intelligence Scale-Revised.* New York: Psychological Corporation.

Westerheide, W. J., Lenhart, L., & Miller, M. C. (1975). *Field test of a services outcome measurement form: Client change.* Oklahoma City: Department of Institutions, Social and Rehabilitation Services.

Woodruff, G., & McGonigel, J. J. (1988). Early intervention team approaches: The trans-disciplinary model. In J. B. Jordan (Ed.), *Early childhood special education: Birth to three* (pp. 163–181). Reston, VA: Council for Exceptional Children.

Yuker, H. E., Block, J. R., & Young, J. H. (1970). *The measurement of attitudes toward disabled persons.* Albertson, NY: Human Resources Center.

10

Neuropsychology

Raymond L. Ownby

Neuropsychologists, especially those who work in health care settings, are correctly regarded as having specialized expertise in the assessment and remediation of a wide range of cognitive problems. Neuropsychologists often assess problems in patients with medical illnesses (see table 10.1). These may range from liver disease to psychiatric disorders. The task of the neuropsychologist is thus to identify the problem, describe it, discuss its etiology, and suggest what can be done about it. A related and sometimes integral issue is whether the problem is caused by or related to biological, often neurological, dysfunction. Such dysfunctions include, but are not limited to, concerns as diverse as attention deficits, language impairments, and visuospatial skills problems.

The contexts in which problems occur may also be quite diverse. Neuropsychologists may function, for example, in many specialized niches in health care, making their work in these diverse settings quite different from site to site. For example, neuropsychologists may routinely assess all patients scheduled for neurosurgery in order to provide a baseline evaluation of their cognitive function. Others might work in clinics for patients with specific illnesses such as diabetes, HIV-related neurological illnesses, or with elderly dementia patients. Still others may work with psychiatric patients or in rehabilitation centers with patients with neurological disorders such as closed head injury or stroke.

This is not to say that neuropsychologists in health care settings function only to provide routine assessments or that their only duties are to assess

---

Table 10.1
Common Problems Neuropsychologists Assess

Neurology and Neurosurgery

    Cerebrovascular accident ("stroke")

    Closed or open head injury

    Pre/postsurgery assessments

    Epilepsy

    Dementing illnesses (including Alzheimer's and Huntington's disease, as well as various other conditions)

Psychiatry

    Depression and memory complaints

    Cognitive problems in patients with various disorders

    Dementing illnesses

    Schizophrenia

    "Organic" mental disorders

Rehabilitation Medicine

    Closed head injury

    Chronic pain

    Spinal cord injuries

Internal Medicine

    Transplantation, e.g., cognitive dysfunction in patients with liver disease

    Diabetes, thyroid problems, and other endocrinological disorders

Pediatrics

    General developmental disabilities

    Specific learning disorders

    Attention-deficit/hyperactivity disorder

---

cognitive abilities. Neuropsychologists often function as consultants, offering recommendations on an enormous number of disparate problems, and often find that assessment of patients' social, emotional, personality, and vocational functioning is an integral aspect of understanding and helping patients. The assessment approaches taken by neuropsychologists in each instance may be different, but in each case the problem is the same: to find out whether patients have cognitive problems and, if so, what they are and what can be done about them.

Neuropsychologists are often asked to answer very difficult questions about clients' functioning. Often, an important aspect of the request for evaluation is only implicitly stated. Although the question is probably imprecise and undoubtedly outmoded, referral sources often ask, "Is it organic?" Historically, clinicians have asked neuropsychologists whether brain damage is a likely cause of a cognitive or emotional problem. This approach to mental disorders was institutionalized even recently in psychiatric nomenclatures that included such vague diagnoses as "organic mood disorder" or "organic psychosis." The diagnosis implies that some form of biological pathology underlies the disorder, but fails to specify what it is. Further, it implies that there are some forms of mood disorder or psychosis that are *not* biological.

The question concerning organicity is based on the outdated, incorrect premise that the consequences of damage to the brain are similar regardless of location, but different depending on the amount of damage. Based on Karl Lashley's work with rats, this mass action approach was a prominent theory of brain function in the 1950s and 1960s (Lashley & Franz, 1917; see also Feinberg & Farah, 1997, for a more detailed review of this subject). In contrast, the localizationist school holds that specific brain functions are served by specific locales in the brain. More recent research on how the brain works supports a modified localizationist school. This school holds that particular areas of the brain are highly specialized for specific functions, but also acknowledges the importance of the way fiber tracts connect specific areas of the brain into large-scale neural networks (Mesulam, 1990). It is well established, for example, that damage to the left hemisphere is likely to be associated with impairments in language function, whereas right hemisphere damage may be associated with impairments in visuospatial skills.

It is important to realize that the association of specific brain areas with specific impairments is not absolute. To illustrate, damage to a part of the anterior left frontal lobe, sometimes called Broca's area, is likely to cause a language impairment characterized by labored speech and loss of the grammatic elements of language (a nonfluent aphasia). The more widespread the damage in this area, the more likely that a nonfluent aphasia will result; however, the precise location of the damage varies widely among patients. Similar types of damage in the area of the temporal lobe called Wernicke's area can result in a language impairment characterized by preservation of the flow of speech but loss of its content (a fluent aphasia). Here again, the association of this cognitive impairment with a specific location is probabilistic, with the precise extent and location of damage varying widely. Interestingly, problems in using a specific word (word-finding difficulties) can be caused by injury to many sites in the brain, with damage in certain sites more likely to cause this impairment. Mesulam (1990) has shown that a large-scale network for language exists in the brain, with specific linguistic functions, such as expressive or receptive language skills, more or less localized to particular areas that are interconnected by fiber tracts.

The question "Is it organic?" is outmoded for a second reason, alluded to above. It is most directly relevant to psychiatry, but has important implications for psychology and for other medical specialties. Psychiatric disorders have traditionally been classified as either functional or organic. This classification presumed that some psychiatric disorders, such as the anxiety disorders or schizophrenia, were caused primarily by learning or life experiences rather than aberrant biological function—they were a "function" of the patient's interactions with the environment. Organic mental disorders, on the other hand, were those clearly associated with structural or functional brain damage, such as depression occurring for the first time after a stroke or psychosis associated with amphetamine abuse.

Over the last few decades, research has accumulated on the genetic, biochemical, and structural bases of those psychiatric disorders previously labeled "functional." This has led many to question the usefulness as well as the precision of the functional/organic dichotomy. In the most recent edition of the *Diagnostic and Statistical Manual* of the American Psychiatric Association (1994), this dichotomy has been eliminated. Mood disorders, for example, that are associated with medical illnesses are called "depression secondary to a medical condition," and psychosis associated with amphetamine ingestion is called "psychosis secondary to amphetamine abuse."

The practical significance of these distinctions for neuropsychologists lies in the importance of clarifying exactly what the referral source wants to know about the patient. The question "Is it organic?"can often be answered "yes," but is of little use to the treating clinician unless he or she is only hoping for justification of his or her clinical pessimism about a difficult patient. (Even when a patient's difficulties can be causally related to a biological etiology, such therapeutic pessimism is unjustified.) If, during the referral process, the question becomes, "Does the patient have attention problems?" the neuropsychologist can often provide a specific and detailed answer by administering specific measures. A possible corollary question, "Were the attention problems the result of a closed head injury sustained in a car accident?" is harder to address but may have important implications for the referral source and the patient.

Neuropsychologists are correctly perceived as having special knowledge of brain-behavior relationships. This knowledge, when applied to an assessment of a client's current problems, may allow the neuropsychologist to make a statement about whether the client is suffering from a neurological disorder or has some other pathology. One application of this use of neuropsychological assessment arises in the evaluation of elderly patients with complaints of memory problems. Neuropsychological assessment may help differentiate memory problems that arise from anoxia due to heart failure from those caused by a dementing illness, such as Alzheimer's disease.

A similarly murky, but often useful, assessment question arises when patients with some problem in personal or vocational functioning wonder whether it may be caused by a head injury or the result of an unrecognized learning disability present since childhood. Neuropsychological assessment can help clarify whether the person's cognitive function is atypical (e.g., by comparing the person's scores on standardized measures) and, if so, whether his or her pattern of abilities is similar to that of others with known disabilities. In an adult with vocational problems, for example, finding attentional deficits and problems in the phonetic skills used in reading might support the diagnosis of a specific learning disability.

The following case demonstrates how unrecognized cognitive deficits arising from a stroke can cause severe vocational problems.

A 67-year-old man was referred by a psychologist treating him for depression at a local HMO. The patient had had a right-hemisphere stroke a few months before, but to all appearances had made an excellent recovery. He had even returned on a part-time basis to his work operating a photographic printing press. The client complained of depression and feeling as though he couldn't do his job any longer, but had difficulty saying just what the problem at work was. This previously strong and well-functioning man appeared to have lost his self-confidence with the onset of his depression. Neuropsychological assessment, however, showed severe deficits in visuospatial skills. Once the deficits were revealed on tests, closer questioning helped clarify what problems the patient encountered at work. Modifications were made in the patient's job duties, and he was able to return to work full-time.

This vignette illustrates the types of problems in which neuropsychological assessment may be useful. Although neurologically-based cognitive deficits are usually difficult to treat, understanding them can permit psychologists to develop plans involving appropriate remedial and compensatory strategies. Implementing these strategies can result in significant improvement in clients' functioning and can sometimes, as in this case, have a critical impact in maintaining or improving vocational and personal functioning.

Diagnosis and Assessment

Approaches to neuropsychological assessment can be characterized by two polar opposites, although most practitioners do not adhere absolutely to one school or the other. These two approaches can be characterized as the battery approach and the process approach. Many variants of each exist, but most neuropsychologists adhere more or less explicitly to one or the other of these schools (Sweet, Moberg, & Westergaard, 1996). Understanding the theory behind each approach may help avoid confusion.

Practitioners of the *battery* school assess patients with a standard set of measures; all patients receive the same battery. This approach is exemplified in the approach to assessment of Reitan and his associates (Reitan & Wolfson, 1985), who may administer the complete *Halstead-Reitan Neuropsychological Test Battery* (HRNTB) to each patient seen. The HRNTB includes measures such as the Category Test (a nonverbal reasoning measure that taps clients' ability to profit from feedback about their behavior), the Tactual Performance Test (a measure of spatial problem solving undertaken with patients blindfolded), as well as motor measures such as the Finger Oscillation Test (speed of tapping a lever with a finger). This battery grew out of empirical research on the types of cognitive deficits displayed by persons with known neurological disease, such as penetrating head injures or brain tumors. Reitan developed the battery at a time when neuroimaging could not provide good information about lesion location. The HRNTB was developed, at least in part, to assist in locating neurological lesions through their association with deficits in specific cognitive functions. Today, practitioners may use it to assess a wide variety of cognitive functions in a standard way.

The *process* approach is most closely identified with Edith Kaplan and her colleagues (see Lezak, 1995, for a discussion). The process approach typically involves choosing assessment measures based on the referral question and deficits to be tested, rather than using a predefined battery of instruments. Although practitioners of this approach may use a number of measures routinely with most patients, there is less emphasis on finding a pattern among performances on a standard set of measures given to the patients. Rather, the process approach emphasizes understanding how patients arrive at the score on the test.

An often-cited example that clarifies the differences between these two approaches concerns the problem-solving behavior of patients with right- or left-hemisphere injuries. While either type of injury may result in deficits in performance on a task such as the Block Design subtest of the WAIS-III, the way in which a patient achieves this score may be quite different. Patients with left-hemisphere injuries may produce a design that preserves its over-all configuration but is scored as incorrect because of neglecting important details. By contrast, patients with right-hemisphere injuries may produce designs that include correct attention to details but that betray a complete loss of the overall idea of the design. Either type of patient may obtain the same psychometric score on the task but with differences in approach that may have important implications for understanding the nature of the patient's problems.

Most neuropsychologists approach assessment with some mixture of these extremes. Many psychologists who use the HRNTB supplement it, for example, with a memory measure, since the HRNTB is notoriously poor in assessing this critical ability domain. Battery-oriented psychologists may also do follow-up testing after the battery has been administered and scored, in order to allow closer assessment of problems found in the initial assessment. On the other hand, many process-oriented neuropsychologists find the use of normed tests helpful in placing their assessments in context. To extend the example above, it is important to know both that the patient takes a particular route to obtaining a poor performance and that the level of performance indicates severe deficits in visuospatial skills. Both forms of information are useful in understanding patients' cognitive problems and planning for their rehabilitation.

Systematic Approach to Assessment

No matter what school of assessment the neuropsychologist espouses, the assessment begins with the referral. Even in routine assessments, a referral is implicit: The neuropsychologist is asked to provide specific information about a patient's problems, and perhaps an opinion about their cause and the best ways to treat them. Clarification of the referral question is thus a criti-cal first step. The question should not be, "Is the problem organic?" but rather, "What are the patient's cognitive or emotional problems, and are they the result of a medical condition?"

Obtaining a background history is critical in making these determinations. Because of the nature of their problems, patients with neurological and psychiatric disorders may not be reliable reporters of their past history or current functioning, so that getting information from a collateral source is especially important. Communication with the referring physician, a common referral source in health care settings, is especially valuable in clarifying the referral problem, obtaining collateral information, and developing rapport, which is useful later when recommendations about treatment are made.

Rationale for the Assessment and Selection of Instruments

The precise way in which neuropsychologists choose assessment instruments is based on a combination of their past experiences, theoretical considerations, and the needs of patients. Neuropsychologists who espouse a standard battery approach may not change their choice of instruments from patient to patient, although many supplement their standard battery with measures directly related to the patient's presenting complaint. A patient with complaints of memory problems may be administered a more extensive set of memory measures to tap this ability domain. For neuropsychologists who take a less standardized approach to assessment, the evaluation may begin with administration of a basic set of measures used with most patients. For example, many neuropsychologists include the Wechsler scale appropriate for the patient's age in almost every assessment. The neuropsychologist may then use supplementary measures to study the ways in which patients complete the tasks in the scale. The evaluator may try to understand why a patient does poorly on the Object Assembly subtest of the WAIS-III by providing alternate puzzles for the patient to solve. These alternates might vary the extent to which a correct solution depends on perceiving the underlying form or matching up lines on the puzzle pieces.

Although a complete assessment may include all the domains listed in table 10.2, many neuropsychologists conduct briefer assessments targeted on specific problems. This may be especially appropriate when the patient's cognitive problem is already recognized and assessed by another clinician, as might be true when a patient is referred by a behavioral neurologist who has already done a cognitive assessment. In this case, thoroughness may be balanced with time constraints. A neurologist, for example, may refer a

Table 10.2

Cognitive Domains Assessed and Examples of Measures Used

General cognitive ability
Wechsler Intelligence Scales (WAIS-III; WISC-III; WPPSI-R)
Stanford-Binet Intelligence Scale, 4th ed.
Woodcock-Johnson Psych-Educational Battery, Cognitive Tests

Executive functions and abstraction
Category test of the HRNTB
Trail-Making Test, Parts A and B
Stroop
Wisconsin Card Sorting Test
Porteus mazes
Subtests of the Wechsler Intelligence Scales

Language
Boston Diagnostic Aphasia Exam
Wechsler Intelligence Scales, Verbal Scale Subtests
Boston Naming Test
Peabody Picture Vocabulary Test

Visual and nonvisual spatial
 Drawing tasks
  Rey Complex Figure Test
  Benton Visual Retention Test
 Manipulation
  Tactual Performance Test of HRNTB
 Nonmotor
  Benton Judgment of Line Orientation
  Benton Face Recognition Test

Learning and memory
California Verbal Learning Test
Rey Auditory Verbal Learning Test
Wechsler Memory Scale-Revised

Perceptual
Tactual Performance Test of the HRNTB
Fingertip Number Writing

Motor
Finger Tapping/Foot Tapping
Purdue Pegboard/Grooved Pegboard

Other measures for specific abilities or to screen for specific problems
Bilateral simultaneous stimulation

Social-emotional functioning
Minnesota Multiphasic Personality Inventory (MMPI)
Personality Inventory for Children (PIC)

patient who has had a stroke for a more definitive assessment of language or visuospatial impairments. Depending on the patient's needs, an assessment of this sort of problem might comprise a brief assessment of general function with more specific measures for language or visuospatial function.

Interpretation of Measures

Although the interpretation of test scores obtained is, to some extent, a clinical art, most neuropsychologists approach interpretation systematically. Both Reitan (Reitan & Wolfson, 1985) and Lezak (1995) suggest that specific principles should be applied in test interpretation.

Level of Performance

This is perhaps the most intuitively appealing (but perhaps misleading) approach to understanding performance during the neuropsychological evaluation. This approach must rely on some reference point to assess the deviation of a score from that point. Reference points may depend on norms derived from large studies, as when a clinician assesses the difference of an IQ score from the population average of 100. This approach can, however, be misleading, since population averages may be inappropriate for specific patients. A low-average IQ score, for example, may be normal for a patient with general developmental disabilities, a history of special education class placement, adaptive behavior deficits, and poor vocational performance. Conversely, a Verbal IQ score in the high-average range may indicate impairment in a patient who is a distinguished legal scholar.

The second approach may be to establish estimated levels of premorbid functioning for the patient. This is done in several ways. The simplest way is to look for internal consistencies in obtained test scores and then evaluate discrepancies based on their deviations from this internal norm. Scores in the superior range on five measures requiring verbal skills, for example, can be contrasted with one in the impaired range. Another way to evaluate deviations in test performance is an informal estimate of premorbid functioning based on educational background and vocational functioning. A low average Performance IQ (tapping visuospatial skills) might mean something far different in a successful architect than in an English teacher.

Others have developed more sophisticated approaches to estimation of premorbid functioning based on regression formulas. These formulas are usually based on such predictor variables as age, gender, geographic residence, years of education, and vocational attainment. Estimates of premorbid general intellectual functioning have also been based on word recognition skills or composites of several types of predictors.

Cutting scores

A number of empirical studies have established cutting scores on neuropsychological instruments to help differentiate normal from abnormal performance. An example of this approach is used in the HRNTB, in which scores on the core battery measures are classed as either normal or impaired. The number of impaired scores is divided by the total number of measures administered to yield the Impairment Index.

Right versus Left Performance

Reitan and his colleagues have emphasized the importance of discrepancies between measures that tap right versus left hemisphere function. This is most reliably interpreted when assessing the relative right- and left-sided performance of individuals on motor tasks. For right-handed individuals, a certain decrement on the left-sided performance is expected when motor speed or strength is assessed relative to the right side. For example, a typical adult may tap his or her right index finger an average of 50 times per trial over five 10-second trials on the Finger Oscillation Test of the HRNTB. Most persons perform about 10 percent less well with their nonpreferred hand, so that a left-handed performance of 30 suggests a decrement in performance on the left hand. In combination with problems in discriminating rhythm patterns or in visuospatial skills (also dependent on the integrity of the right cerebral hemisphere) this finger-tapping score might suggest right hemisphere dysfunction.

Double Dissociation

In this approach to test interpretation, the neuropsychologist tries to isolate a single impaired ability across several measures. A simple analogy might be a Venn diagram, in which the overlap among several cognitive domains is related to a patient's poor performance on some measures and good performance on others.

This strategy is likely to be used by process-approach clinicians as a means of hypothesis testing during assessment. A simple example might be when the neuropsychologist is confronted with a Verbal IQ score of 65. He or she might hypothesize that the patient has verbal skills deficits and, possibly, mildly impaired general intellectual ability. This interpretation might be strengthened by impaired performances on measures of verbal fluency or naming. It would be weakened, however, by a score of 120 on the Peabody Picture Vocabulary Test—Revised. Recognizing this discrepancy, the neuropsychologist might refine his or her hypothesis and venture that the patient has *expressive* language deficits. This hypothesis could be tested further by administering other measures of language and general intellectual skills that do not depend on expressive speech. Performances on these measures could then be used to further refine the neuropsychologist's hypotheses about the patient's functioning, perhaps leading to still further testing and refinement.

Pattern Analysis

In this approach, the neuropsychologist integrates a distinct group of strengths and weaknesses on neuropsychological measures, formulating a pattern that may be characteristic of a particular disorder. An illustration of the value of this approach might arise in the evaluation of a child referred for poor academic achievement. In one case, test scores might show deficiencies in auditory perceptual and word recognition skills, consistent with a specific reading disability. In another case, test scores might show that these skills are intact but that the child is behaviorally impulsive, for example, performing poorly on the Mazes subtest of the WISC-III. If additional data showed that the child was unusually active and had difficulty regulating his or her behavior in the classroom, the neuropsychologist might hypothesize that the child's poor school achievement might be related to attention-deficit/hyperactivity disorder. In each case, the overall analysis of a pattern of neuropsychological impairment leads to a different conclusion.

The Neuropsychological Report

More than most other psychological specialties, clinical neuropsychology is assessment-oriented. The result of the assessment is usually a written report, often provided in the context of a verbal consultation. Since the written report is the most concrete outcome of the long and often complicated assessment process, it is critical that the report accurately reflect and summarize the evaluation. It should provide a clear statement of the assessment problem, what the neuropsychologist did to address that problem, what the results were, and what ought to be done about the problem. As I have outlined elsewhere (1997), the report is usually organized in the following sections:

Identifying information. This section of the report establishes the identity of the person assessed. It usually includes at least the patient's name, date of birth, hospital or other identification number, and the date of the report.

Referral information. This section usually includes background information and a brief explanation of the reason for the assessment. Information that is important to understanding the patient's functioning or the reason for referral should be presented here. Such information might include a brief synopsis of the patient's medical history as it is relevant to the assessment problem or information about proposed medical procedures pertinent to the evaluation. Results of previous evaluations could also be placed here so that comparisons can be made with results obtained in the current evaluation. The implications of previous findings and why reevaluation is undertaken might also be discussed here. Only one thing is critical in this section: It should clearly state the question or questions that the assessment is to answer.

Assessment information. This section provides details about the assessment. Usually, the neuropsychologist provides a brief paragraph about measures administered during the assessment. Some neuropsychologists prefer to list every measure administered during evaluation, although those who use well-known batteries may simply note that fact. The rest of this section provides an explanation of test results and their meaning. A key concept is to reference test scores to easily understood terms that are clearly explained. Rather than merely report a score on a scale of a personality measure, for example, the score might be integrated with observations of the patient to support the idea that the patient presents a specific problem, such as depression. Other key ideas can be presented in this way to provide a coherent account of how the neuropsychologist approached the assessment and what he or she found out. This section of the report should conclude with a paragraph summarizing the key ideas of the assessment.

Conclusions and recommendations. In this section, the neuropsychologist draws broad conclusions from the assessment results and provides a specific answer to the assessment question. The neuropsychologist integrates the key ideas described in the results section into an overall picture of the patient's functioning. From this overall picture, the psychologist should provide conclusions in the form of answers to the assessment questions. The conclusions then in turn lead to a set of detailed recommendations for patient management. For example, if the assessment showed that the patient had a memory disorder, recommendations might discuss ways of helping the patient deal with the problem (such as making lists or using small notes as reminders about important activities). Recommendations might also include referrals for counseling, psychotherapy, or cognitive remediation (see next section) as are appropriate.

Cognitive Remediation

Recently, neuropsychologists have become interested not only in assessing patients' cognitive problems but also treating them. This field has come to be called cognitive remediation or cognitive rehabilitation. Neuropsychologists interested in this area of treatment work with patients with specific cognitive problems to help them better cope and, in some instances, to improve the function itself.

Cognitive remediation is not a new field, although it is fairly new as part of clinical neuropsychology. Speech pathologists, for example, have worked for many years with patients with neurological insults and helped develop both specific instruments to assess communication and other cognitive disorders and interventions aimed at improving the communicative competence of patients with diverse neurological injuries. Special educators long ago developed special teaching techniques for children with innate or acquired cognitive problems. Speech pathologists and neuropsychologists have also worked to improve cognitive function in other areas less directly related to speech and language disorders, such as visuospatial or memory skills. Interventions for treating cognitive disorders can be divided into two main types: compensatory and remedial.

Compensatory Interventions

These interventions help patients deal with lost or altered cognitive functions by finding "work arounds." A patient with significant loss of expressive language (as might occur with an anterior left hemisphere stroke) may not be able to regain the capacity to express him- or herself orally, but will retain the capacity to point. Patients with this pattern of motor speech loss can be helped to express themselves with a device called a communication board. These boards typically include squares on which frequently used words, as well as the alphabet, are written. The patient can communicate with others by pointing to words or letters. More recently, the availability of small computers has expanded the use of this approach by integrating an electronic version of the communication board with speech synthesis technology. Rather than merely pointing at what he or she wants to say, the patient presses the keyboard and the word or sentence is "spoken" by an electronic voice.

A very common problem in individuals who have experienced anoxia (a period of reduced oxygen delivery to the brain, as may occur during a heart attack) is poor memory. Cells in the hippocampus, a brain structure critical in the consolidation of new memories, are extremely sensitive to oxygen deprivation for even short periods. Persons who have experienced anoxic events thus may have specific deficits in short-term memory in the absence of more grossly obvious cognitive problems. Patients who previously could easily remember a list of five to ten items at the grocery store now may arrive at the store unsure of why they are there. These patients can be taught a variety of simple yet effective techniques. They may be taught, for example, to rehearse items they are to remember so as to improve their capacity to remember them. They can be coached to make lists or to leave reminding notes in prominent places where they are likely to see them. Research in cognitive psychology has been applied to developing specific techniques in memory rehabilitation (Glisky, 1997). These then, are a few of the many ways of helping patients cope with cognitive problems.

Remedial Strategies

While more controversial as to its effectiveness, some neuropsychologists have tried to find ways of actually improving the affected function in patients with cognitive disorders. Speech pathologists have long known, for example, that stimulation of language abilities may speed and perhaps enhance recovery of function (Davis, 1992). The precise mechanisms for recovery of function after neurological injury are unclear, but range across such diverse factors as reduction of inflammation after the injury to reorganization of the neurological circuits subserving language (Kertesz, 1997). It is not clear, however, whether cognitive interventions actually improve the function of underlying neural structures, so that the theoretical rationale underlying this approach, while promising, is unproven.

Controversies

As with most other areas of psychology, clinical neuropsychology has been influenced by diverse economic and political forces, creating controversies in the areas of training, credentialing, and service provision. Other controversies exist in the areas of approaches to assessment and the use of service extenders, such as technicians or psychometrists.

Training

A consensus may be emerging about what is appropriate training for independent practice as a neuropsychologist. Although models exist for specific predoctoral training as a neuropsychologist, most practicing neuropsychologists agree that specific training in clinical neuropsychology should be postdoctoral. Predoctoral education and training should comprise a strong background in assessment (including measurement and test construction theory along with practical experience) and psychopathology as well as in research methods and statistics. Since most neuropsychologists have been trained as clinical psychologists, many espouse predoctoral training in clinical psychology as the appropriate prerequisite for postdoctoral training in neuropsychology. Counseling psychologists with strong backgrounds in assessment and psychopathology may also be eligible for postdoctoral training in neuropsychology. As with clinical psychologists, counseling psychologists who are interested in pursuing postdoctoral training in clinical neuropsychology should be able to present evidence of good performance in courses in physiological psychology, assessment, and other courses related to the biological bases of behavior. The training that many counseling psychologists receive in vocational assessment may be an asset for them, especially if pursuing a career as a neuropsychologist in a rehabilitation setting.

Credentialing

At present, a consensus is emerging that the minimum level of training required for independent practice of clinical neuropsychology is a doctoral degree in psychology and at least one postdoctoral year of supervised training in neuropsychology. Standards for accreditation of postdoctoral fellowships are emerging. At this juncture, there is no formal credential for practice as a neuropsychologist. Advanced practitioners may qualify for the Diplomate in Clinical Neuropsychology awarded by the American Board of Professional Psychology (ABPP) or the American Board of Clinical Neuropsychology (ABCN). Some managed care organizations have moved to allow only board-certified practitioners privileges in their organizations; it is possible that in the future neuropsychologists may be required to have the diplomate awarded by the ABPP or ABCN to participate in some reimbursement programs.

Service Provision

Recent changes in rules concerning Medicare reimbursement for services have had an impact on clinicians in many settings. Whether neuropsychologists may bill for services not provided directly is controversial, especially in teaching institutions where tests may have been administered by trainees. Medicare rules now require that services be closely supervised by the clinician who bills for the services. This may reduce time available for other clinical and research activities.

Approaches to Assessment

Finally, a longstanding area of controversy in neuropsychology concerns how assessments are done and what they comprise. The different schools of neuropsychological assessment were discussed above. At times, adherents of each school have argued that adherents of the other school neglect important issues in their approach. Neuropsychologists who advocate for the flexible battery approach to assessment have argued that battery-oriented assessments may not reveal critically important information about the processes by which patients arrive at answers to questions posed by assessment tasks. These clinicians might argue that the information lost in the battery-oriented assessment would provide essential information about how to help the patient. In contrast, battery-oriented clinicians might point out that process-oriented clinicians sacrifice validity through the use of poorly-normed instruments whose interpretation is susceptible to clinician bias. Selection of instruments to assess problems the clinician suspects are there, while not assessing other ability domains, leads to the possibility of confirmatory test-ing—the clinician may only investigate problems that he or she already thinks are there, and then, unsurprisingly, finds precisely that problem. The process-oriented assessment also does not allow for the collection of stan-dardized data on neuropsychological conditions. Thus, assessment results cannot be compared across conditions.

A related controversy is the use of technicians or psychometrists for administration of tests. Process-oriented clinicians are less likely than bat-tery-oriented clinicians to rely on such service extenders. Here again, process-oriented clinicians may argue that important information is lost when clinical impressions are not available to the neuropsychologist report-ing the assessment. Battery-oriented clinicians might respond that well-trained psychometrists may be keen clinical observers whose services allow doctorally-trained neuropsychologists to spend more time in tasks such as data interpretation, patient interview, and research.

Summary

This chapter has provided a brief overview of the applications of clinical neuropsychology in health care settings. Although neuropsychologists use a wide variety of assessment techniques in an enormous number of set-tings, their tasks are usually the same: to determine whether a cognitive problem exists, what might cause it, and what can be done about it. Neuropsychological assessment requires an understanding of the principles of brain-behavior relations and an appreciation of the complexity of the ways that normal and damaged brain structures may interact. Answers to the assessment questions are usually communicated to the referral source in a written report, often accompanied by face-to-face consultation.

Neuropsychologists may also provide cognitive remediation services, in which patients are helped to deal with their cognitive problems by learning ways of dealing with them. Some neuropsychologists are working to devel-op ways in which the actual impaired abilities of patients can be improved. Although most persons who pursue training in clinical neuropsychology have been trained in clinical psychology, counseling psychologists with strong backgrounds in assessment and the neural bases of behavior may find neuropsychological training available to them. Overall, clinical neuropsy-chology is a challenging field in which psychologists can make important contributions to patient evaluation, treatment approaches, and research.

Suggested Resources

The student of neuropsychology is fortunate in having a number of excellent textbooks to consult. *Neuropsychological Assessment* (Lezak, 1995), now in its third edition, is perhaps the best known. Lezak presents a basic review of brain-behavior relations and the importance of these relations to neuropsychological assessment. The strength of this book, however, is its coherent and encyclopedic survey of measures used in neuropsychological assessment. The book can serve as both a textbook and a reference.

At another level of sophistication is Heilman and Valenstein's (1993) *Clinical Neuropsychology.* This edited book comprises chapters on most important topics in human neuropsychology at a level suitable for the serious student. Kolb and Whishaw's (1994) *Fundamentals of Human Neuropsychology* provides a broad overview of basic and clinical neuropsychology. It represents an excellent textbook for advanced undergraduate and graduate students. *Neuropsychology: A Clinical Approach* (Walsh, 1994) is a similar review of topics in clinical neuropsychology at a slightly more advanced graduate level.

The recently published *Behavioral Neurology and Neuropsychology,* edited by Feinberg and Farah (1997b), integrates presentations on behavioral neurology and clinical neuropsychology. It also provides a brief introduction to computational methods for simulating neuropsychological phenomena. It is likely to be especially useful to neuropsychologists interested in the cognitive phenomena associated with neurological disorders.

Discussion Questions

1. What evidence supports the mass action and localizationist theories of brain function? Why is the approach that emphasizes the importance of large-scale neural networks more accurate?
2. What are the essential differences between the battery and process-oriented approaches to neuropsychological assessment? What are the strengths and weaknesses of each? Suggest clinical situations in which one or the other might be preferable.
3. What are basic strategies for interpreting data from a neuropsychological evaluation? How might you apply these strategies in interpreting test data in the assessment of a patient who has experienced an anoxic episode?

With a patient suspected of having a dementing condition? With a patient suspected of having psychiatric symptoms caused by a medical condition?

4. What types of training should a psychologist have as a preliminary to more advanced training in clinical neuropsychology? What level of training is appropriate for independent practice as a neuropsychologist?

5. What types of information are important to include in the report of a neuropsychological evaluation?

6. Suggest several compensatory strategies that could be implemented with a patient with memory problems. What might be remedial strategies for this patient?

7. Describe several current controversies in the area of clinical neuropsychology.

References

American Psychiatric Association. (1994). *Diagnostic and statistical manual* (4th ed.). Washington, DC: Author.

Davis, G. A. (1992). *A survey of adult aphasia and related language disorders* (2nd ed.). Englewood Cliffs, NJ: Prentice-Hall.

Feinberg, T. E., & Farah, M. J. (1997a). The development of modern behavioral neurology and neuropsychology. In T. E. Feinberg, & M. J. Farah (Eds.), *Behavioral neurology and neuropsychology* (pp. 3–23). New York: McGraw-Hill.

Feinberg, T. E., & Farah, M. J. (1997b). *Behavioral neurology and neuropsychology.* New York: McGraw-Hill.

Glisky, E. L. (1997). Rehabilitation of memory dysfunction. In T. E. Feinberg, & M. J. Farah (Eds.), *Behavioral neurology and neuropsychology* (pp. 491–495). New York: McGraw-Hill.

Heilman, K. M., & Valenstein, E. (1993). *Clinical neuropsychology* (3rd ed.). New York: Oxford University.

Kertesz, A. (1997). Recovery of aphasia. In T. E. Feinberg, & M. J. Farah (Eds.), *Behavioral neurology and neuropsychology* (pp. 167–182). New York: McGraw-Hill.

Kolb, B., & Whishaw, I. Q. (1994). *Fundamentals of human neuropsychology* (3rd ed.). San Francisco: Freeman.

Lashley K. S., & Franz, S. I. (1917). The effects of cerebral destruction upon habit-formation and retention in the albino rat. *Psychobiology, 1,* 71–139.

Lezak, M. D. (1995). *Neuropsychological assessment* (3rd ed.). New York: Oxford University.

Mesulam, M-M. (1990). Large scale neurocognitive networks and distributed processing for attention, language, and memory. *Annals of Neurology, 28,* 597–613.

Ownby, R. L. (1997). *How to write psychological reports* (3rd ed.). New York: John Wiley & Sons.

Reitan, R. M., & Wolfson, D. (1985). *The Halstead-Reitan neuropsychological test battery.* Tucson, AZ: Neuropsychology.

Sweet, J. J., Moberg P. J., & Westergaard, C. K. (1996). Five-year follow-up survey of practices and beliefs of clinical neuropsychologists. *The Clinical Neuropsychologist, 10,* 202–221.

Walsh, K. W. (1994). *Neuropsychology: A clinical approach.* 3rd ed.). New York: Churchill Livingstone.

11

Eating Disorders

Cynthia R. Kalodner

Anorexia nervosa and bulimia nervosa are eating disorders that affect a relatively small percentage of women and an even smaller percentage of men. Despite their low prevalence, these disorders receive a great deal of attention in the media. This media attention may result from the current societal obsession with thinness and the pervasive pressure to be thin. Concern about body image and weight coupled with biological and psychological risk factors can be influential in the development of eating disorders as well as less severe eating problems during adolescence and early adulthood.

These disorders are worthy of consideration in a text on the role of counseling psychology in health care because eating disorders are psychological problems that often require collaboration between mental health professionals and physicians (especially primary care practitioners, pediatricians, and psychiatrists). Referrals from physicians to mental health workers often occur when medical professionals suspect that an eating disorder may be present. Formal diagnosis of eating disorders is usually conducted by psychologists or psychiatrists. It is also important for mental health providers to refer individuals with eating disorders to physicians for an evaluation of physical health and nutritional status. The referral for physical evaluation may become a therapeutic issue framed by the therapist as a part of the recovery process. Treatment for serious eating disorders may require hospitalization, which allows psychologists to work with other health care professionals. Teams of professionals work together to provide coordinated and comprehensive care. These teams often include mental health workers (psychologists, social workers, counselors), physicians, psychiatric nurses, and other allied health professionals, such as occupational and recreational therapists. Dentists and dietitians are often essential to the effective identification and treatment of eating disorders.

Definitions

It is important to know the defining criteria for eating disorders. The *DSM-IV* (American Psychiatric Association, 1994) includes two major categories of eating disorders: anorexia nervosa and bulimia nervosa. In addition, eating disorder not otherwise specified (NOS) is used when an individual does not meet the criteria for either anorexia or bulimia but has a significant eating problem. Binge-eating disorder is an eating disorder NOS, characterized by binge-eating without regular use of compensatory behavior. (See table 11.1 for the diagnostic criteria for anorexia nervosa, table 11.2 for bulimia nervosa, and table 11.3 for the research criteria for binge-eating disorder.)

Table 11.1
Diagnostic Criteria for Anorexia Nervosa

A. Refusal to maintain body weight at or above a minimally normal weight for age and height (e.g., weight loss leading to maintenance of body weight less than 85% of that expected; or failure to make expected weight gain during period of growth, leading to body weight less than 85% of that expected).

B. Intense fear of gaining weight or becoming fat, even though underweight.

C. Disturbance in the way in which one's body weight or shape is experienced, undue influence of body weight or shape on self-evaluation, or denial of the seriousness of the current low body weight.

D. In postmenarcheal females, amenorrhea, i.e., the absence of at least three consecutive menstrual cycles. (A woman is considered to have amenorrhea if her periods occur only following hormone, e.g., estrogen, administration.)

Type

Restricting Type: During the current episode of Anorexia Nervosa, the person has not regularly engaged in binge-eating or purging behavior (i.e., self-induced vomiting or the misuse of laxatives, diuretics, or enemas)

Binge-Eating/Purging Type: During the current episode of Anorexia Nervosa, the person has regularly engaged in binge-eating or purging behavior (i.e., self-induced vomiting or the misuse of laxatives, diuretics, or enemas)

From APA, 1994, pp. 544–545.

Table 11.2
Diagnostic Criteria for Bulimia Nervosa

A. Recurrent episodes of binge eating. An episode of binge eating is characterized by both of the following:

    (1) eating, in a discrete period of time (e.g., within any 2-hour period), an amount of food that is definitely larger than most people would eat during a similar period of time and under similar circumstances

    (2) a sense of lack of control over eating during the episode (e.g., a feeling that one cannot stop eating or control what or how much one is eating)

B. Recurrent inappropriate compensatory behavior in order to prevent weight gain, such as self-induced vomiting; misuse of laxatives, diuretics, enemas, or other medications; fasting; or excessive exercise.

C. The binge eating and inappropriate compensatory behaviors both occur, on average, at least twice a week for 3 months.

D. Self-evaluation is unduly influenced by body shape and weight.

E. The disturbance does not occur exclusively during episodes of Anorexia Nervosa.

Type

Purging Type: During the current episode of Bulimia Nervosa, the person has regularly engaged in self-induced vomiting or the misuse of laxatives, diuretics, or enemas.

Nonpurging Type: During the current episode of Bulimia Nervosa, the person has used other inappropriate compensatory behaviors, such as fasting or excessive exercise, but has not regularly engaged in self-induced vomiting or the misuse of laxatives, diuretics, or enemas.

From APA, 1994, pp. 549–550.

A major advancement in the current edition of the *DSM* concerns the subtyping of anorexia and bulimia. Anorexia is subtyped as restricting type or binge-eating/purging type. Bulimia is subtyped as purging or nonpurging type. These subtypes are important since they eliminate double diagnoses and confusion when an individual is of very low weight and reports binge-eating. Purging methods include vomiting or the use of laxatives, diuretics, and enemas. Restricting methods involve excessive exercise or fasting.

When using the *DSM-IV* criteria to assess an individual for the presence of an eating disorder, it is necessary to begin with the criteria for anorexia, since the diagnosis of bulimia is inappropriate if the criteria for anorexia are met (see table 11.1). An individual who has a very low weight, reports a fear of gaining weight, has an inaccurate perception of body shape, and has

---

Table 11.3
Research Criteria for Binge-Eating Disorder

A. Recurrent episodes of binge eating. An episode of binge eating is characterized by both of the following:

    (1) eating, in a discrete period of time (e.g., within any 2-hour period), an amount of food that is definitely larger than most people would eat during a similar period of time and under similar circumstances

    (2) a sense of lack of control over eating during the episode (e.g., a feeling that one cannot stop eating or control what or how much one is eating)

B. The binge-eating episodes are associated with three (or more) of the following:

    (1) eating much more rapidly than normal

    (2) eating until feeling uncomfortably full

    (3) eating large amounts of food when not feeling physically hungry

    (4) eating alone because of being embarrassed by how much one is eating

    (5) feeling disgusted with oneself, depressed, or very guilty after overeating

C. Marked distress regarding binge eating is present.

D. The binge eating occurs, on average, at least 2 days a week or 6 months.

. . .

E. The binge eating is not associated with the regular use of inappropriate compensatory behaviors (e.g., purging, fasting, excessive exercise) and does not occur exclusively during episodes of Anorexia Nervosa or Bulimia Nervosa.

From APA, 1994, p. 731.

---

missed three menstrual periods meets the criteria for anorexia. In addition, if she* engages in binge-eating and purging, the binge-eating/purging subtype applies.

A case example may help to clarify the differential diagnosis of anorexia and bulimia. A young woman was accompanied by her mother for evaluation at an inpatient eating disorders unit. The mother reported that her daughter had begun dieting several months ago and that the dieting had become extreme. She wasn't sure if her daughter needed to stay in the hospital. At the mention of staying in the hospital, the young woman burst into tears and said that she wouldn't stay. The woman appeared to be very thin and when questioned, she reported that she was eating "lots of salad with nonfat dressing and some nonfat yogurt" for lunch and dinner. The student reported that she was worried about being fat and insisted that she needed to

---

*Since anorexia nervosa and bulimia nervosa are far more common in females than in males, the feminine pronoun will be used to refer to individuals with either disorder.

lose at least 10 more pounds. She did not believe that she had any kind of problem since she never vomited. She reported that she exercised two hours a day, alternating between using a treadmill and swimming. During the evaluation, the client reported that she had not had a menstrual period in five months. She initially refused to be weighed, but agreed after the intake session to be weighed if her mother promised not to make her stay at the hospital. She weighed 105 pounds, and she was 5'6". This individual meets the criteria for anorexia, restricting type.

In the case of bulimia, the individual is subtyped as either purging or nonpurging, depending on the type of inappropriate compensatory behavior used. The purging subtype uses vomiting or laxatives, diuretics, and enemas, while the nonpurging subtype engages in fasting or excessive exercise. The following case example highlights the use of the diagnostic criteria for bulimia.

A college student reported to the counseling center in response to an advertisement for an eating disorders group. She reported that she had been binge-eating and purging since her senior year in high school, but that she is doing it daily now and is afraid that she can't stop. She described her binges as something that just seems to happen most nights after she eats a normal dinner and has been studying for a short time. She drives to a fast food restaurant and orders several sandwiches, fries, and two milkshakes and begins eating on her way home. Eating seems out of her control and once she starts she cannot stop until all the food in finished, and then she immediately vomits in the hall bathroom. This description fits with the criteria for bulimia, purging type.

Distinguishing between the binge-eating/purging type of anorexia and the purging type of bulimia is a matter of weight and amenorrhea. Individuals who are of very low body weight who engage in binge-eating and purging and have missed three consecutive menstrual cycles fit the current criteria for anorexia, binge-eating/purging type.

In addition to understanding anorexia and bulimia, it is important to attend to the subclinical presentations that are assigned to the eating disorders NOS category. Eating problems seem to exist on a continuum with anorexia and bulimia as endpoints on that continuum (Ruderman & Besbeas, 1992; Scarano & Kalodner, 1994). Figure 11.1 demonstrates a possible conceptualization of points on the continuum and how they relate to anorexia and bulimia. The continuum allows description of various levels of eating problems that are significant clinically. It may not be unusual for counselors

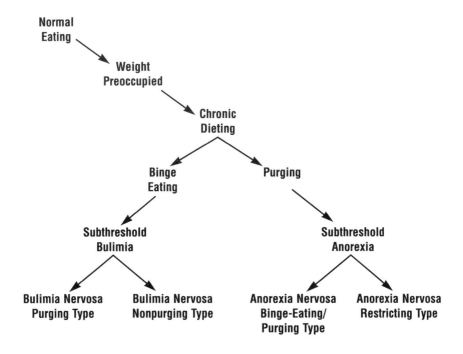

Figure 11.1. The continuum of eating disturbances and disorders.

to have clients who are preoccupied about their weight, are chronic dieters, or engage in subclinical anorexia or bulimia. Furthermore, being attentive to these nuances of diagnosis is important due to both research and treatment implications, since some characteristics of patients with eating disorders NOS may be similar to those found in individuals with bulimia or anorexia.

Epidemiology

As the previous section indicates, it is necessary to distinguish between anorexia, bulimia, and eating disorders NOS. Fairburn and Beglin (1990) reported a prevalence rate for bulimia of about 1 percent, which is in line with the *DSM-IV*, which reports a prevalence rate of 1–3 percent in adolescent and young females (APA, 1994). Anorexia is a less common disorder, with the prevalence ranging from .05–1.0 percent (APA, 1994). Subclinical anorexia and bulimia (which would be classified as eating disorders NOS) are more common, especially among college-aged women (Kalodner &

Scarano, 1992; Mintz & Betz, 1988). Subclinical bulimia is reported in 17–27 percent of college women, while other groups on the continuum (including chronic dieters, binge-eaters, purgers), range from 10–14 percent (Kalodner & Scarano, 1992; Mintz & Betz, 1988). In Fairburn and Beglin's summary of the prevalence of key features of eating disorders of females between 14 and 40 years of age, binge-eating was reported by 35.8 percent of respondents, strict dieting or fasting by 29 percent, self-induced vomiting by 8 percent, and laxative misuse by 6 percent. These data are important since they highlight the high prevalence of binge-eating and use of unhealthy weight control strategies among individuals who may not meet *DSM* criteria for an eating disorder.

There is a much higher prevalence of eating disorders in women relative to men, with 90 percent of cases of anorexia and bulimia occurring in females (APA, 1994). Reports of eating disorders in males do exist (e.g., Andersen, 1990), and some researchers have noted that eating problems in males are becoming more prevalent, especially among some special groups of men, such as wrestlers (Enns, Drewnowski, & Grinker, 1987).

Adolescence is a critical time for the development of eating disorders NOS, which may serve as a precursor to anorexia and bulimia. For females, body dissatisfaction increases with the onset of adolescence that may be, in part, a result of physical changes during puberty, especially an increase in body fat (Brooks-Gunn, 1987; Gralen, Levine, Smolak, & Muren, 1990). Adolescents seem to misperceive their weight and body size, defining themselves as overweight when they are not (cf. Killen et al., 1987). Such misperceptions may lead them to engage in unhealthy weight regulation practices, such as chronic dieting and purging. Almost 70 percent of a sample of female high school students reported that they were presently trying to lose weight (Rosen, Tacy, & Howell, 1990). Alarmingly, this concern about weight and body shape is also evident in children; 30 percent of 9-year-olds reported worrying that they were too fat, and 9 percent reported purging behavior to control weight (Mellin, Irwin, & Scully, 1992).

Associated Psychological Features

Eating disorders are often concurrent with other psychological issues. Depressive symptoms may be found in individuals with anorexia and bulimia, while obsessive-compulsive issues are more often associated with anorexia (APA, 1994). A genetic link between depression and eating disorders is still being explored. First-degree relatives of women with eating disorders have a greater than expected chance of having an eating disorder or an affective disorder (Gershon, Schreiber, & Hamovit, 1984; Hudson, Pope, Jonas, & Yurgelun-Todd, 1983). In addition, the *DSM-IV* indicates that one-third to one-half of all individuals with bulimia also meet the criteria for a personality disorder (APA, 1994). To be sure that associated issues are addressed in treatment, a global assessment of psychological functioning is recommended as a part of all clinical work with individuals who describe concerns with eating-related problems.

Comorbidity of eating disorders with substance abuse is also an issue. The prevalence of comorbid substance abuse in women requesting treatment for an eating disorder ranges from under 3 percent to over 59 percent, with a median of 22 percent (Holderness, Brooks-Gunn, & Warren, 1994). The *DSM-IV* reports that a third of individuals with bulimia also meet criteria for substance abuse or dependence. In considering this, it is advisable to assess for both eating disorders and substance abuse in individuals seeking treatment for either, since treatment issues may be further complicated by this dual diagnosis.

Physical Health Issues Associated with Eating Disorders

Eating disorders are associated with a variety of physical health problems and medical complications. In anorexia, the medical issues that arise are the result of starvation and malnutrition. In bulimia, medical issues usually develop as a consequence of the methods of purging used.

Anorexia nervosa is associated with 10 percent mortality rate (higher than most other psychiatric problems). Death may occur due to starvation, suicide, or electrolyte imbalance (APA, 1994). The physical symptoms of anorexia nervosa may affect most major organ systems and have serious implications for both cardiovascular and renal functioning. Starvation itself may be the cause of several medical problems, such as constipation, abdominal pain, cold intolerance, lethargy, and excess energy (APA, 1994).

The medical complications associated with bulimia are related to the methods of compensation used to avoid the weight gain associated with binge-eating. Metabolic complications (i.e., low serum chloride, potassium, magnesium) are associated with vomiting and laxative and diuretic abuse.

Vomiting is also responsible for dental erosion, pharyngeal/esophageal inflammation, and esophageal and gastric tears. An additional warning about the use of syrup of ipecac is important—when it is used repeatedly to induce vomiting, it may accumulate and become cardiotoxic. In addition, chronic laxative use may lead to dependence on laxatives to stimulate colon functioning. Diuretic use is associated with dehydration that can lead to loss of kidney function.

It is beyond the scope of this chapter to provide details on issues related to the medical complications of eating disorders. For complete information on this topic, see Mitchell, Pomeroy, and Adson (1997) or Sansone and Sansone (1994). Consultation with medical professionals is essential when working with individuals with anorexia and may be necessary when treating individuals with bulimia, since many of the medical complications described above can rapidly become life-threatening.

Eating Disorders in Ethnic Minorities

Until recently, eating disorders were typically described as a Western cultural phenomenon facing primarily middle- to upper-class white females. There is evidence, however, that symptoms of eating disorders exist among various ethnic and cultural minority groups in the United States (see Kalodner, 1996). Three comprehensive reviews of the literature (Davis & Yager, 1992; Dolan, 1991; Pate, Pumariega, Hester, & Garner, 1992) support the cross-cultural prevalence of eating disorders and provide examples of eating disorders in other cultures both within and outside the United States. The assumption that eating disorders do not exist in non-white females may lead professionals to miss early warning signs.

Assessment

The *DSM-IV* criteria described earlier must be met for the diagnoses of anorexia nervosa, bulimia nervosa, and other forms of eating problems. Assessment of eating disorders and associated issues may be accomplished through interviews, self-reports of behaviors, attitudes and thoughts, and through self-monitoring and behavioral observation.

An advantage of using interviews is that a greater understanding of the breadth and depth of the eating behavior and its associated psychological issues is obtained. The utility of interviews may be limited because they require more than an hour to complete and specialized training for the inter- viewer. The Eating Disorder Examination (EDE), now in its 12th edition (Fairburn & Cooper, 1993), is an example of a structured interview designed to assess the specific psychopathology of eating disorders. Overeating (binge-eating) and extreme methods of weight control and restraint, eating concern, shape concern, and weight concern are assessed. Significant corre- lations between the EDE and self-report measures indicate that once a diag- nosis of bulimia is established, self-reports could be used to assess progress and measure treatment outcome (Loeb, Pike, Walsh, & Wilson, 1994). However, the EDE may be preferred to assess the more psychological con- structs of restraint and eating concern, since the self-report measures of these constructs correlate only modestly with the EDE interview.

Due to their ease of administration, various self-report measures are used frequently in both clinical and research settings. Two recommended self- report assessment tools are the Eating Attitudes Test (EAT-26; Garner, Olmsted, Bohr, & Garfinkel, 1982) and Eating Disorders Inventory-2 (EDI- 2; Garner, 1991). These measures are not designed to provide a diagnosis of a particular type of eating disorder but rather to elucidate the associated psy- chological variables. The EAT-26 is used frequently as a screening instru- ment for maladaptive eating attitudes and behaviors. In addition, there is a children's version of the Eating Attitudes Test (ChEAT; Maloney, McGuire, & Daniels, 1988), used to assess abnormal eating attitudes and behaviors in children in grades 3 through 6.

The EDI-2 (Garner, 1991) yields 11 subscales, including: drive for thin- ness, bulimia, body dissatisfaction, ineffectiveness, perfectionism, interper- sonal distrust, interoceptive awareness, maturity fears, asceticism, impulse regulation, and social insecurity. The brief descriptions in table 11.4 denote the psychological issues associated with eating disorders that have important ramifications for treatment. The EDI and EDI-2 are probably the most well known and frequently used of the self-report measures. Crowther and Sherwood (1997) provide other useful information on self-report measures.

Self-monitoring (use of eating diaries) may be a useful adjunct to thera- py along with serving as an assessment tool. Detailed information can be included, such as the frequency and content of meals, snacks, and binges, and whether the client vomited or used laxatives or diuretics. Clients may also be asked to record antecedent thoughts or feelings that can be used in

---

Table 11.4

Description of the Subscales of the Eating Disorders Inventory-2

Drive for thinness assesses thoughts and behaviors regarding dieting and preoccupation with weight and thinness.

Bulimia concerns thoughts and behaviors associated with binge-eating, including loss of control, secrecy, and vomiting.

Body dissatisfaction assesses thoughts of dissatisfaction with various body parts (i.e., stomach, thighs, hips) and body shape.

Ineffectiveness assesses feelings of inadequacy, insecurity, and aloneness.

Perfectionism assesses the need for outstanding performance and the pursuit of high goals.

Interpersonal distrust assesses feelings of trust in others (e.g., openness about feelings).

Interoceptive awareness concerns the ability to identify and understand feelings.

Maturity fears expresses the desire to be younger.

Asceticism concerns the desire to be self-disciplined and engage in self-denial.

Impulse regulation concerns the ability to control own thoughts and behavior (e.g., have strange thoughts or feelings).

Social insecurity concerns anxiety in interpersonal settings.

---

planning treatment strategies. Behavioral observation, usually conducted by a friend or family member or other person selected by the client, is used less frequently but may provide more precise information about eating behavior than self-monitoring.

Intervention: An Introduction

There are a tremendous number of interventions designed for treating eating disorders, only some of which have been the focus of controlled outcome research. As a result, there is a lack of consensus about the "best" treatment for bulimia (Herzog, Keller, Strober, Yeh, & Pai, 1992) and an insufficient amount of evidence to provide empirically-based suggestions for treatment of anorexia (Goldner & Birmingham, 1994; Herzog et al., 1992). In a survey of clinicians participating in two International Conferences on Eating Disorders, psychologists and physicians were likely to endorse treatments for anorexia that have not yet been demonstrated to be efficacious, although these treatments had been studied and supported for treatment of bulimia

(Herzog et al., 1992). Not surprisingly, medical doctors were more likely than psychologists to endorse drugs as a treatment for anorexia and bulimia in depressed individuals (Herzog et al., 1992). The issue of medication as an adjunct to psychological intervention and recommendations regarding medication are discussed later in this chapter.

Anorexia, bulimia, and eating disorders NOS are disorders that share many features; therefore, it makes sense that there are features of treatment that address these common themes regardless of the type of eating disorder. However, since there are also meaningful differences between anorexia and bulimia, there are aspects of treatment that should differ. For example, Garner, Vitousek, and Pike (1997) point out that the topic of weight is entirely different in treatment of anorexia and bulimia. In the cognitive-behavioral approach to treatment of bulimia, patients are informed that, in most cases, treatment has little or no effect on weight; therefore, they can eat much more than they think without gaining weight. Since weight gain is a major goal in the treatment of anorexia, however, this argument is not usable. When treating anorexia, the fear of weight gain must be addressed while the client is actually gaining weight.

Garner and Needleman (1997) provide a flowchart to assist clinicians in decision-making regarding treatment. The chart uses a series of questions to recommend treatment approaches based on the client's presenting concerns. For example, the chart indicates that a patient who is not in physical danger and has a moderate to severe eating disorder should be treated by individual cognitive-behavioral therapy. Patients who are emaciated, experiencing physical complications, or who are a suicide risk should be hospitalized for psychological treatment along with medical stabilization and weight restoration (if necessary). Treatments included in the flowchart are hospitalization, day treatment, family therapy, self-help/education, individual cognitive-behavioral therapy, medication, interpersonal therapy, and a longer-term integration of cognitive-behavioral approaches, psychodynamic therapy, interpersonal therapy, and family therapy.

As noted above, the extant empirical literature allows us to draw few conclusions regarding what constitutes effective treatment for anorexia. Garner and colleagues (1997) describe a cognitive-behavioral program for treating anorexia that contains some components of the empirically validated program for treatment of bulimia and addresses issues specific to anorexia, such as the effects of starvation and the need for weight gain. Although there are case studies that document the efficacy of this type of intervention, there are no large-scale clinical trials at present. Specific issues that require attention in the treatment of anorexia include (Goldner & Birmingham, 1994):

- medical stabilization
- establishment of therapeutic alliance
- weight restoration
- promotion of healthy eating attitudes, behaviors, and activity levels
- psychotherapeutic treatment
- family and community interventions

In the following pages, two different empirically validated interventions for bulimia are presented. These include cognitive-behavioral therapy and interpersonal therapy. The level of detail necessary to conduct therapy is not provided. For such information, readers are encouraged to read the sources cited and to obtain supervision from clinicians experienced in working with these disorders.

Individual Approaches

Considerable research focuses on cognitive-behavioral approaches; in fact, cognitive-behavioral therapy is described as a treatment of choice for bulimia (Wilson & Fairburn, 1993; Wilson, Fairburn, & Agras, 1997). A primary focus is to change cognitive distortions related to body image and other maladaptive cognitions that seem to exist in individuals with bulimia (e.g., perfectionism and low self-esteem). With modifications, cognitive-behavioral therapy may be successfully used to treat binge-eating disorder. Cognitive-behavioral therapy attempts to modify behaviors by:

- using strategies such as self-monitoring and stimulus control
- educating patients about body weight regulation and the hazards of purging
- presenting nutritional information

Interpersonal therapy also has empirical support. Two controlled treatment outcome studies demonstrate the effectiveness of interpersonal therapy for the treatment of bulimia (Fairburn et al., 1991; Fairburn, Kirk, O'Connor, & Cooper, 1986). Interpersonal therapy, originally developed to address depression, focuses on a detailed analysis of the interpersonal context within which the eating disorder developed and has been maintained

(Fairburn, 1997; Fairburn et al., 1991). The eating disorder is understood as an interpersonal issue, and treatment addresses these interpersonal problems; no attention is given to eating habits or behavior.

Fairburn and colleagues (1991) compared cognitive-behavioral therapy with a behavioral version (behavior therapy; all cognitive components removed) of cognitive-behavioral therapy treatment and with interpersonal therapy treatments for bulimia. Although clients rated the three approaches as equally credible forms of therapy, the researchers concluded that cognitive-behavioral therapy was more effective than behavior therapy or interpersonal therapy for treatment of bulimia. Interestingly, interpersonal therapy was as effective as cognitive-behavioral therapy in modifying loss of control over eating, although interpersonal therapy does not target eating problems specifically. Interpersonal therapy was less effective in dealing with disturbed attitudes toward weight and shape, attempts to diet, and use of vomiting. Cognitive-behavioral therapy was judged to be superior to behavior therapy, although behavior therapy was effective in reducing overeating, vomiting, and general psychiatric symptoms. A follow-up report four, eight, and twelve months after treatment indicated both cognitive-behavioral therapy and interpersonal therapy were efficacious treatments for bulimia, although they seemed to effect change in different ways (Fairburn, Jones, Peveler, Hope, & O'Connor, 1993). These results suggest that treatment effects were substantial, were reflected in all aspects of functioning, and were well-maintained. Although interpersonal therapy was inferior to cognitive-behavioral therapy at the end of treatment, at follow-up this did not continue to be true. The proportion of clients who had a positive outcome as a result of therapy during the subsequent 12-month follow-up was equivalent (cognitive-behavioral therapy and interpersonal therapy). Improved interpersonal functioning thus appears to be an efficacious way to treat bulimia.

Family Therapy

There is more literature on family therapy for anorexia nervosa than there is on bulimia, although a great deal of literature is descriptive and evaluations of the efficacy of family interventions have not been studied to the same extent as individual and group interventions. According to Garner and Needleman's (1997) flowchart, family therapy is the treatment of choice for patients who are 18 years old or younger and who live at home.

Families of individuals with anorexia have been described as having characteristics of enmeshment, overprotectiveness, and rigidity. Enmeshment and overprotectiveness refer to boundaries that are not well established and often leave the person with anorexia feeling as though she cannot separate herself from her family. Rigidity within the family system involves the persistence in behaviors that are not adaptive. There are also issues around conflict, typically involving the family's inability to tolerate disagreement and avoidance of topics that are likely to spark controversy.

In family therapy, it is essential to treat the entire family as a unit, rather than allow the individual with anorexia to be the identified patient. Families are often in a great deal of distress over the low weight and food refusal of the person with anorexia. Since consistent weight gain is an important part of treatment for the anorexia, this aspect of treatment must be addressed with the entire family. While it is the responsibility of the person with anorexia to gain weight, parents and family are encouraged to assist by allowing her to eat foods of her choosing.

Group Therapy

Groups provide a promising modality for the treatment of bulimia, in that they help to reduce the secrecy and shame associated with eating disorders, supply a place for reality-testing of distorted beliefs and self-perceptions among others who are also facing eating disorders, and provide an interpersonal context to facilitate links between eating disorders and interpersonal relationships (Fettes & Peters, 1992; Oesterheld, McKenna, & Gould, 1987). In a meta-analysis of group treatment for bulimia, Fettes and Peters concluded that about a quarter of participants in group therapy are completely abstinent from bulimic symptoms after receiving nine hours of group therapy. The abstinence rate was maintained or increased in the year following treatment. Oesterheld and colleagues noted that the percentage reduction in binge/purge episodes varies between 52 percent and 97 percent at the end of group treatment.

Approaches to group work with clients who have eating disorders vary considerably. Most often, groups are active and symptom- and affect-focused (Oesterheld et al., 1987). Common features include a focus on the here-and-now, use of journals, cognitive restructuring, incremental goal-setting, and support (Oesterheld et al., 1987). Interestingly, group treatment in combination with additional therapy was found to be more effective than group therapy alone (Fettes & Peters, 1992). No particular type of group treatment has consistently demonstrated better results than others (Polivy & Federoff, 1997). It is likely that the nonspecific factors of group interventions (e.g., universality, interpersonal learning, and other therapeutic factors; Yalom, 1995) contribute to the power of group treatment (Polivy & Federoff, 1997).

Due to some of the difficulties in doing group work with individuals who have anorexia, considerably less is known about these group interventions. Since the 1980s, group studies have focused almost exclusively on bulimic individuals (Polivy & Federoff, 1997). Hall (1985) noted that in group treatment, anorexics are often withdrawn, anxious, rigid, and egocentric; they are preoccupied with body weight and food and have extreme difficulty identifying and expressing feelings. Group work can be one of the most demanding and anxiety-provoking and least rewarding of the psychotherapies in use for anorexia (Hall, 1985). Consequently, some therapists do not use group approaches at all for the treatment of anorexia. Nevertheless, Hall provides some direction about selection, group composition, group process, and other issues.

There is a growing body of literature on the use of groups with eating disorders NOS. McNamara's (1989) group intervention for repeat dieters is an example. This structured group program was designed to replace dieting with healthier eating and regular, moderate exercise and to increase body esteem by encouraging self-acceptance. Eating behaviors and weight preoccupation were also addressed, in addition to psychological issues common in chronic dieters, such as perfectionism, assertiveness, and depression. Polivy and Herman (1992) developed a similar program called "undieting," aimed at reducing dieting behavior in overweight women. The undieting program led to a significant reduction on various EDI subscales, indicating that the program was able to reduce some maladaptive attitudes and behaviors related to body and weight issues.

Support Groups

Support or self-help groups are common in the treatment of eating disorders. Enright, Butterfield, and Berkowitz (1985) indicated that support groups are usually free of charge, held in a nontherapy setting, and are often led by persons who have recovered from an eating problem rather than a mental health professional. A support group may be the first contact a person with an eating problem makes for help. Many self-help groups are associated with national organizations such as Anorexia Nervosa and Associated Disorders. National organizations may also provide newsletters, telephone hotlines, Web sites, and consultation to parents and professionals. Some support groups have a speaker and limited discussions, while others are more loosely defined and open to whatever topics are presented by members. There is tremendous variation in the kinds of support groups offered and little empirical evidence to indicate which kinds of groups are of most benefit with various kinds of eating problems. It is also not known how support groups meet the needs of individuals at different stages of recovery. Clearly, more research would help elucidate these important questions.

Despite the dearth of empirical data, referrals to support groups may be useful as an adjunct to counseling or as continued support after formal therapy has ended. Mental health professionals may benefit from learning about the kinds of groups available in their community.

Education

The importance of nutritional education in working with individuals who have anorexia, bulimia, or eating disorders NOS cannot be overlooked. Rock and Yager (1987) and O'Connor, Touyz, and Beaumont (1988) provide basic information on nutrition as it applies to eating disorders. The impact of nutrition on eating behavior and health is not typically part of the educational experience of the majority of mental health professionals. For example, few counselors know that zinc deficiencies are common in patients with anorexia. Zinc deficiencies alter taste thresholds for bitter and sour tastes and reduce appetite. In working with anorexia patients who use what seems to be a great deal of lemon juice, it can be hypothesized that this may be due to lack of zinc. To provide comprehensive care, it is important for mental health providers to consult with registered dietitians and physicians, thus ensuring that treatment issues relevant to health and nutritional status are addressed.

Prevention

A key issue in the field of eating disorders is prevention. Unfortunately, the first long-term controlled prevention program was not successful in influencing eating attitudes and habits in adolescent girls. Killen and colleagues' (1993) intervention was developed and implemented with sixth- and seventh-grade girls and included lessons addressing weight gain as a normal and necessary part of growth in females, excessive dieting as an ineffective long-term weight control strategy that may lead to weight dysregulation, methods adolescents can use to counteract the cultural pressures promoting dieting and a thin body, and adaptation of more healthful nutrition practices and realistic physical activity programs. Although there were gains in knowledge after participating in the 18-session program, there were no significant changes in eating attitudes or weight reduction practices. Killen and colleagues suggested that this type of program may be more effective as a secondary prevention program aimed at high-risk adolescents who are already expressing weight concerns or body image dissatisfaction.

Controversies

Sexual Abuse

The causal relationship between sexual abuse and eating disorders is a topic that has received a great deal of attention. Disagreement seems to focus on the specificity of the risk: Does sexual abuse constitute a specific risk for eating disorders or is sexual abuse a risk for any psychiatric problem? (Kearney-Cooke & Striegel-Moore, 1994). Controlled studies have shown that childhood sexual abuse is associated with increased risk for a variety of psychiatric problems, including eating disorders (Pope & Hudson, 1992; Welch & Fairburn, 1994). A study by Welch and Fairburn indicated that sexual abuse is not a risk factor specific to the development of bulimia. However, Kearney-Cooke and Striegel-Moore provide a strong argument in support of the specificity link. Using a trauma conceptualization, Root (1991) describes a link between eating disorders and childhood sexual abuse and rape.

Several psychological factors are associated with both eating disorders and sexual abuse, such as diminished self-esteem, self-blame, dissociation, issues with control, and personality disorders (Waller, Everill, & Calam, 1994). The dissociation link is a particularly interesting one (cf. Heatherton & Baumister, 1991), since it posits that dissociation may be a part of the binge-eating experience as well as part of the repression of memories of sexual abuse (Waller et al., 1994). The issue of the link between sexual abuse and eating disorders, however, remains a topic of continued attention.

Pharmacotherapy

Drug treatment recommendations differ for bulimia and anorexia. It can be concluded from the literature that medication should not be the exclusive mode of treatment for either disorder. At present, there is no evidence that antidepressants or other medications are effective treatments for anorexia (Garfinkel & Walsh, 1997; Leach, 1995). Furthermore, the side effects of antidepressant medications are especially problematic with anorexia. In contrast, bulimia has been responsive to treatment with antidepressant medications. Antidepressants were described as useful, independent of the presence of depression, in the practice guidelines for eating disorders published by the American Psychiatric Association (APA, 1993). Garfinkel and Walsh (1997) state that since there is no demonstrated efficacy of a particular antidepressant over others, choice of a particular medication should be based on minimizing side effects. At the same time, medications should be viewed as a part of a comprehensive treatment package and should not be prescribed without attention to the psychological issues that are addressed in individual, group, or family therapy.

Influence of the Media

Sociocultural pressures are often cited as an important contributor to the development of eating disorders (Streigel-Moore, Silberstein, & Rodin, 1986), and the media is often blamed for perpetuating and furthering these sociocultural pressures to be thin. Most research has addressed the effects of the media on individuals already suffering from eating disorders; however, it seems that vulnerability to media influences is not limited to those individuals experiencing eating disordered behavior. Irving (1990) noted lower self-evaluation in both individuals with eating disorders and female college students without eating disorders. Murray, Touyz, and Beumont (1996) found that female controls were as likely to be influenced by the media as women currently in treatment for eating disorders. A study designed to assess the immediate impact of very brief exposure to media on the self-consciousness and anxiety of male and female college students also found that there is a negative impact of media presentations of thin models on non-eating-disordered college women (Kalodner, 1997).

Body-image was described as "elastic" by Myers and Biocca (1992), meaning that body-image is unstable and can be manipulated by social cues. Might it also be possible to influence women to feel more positively about their body? Can we teach young women to decrease the comparisons they make with images in magazines and on television? Thinking more critically about the ideals promoted by the media may help to lessen the impact of the message (Murray et al., 1996). It seems as though women, regardless of their eating disorder status, experience societal pressure, expressed in the media, to be thin. Perhaps the degree of media influence should be studied as a potential risk factor for the development of serious eating disorders.

Summary

Eating disorders are a part of our society, perhaps because our society continues to focus on the importance of thinness and dieting. This impact, along with other biological and psychological risk factors, may be influential in the development of eating disorders and less severe eating problems, particularly among women during adolescence and early adulthood. Much is not known about eating disorders, particularly in the area of treatment for anorexia. Effective prevention programs have not been developed, although it is clear that they are necessary. We need to know more about risk factors with additional attention to those factors that protect individuals from progressing along the eating disorders continuum. Professionals from psychological, medical, and allied health fields working together may be taking a step toward achieving these goals.

Suggested Resources

Current information about eating disorders is available in two journals devoted to this topic. *The International Journal of Eating Disorders* and *Eating Disorders: The Journal of Treatment and Prevention* contain clinical information and research on various aspects of eating disorders.

Two book chapters detail the medical complications of eating disorders:

- "Managing Medical Complications" (Mitchell, Pomeroy, & Adson, 1997)

- "Bulimia Nervosa: Medical Complications" (Sansone & Sansone, 1994).

The multicultural impact of eating disorders is discussed in the following:

- "Transcultural Aspects of Eating Disorders: A Review" (Davis & Yager, 1992)
- "Cross-Cultural Aspects of Anorexia Nervosa and Bulimia: A Review" (Dolan, 1991)
- "Eating Discorders from a Multicultural Perspective" (Kalodner, 1996)
- "Cross-Cultural Patterns in Eating Disorders: A Review" (Pate, Pumariega, Hester, &, Garner, 1992).

For more information on assessment, especially interviews, self-report measures, and self-monitoring, see "Assessment" by Crowther and Sherwood (1997).

There are a tremendous number of resources for treatment of eating disorders:

- A flowchart to assist clinicians in decision-making regarding treatment is presented in "Sequencing and Integration of Treatments" (Garner & Needleman, 1997).
- Cognitive-behavioral therapy treatment information is provided in "Cognitive-Behavioral Therapy for Binge Eating and Bulimia Nervosa: A Comprehensive Treatment Manual" (Fairburn, Marcus, & Wilson, 1993) and "Cognitive-Behavioral Therapy for Bulimia Nervosa" (Wilson, Fairburn, & Agras, 1997).
- Procedures for interpersonal therapy are detailed in "Interpersonal Psychotherapy for Bulimia Nervosa" (Fairburn, 1997).
- Family therapy with anorexia patients is discussed by Dare and Eisler (1997) and Sargent, Liebman, and Silver (1985); Schwartz, Barrett, and Saba (1985) discuss family therapy for bulimia.
- A review of treatment groups for bulimia is presented in a table in "Experimental Group Research: Can the Cannon Fire?" (Bednar & Kaul, 1994).
- Readers interested in more information on group work with anorexia are encouraged to read "Group Psychotherapy for Anorexia Nervosa" (Hall, 1985).

Discussion Questions

1. What are the psychological issues often associated with anorexia and bulimia?
2. Why is it problematic to assume that eating disorders exist only in white females?
3. How can interviews and self-report measures be used to provide a comprehensive assessment of a patient with an eating disorder?
4. Describe key features of the treatments that have been demonstrated to be effective for bulimia.
5. Why does group therapy seem to an especially promising modality to treat bulimia?
6. How are treatments for anorexia and bulimia similar? How do they differ?
7. What are the current recommendations regarding drug treatments for eating disorders?

References

American Psychiatric Association (1994). *Diagnostic and statistical manual of mental disorders* (4th ed.). Washington DC: Author.

American Psychiatric Association (1993). Practice guidelines for eating disorders. *American Journal of Psychiatry, 150,* 212–228.

Andersen, A. E. (1990). *Males with eating disorders.* New York: Brunner/Mazel.

Bednar, R. L., & Kaul, T. J. (1994). Experiential group research: Can the cannon fire? In A. E. Bergin, & S. L. Garfield (Eds.), *Handbook of psychotherapy and behavior change* (4th ed., pp. 631–663). New York: Wiley.

Brooks-Gunn, J. (1987). Pubertal processes and girls' psychological adaptation. In R. M. Lerner, & T. T. Foch (Eds.), *Biological psychosocial interactions in early adolescence* (pp. 123–153). Hillsdale, NJ: Earlbaum.

Crowther, J. H., & Sherwood, N. E. (1997). Assessment. In D. M. Garner, & P. E. Garfinkel (Eds.), *Handbook of treatment for eating disorders* (2nd ed., pp. 34–49). New York: Guilford.

Dare, C., & Eisler, I. (1997). Family therapy for anorexia nervosa. In D. M. Garner, & P. E. Garfinkel (Eds.), *Handbook of treatment for eating disorders* (2nd ed., pp. 307–324). New York: Guilford.

Davis, C., & Yager, J. (1992). Transcultural aspects of eating disorders: A review. *Culture, Medicine, & Psychiatry, 16,* 377–394.

Dolan, B. (1991). Cross-cultural aspects of anorexia nervosa and bulimia: A Review. *International Journal of Eating Disorders, 10,* 67–78.

Enns, M. P., Drewnowski, A., & Grinker, J. A. (1987). Body composition, body size estimation and attitudes towards eating in male college athletes. *Psychosomatic Medicine, 49,* 56–64.

Enright, A. B., Butterfield, P., & Berkowitz, B. (1985) Self-help and support groups in the management of eating disorders. In D. M. Garner, & P. E. Garfinkel (Eds.), *Handbook of psychotherapy for anorexia nervosa and bulimia* (pp. 491–512). New York: Guilford.

Fairburn, C. G. (1997). Interpersonal psychotherapy for bulimia nervosa. In D. M. Garner, & P. E. Garfinkel (Eds.), *Handbook of treatment for eating disorders* (2nd ed., pp. 278–294). New York: Guilford.

Fairburn, C. G., & Beglin, S. J. (1990). Studies of the epidemiology of bulimia nervosa. *American Journal of Psychiatry, 147,* 401–408.

Fairburn, C. G., & Cooper, Z. (1993). The Eating Disorder Examination. In C. G. Fairburn, & G. T. Wilson (Eds.), *Binge eating: Nature, assessment and treatment* (pp. 317–360). New York: Guilford.

Fairburn, C. G., Jones, R., Peveler, R. C., Carr, S. J., Solomon, R. A., O'Connor, M., Burton, J., & Hope, R. A. (1991). Three psychological treatments for bulimia nervosa: A comparative trial. *Archives of General Psychiatry, 48,* 463–469.

Fairburn, C. G., Jones, R., Peveler, R. C., Hope, R. A., & O'Connor, M. (1993). Psychotherapy and bulimia nervosa: Longer-term effects of interpersonal psychotherapy, behavior therapy, and cognitive behavior therapy. *Archives of General Psychiatry, 50,* 419–428.

Fairburn, C. G., Kirk, J., O'Connor, M., & Cooper, P. J. (1986). A comparison of two psychological treatments for bulimia nervosa. *Behaviour Research and Therapy, 24,* 629–643.

Fairburn, C. G., Marcus, M. D., & Wilson, G. T. (1993). Cognitive-behavioral therapy for binge eating and bulimia nervosa: A comprehensive treatment manual. In C. G. Fairburn, & G. T. Wilson (Eds.), *Binge eating: Nature, assessment and treatment* (pp. 361–404). New York: Guilford.

Fettes, P. A., & Peters, J. M. (1992). A meta-analysis of group treatment for bulimia nervosa. *International Journal of Eating Disorders, 11*(2), 97–110.

Garfinkel, P. E., & Walsh, B. T. (1997). Drug therapies. In D. M. Garner, & P. E. Garfinkel (Eds.), *Handbook of treatment for eating disorders* (2nd ed., pp. 372–380). New York: Guilford.

Garner, D. M. (1991). *Eating Disorder Inventory-II.* Odessa, FL: Psychological Assessment Resources.

Garner, D. M., & Needleman, L. D. (1997). Sequencing and integration of treatments. In D. M. Garner, & P. E. Garfinkel (Eds.), *Handbook of treatment for eating disorders* (2nd ed., pp. 50–63). New York: Guilford.

Garner, D. M., Olmsted, M. P., Bohr, Y., & Garfinkel, P. E. (1982). The Eating Attitudes Test: Psychometric features and clinical correlates. *Psychological Medicine, 12,* 871–878.

Garner, D. M., Vitousek, K. M., & Pike, K. M. (1997). Cognitive-behavioral therapy for anorexia nervosa. In D. M. Garner, & P. E. Garfinkel (Eds.), *Handbook of treatment for eating disorders* (2nd ed., pp. 94–144). New York: Guilford Press.

Gershon, E. S., Schreiber, J. L., & Hamovit, J.R. (1984). Clinical findings in patients with anorexia nervosa and affective illness in their relatives. *American Journal of Psychiatry, 141,* 1419–1422.

Goldner, E. M., & Birmingham, C. L. (1994). Anorexia Nervosa: Methods of treatment. In L. Alexander-Mott, & D. B. Lumsden (Eds.), *Understanding eating disorders* (pp. 135–157). Washington DC: Taylor & Francis.

Gralen, S. J., Levine, M. P., Smolak, L., & Muren, S. K. (1990). Dieting and disordered eating during early and middle adolescence: Do the influences remain the same? *International Journal of Eating Disorders, 9,* 501–512.

Hall, A. (1985). Group psychotherapy for anorexia nervosa. In D. M. Garner, & P. E. Garfinkel (Eds.), *Handbook of psychotherapy for anorexia nervosa and bulimia* (pp. 213–239). New York: Guilford.

Heatherton, T. F., & Baumister, R. F. (1991). Binge eating as escape from self-awareness. *Psychological Bulletin, 110,* 86–108.

Herzog, D. B., Keller, M. B., Strober, M., Yeh, C., & Pai, S. (1992). The current status of treatment for anorexia nervosa and bulimia nervosa. *International Journal of Eating Disorders, 12*(2), 215–220.

Holderness, C. C., Brooks-Gunn, J., & Warren, M. P. (1994). Co-morbidity of eating disorders and substance abuse review of the literature. *International Journal of Eating Disorders, 16*(1), 1–34.

Hudson, J. I., Pope, H. G., Jonas, J. M., & Yurgelun-Todd, D. (1983). Family history of anorexia nervosa and bulimia. *British Journal of Psychiatry, 142,* 133–138.

Irving, L. M. (1990). Mirror images: Effects of the standard of beauty on the self- and body-esteem of women exhibiting varying levels of bulimic symptoms. *Journal of Social and Clinical Psychology, 9*(2), 230–242.

Kalodner, C. R. (1996). Eating disorders from a multicultural perspective. In J. L. DeLucia-Waack (Ed.), *Multicultural counseling competencies: Implications for training and practice* (pp. 197–216). Alexandria, VA: Association for Counselor Education and Supervision.

Kalodner, C. R. (1997). Media influences on male and female non-eating disordered college students: A significant issue. *Eating Disorders: The Journal of Treatment and Prevention, 5,* 47–57.

Kalodner, C. R., & Scarano, G. M. (1992). A continuum of nonclinical eating disorders: A review of behavioral and psychological correlates and suggestions for intervention. *Journal of Mental Health Counseling, 14*(1), 30–41.

Kearney-Cooke, A., & Striegel-Moore, R. H. (1994). Treatment of childhood sexual abuse in anorexia nervosa and bulimia nervosa: A feminist psychodynamic approach. *International Journal of Eating Disorders, 15,* 305–319.

Killen, J. D., Taylor, C. B., Hammer, L. D., Litt, I., Wilson, D. M., Rich, T., Hayward, C., Simmonds, B., Kraemer, H., Varady, A. (1993). An attempt to modify unhealthful eating attitudes and weight regulation practices of young adolescent girls. *International Journal of Eating Disorders, 13*(4), 369–384.

Killen, J. D., Taylor, C. B., Telch, M. J., Saylor, K. E., Maron, D. J., & Robinson, T. N. (1987). Depressive symptoms and substance abuse among adolescent binge eaters and purgers: A defined population study. *American Journal of Public Health, 77,* 1539–1541.

Leach, A. M. (1995). The psychopharmacotherapy of eating disorders. *Psychiatric Annals, 25,* 628–633.

Loeb, K. L., Pike, K. M., Walsh, B. T., & Wilson, G. T. (1994). Assessment of diagnostic features of bulimia nervosa: Interview versus self-report format. *International Journal of Eating Disorders, 16*(1), 75–81.

Maloney, M. J., McGuire, J. B., & Daniels, S. R. (1988) Reliability testing of a children's version of the Eating Attitudes Test. *American Academy of Child and Adolescent Psychiatry, 27,* 541–543.

McNamara, K. (1989). A structured group program for repeat dieters. *Journal for Specialists in Group Work, 14,* 141–150.

Mellin, L. M., Irwin, C. E., Jr., & Scully, S. (1992). Prevalence of disordered eating in girls: A survey of middle-class children. *Journal of the American Dietetic Association, 92,* 851–853.

Mintz, L. B., & Betz, N. E. (1988). Prevalence and correlates of eating behaviors among college women. *Journal of Counseling Psychology, 35,* 463–471.

Mitchell, J. E., Pomeroy, C., & Adson, D. E. (1997). Managing medical complications. In D. M. Garner, & P. E. Garfinkel (Eds.), *Handbook of treatment for eating disorders* (2nd ed., pp. 383–393). New York: Guilford.

Murray, S. H., Touyz, S. W., & Beumont, P. J. V. (1996). Awareness and perceived influence of body ideas in the media: A comparison of eating disorder patients and the general community. *Eating Disorders: The Journal of Treatment & Prevention, 4*(1), 33–46.

Myers, P. N., Jr., & Biocca, F. A. (1992). The elastic body image: The effect of television advertising and programming on body image distortions in young women. *Journal of Communications, 42*(3), 108–133.

O'Connor, M., Touyz, S., & Beumont, P. (1988). Nutritional management and dietary counseling in bulimia nervosa: Some preliminary observations. *International Journal of Eating Disorders, 7*(5), 657–662.

Oesterheld, J. R., McKenna, M. S., & Gould, N. B. (1987). Group psychotherapy of bulimia: A critical review. *International Journal of Group Psychotherapy, 37*(2), 163–185.

Pate, J. E., Pumariega, A. J., Hester, C., & Garner, D. M. (1992). Cross-cultural patterns in eating disorders: A review. *Journal of the American Academy of Child and Adolescent Psychiatry, 31,* 802–809.

Polivy, J. E., & Federoff, I. (1997). Group Psychotherapy. In D. M. Garner, & P. E. Garfinkel (Eds.), *Handbook of treatment for eating disorders* (2nd ed., pp. 462–475). New York: Guilford.

Polivy, J. E., & Herman, C. P. (1992). Undieting: A program to help people stop dieting. *International Journal of Eating Disorders, 11*(3), 261–268.

Pope, H. G. Jr., & Hudson, J. I. (1992). Is childhood sexual abuse a risk factor for bulimia nervosa? *American Journal of Psychiatry, 149,* 455–463.

Rock, C. L., & Yager, J. (1987). Nutrition and eating disorders: A primer for clinicians. *International Journal of Eating Disorders, 6*(2), 267–280.

Root, M. P. P. (1991). Persistent, disordered eating as a gender-specific, post-traumatic stress response to sexual assault. *Psychotherapy, 28,* 96–102.

Rosen, J. C., Tacy, B., & Howell, D. (1990). Life stress, psychological symptoms and weight reduction in adolescent girls: A prospective analysis. *International Journal of Eating Disorders, 9,* 17–26.

Ruderman, A. J., & Besbeas, M. (1992). Psychological characteristics of dieters and bulimics. *Journal of Abnormal Psychology, 101*(3), 383–390.

Sansone, R. A., & Sansone, L. A. (1994). Bulimia nervosa: Medical complications. In L. Alexander-Mott, & D. B. Lumsden (Eds.), *Understanding eating disorders* (pp. 181–201). Washington DC: Taylor & Francis.

Sargent, J., Liebman, R., & Silver, M. (1985). Family therapy for anorexia nervosa. In D. M. Garner, & P. E. Garfinkel (Eds.), *Handbook of psychotherapy for anorexia nervosa and bulimia* (pp. 257–279). New York: Guilford.

Scarano, G. M., & Kalodner, C. R. (1994). A description of the continuum of eating disorders: Implications for intervention and research. *Journal of Counseling & Development, 72,* 356–361.

Schwartz, R. C., Barrett, M. J., & Saba, G. (1985). Family therapy for Bulimia. In D. M. Garner, & P. E. Garfinkel (Eds.), *Handbook of psychotherapy for anorexia nervosa and bulimia* (pp. 280–310). New York: Guilford.

Striegel-Moore, R. H., Silberstein, L. R., & Rodin, J. (1986). Toward and understanding of risk factors for bulimia. *American Psychologist, 41*(3), 246–263.

Waller, G., Everill, J., & Calam, R. (1994). Sexual abuse and the eating disorders. In L. Alexander-Mott, & D. B. Lumsden (Eds.), *Understanding Eating Disorders* (pp. 135–157). Washington DC: Taylor & Francis.

Welch, S. L., & Fairburn, C. G. (1994) Sexual abuse and bulimia nervosa: Three integrated case control comparisons. *American Journal of Psychiatry, 151,* 402–407.

Wilson, G. T., & Fairburn, C. G. (1993). Cognitive treatments for eating disorders. *Journal of Consulting and Clinical Psychology, 61,* 261–279.

Wilson, G. T., Fairburn, C. G., & Agras, W. S. (1997). Cognitive-behavioral therapy for bulimia nervosa. In D. M. Garner, & P. E. Garfinkel (Eds.), *Handbook of treatment for eating disorders* (2nd ed., pp. 67–93). New York: Guilford.

Yalom, I. D. (1995). *The theory and practice of group psychotherapy* (4th ed.). New York: Basic.

III
SPECIAL POPULATIONS

12

Health Counseling for Children and Adolescents in Medical Settings

Marilyn Stern
Bonnie J. McIntosh
Sloan L. Norman

The mental health specialty of child health psychology evolved in large part because practitioners of both pediatric medicine and child psychology recognized that issues related to children dealing with medical stressors were not being adequately addressed by either of these two fields (Roberts & McNeal, 1995). Thus, the knowledge base essential to the interdisciplinary field of child health psychology must include a basic understanding of the medical stressors being experienced by the child as well as the clinical concerns related to working with children and adolescents. One key to the role of psychologists working within a health setting is evaluating how well patients are coping with or adapting to their illness. In the case of child health psychology, this becomes a concern with how well otherwise normally functioning children deal with what might be regarded as a more extreme stressor. This perspective fits within the philosophical orientation from which counseling psychologists operate, focusing on normal, developmental, and systemic processes as opposed to pathology (Altmaier, 1990).

On a systemic level, working effectively with children requires a basic knowledge of the familial, school, and cultural systems that impact children's lives. Those working with children in the medical setting must also be aware of the organizational complexities of the medical environment and the manner in which they interact with these contextual factors in affecting the patient's functioning. Underlying an understanding of systemic factors and fundamental to the knowledge base of child health psychologists is developmental psychology as it pertains to children and adolescents facing medical challenges (Peterson & Harbeck, 1988).

Child health psychologists work in a broad range of settings, including pediatric hospital units, outpatient clinics, intensive care units, and private practice settings. Physical and health-related concerns are among the presenting problems encountered in each of these settings, but they are most likely to be seen by child health psychologists working in hospitals (Roberts, 1986). In order to maintain the focus on the unique aspects of the provision of services offered by child health psychologists, our discussion will be primarily limited to those issues relevant to working within a traditional medical setting. Within this context, the chapter will focus on developmental and systemic issues relevant to working with a pediatric population and how these issues impact methods of assessment and intervention used to assist children and families in adapting to medical stressors.

Population

Counseling psychologists working with children must have a basic theoretical and practical understanding of the major substages of childhood in order to adequately address the emotional, educational, and social developmental needs of the youngest members of our society. Stern and Newland (1994) briefly outlined the major characteristics related to physical, social, and cognitive development associated with each of these substages. In helping children and adolescents learn to adjust to their illness and more effectively manage the stressors associated with the medical environment, psychologists working in this arena must possess a solid foundation in the basic theories of development, that is, cognitive development à la Piaget, psychosocial development à la Erikson, moral development à la Kohlberg, and normal development à la Gesell (see Roberts, 1986). These psychologists must additionally have a thorough understanding of how youth conceptualize illness.

Concepts of Illness

A review of studies examining how children's concepts of physical illness develop as a function of their cognitive development concluded that their concepts of illness seem to evolve in a progressive, systematic manner that is essentially congruent with Piaget's theory of cognitive development (Burbach & Peterson, 1986). Perhaps the most complete model to describe this process is the one proposed by Bibace and Walsh (1979; Bibace, Schmidt, & Walsh, 1994). Although cognitive development corresponds strongly to age, the ages associated with each stage are to some degree arbitrary and will vary from individual to individual. Additional factors that have been shown to affect children's progression from stage to stage include family history, family life stage, and previous experience with health and illness (Koocher & MacDonald, 1992). See table 12.1 for a summary of key psychosocial and cognitive factors related to the development of children's understanding of illness as a function of developmental stage.

Infancy and toddlerhood (birth to 3 years). According to Piaget (Piaget & Inhelder, 1969), during this time period most children are moving from the sensorimotor to early phases of the preoperational stage of cognitive development. Characteristic of this period is a strong egocentric orientation that severely limits children's understanding of what illness is and how it may relate to their treatment (Koocher & MacDonald, 1992). This period is consistent with what Bibace and Walsh (1979; Bibace et al., 1994) refer to as the stage of *incomprehension,* a substage often excluded in models describing how children develop their conceptualization of illness. Yet, those working with this age group need to be cognizant of the important psychosocial developmental tasks associated with infancy and toddlerhood, including establishing a sense of trust, developing language skills, and developing a sense of autonomy through exploring one's environment. These critical domains of development have been shown to be at risk when a child is dealing with a chronic, ongoing illness that involves repeated hospital stays.

Early childhood (3 to 6 years). At this age children are usually within the preoperational stage of cognitive development, during which they engage in magical thinking and infer causal relationships using perceptual rather than logical connections (Piaget & Inhelder, 1969). Illness is viewed as being caused by some specific external force, but children are unable to articulate a causal link between that force and their internal experiences. Bibace and colleagues (Bibace & Walsh, 1979; Bibace et al., 1994) categorize children in this age group as moving from a stage of *phenomenism* to *contagion* in their conceptualization of physical illness. In phenomenism, the cause may be a sight, a sound, or some other sensory phenomenon, such as cold weather, that children may have come to associate with their own experience of illness. During

Table 12.1. Psychosocial and Cognitive Developmental Factors Related to Children's Conceptualization of Illness

Developmental Stage	Psychosocial Developmental Tasks	Cognitive Developmental Stage	Conceptualization of Illness
Infancy & Toddlerhood (age 0–3)	Basic trust Language skills Autonomy and exploration of environment	*Sensorimotor* Egocentrism Little understanding of events as external to oneself	*Incomprehension* No understanding of causes of illness
Early Childhood (age 3–6)	Initiating and enjoying activities/play Beginning peer relationships	*Preoperational* Magical/intuitive thinking Causal relationships inferred based on perceptions rather than logic	*Phenomenism* Sensory phenomenon viewed as cause of illness *Contagion* Events viewed as cause of illness
Later Childhood (age 6–12)	Competence and pleasure derived from completing tasks Cooperation and self-control in peer relationships	*Concrete operational* Able to differentiate internal and external experiences Logic is applied to concrete objects	*Contamination* Physical contact viewed as cause of illness *Internalization* Ingested germs viewed as cause of illness
Adolescence (age 12–18)	Identity development Independence and control Sexual development Vocational development	*Formal operational* Logical thinking applied to abstract concepts Able to simultaneously consider different outcomes	*Physiological* Internal processes viewed as mediating the relationship between external cause and internal symptoms *Psychophysiological* Psychological factors viewed as contributing to physical well-being

contagion, the causal agent is more often seen as involving events that are repeatedly either temporally or spatially associated with the illness. For example, without having any clear understanding of germs as a causal agent, children at this stage might attribute their illness simply to being around other children. Psychosocially, early childhood is the stage at which children begin to develop a sense of self-competence, particularly around their ability to form relationships with peers. Clearly, any illness that interferes with the development of these important relationships and at the same time elicits parental overprotection may inhibit the child's social development.

Later childhood (6 to 12 years). At this age, children are in the concrete operations stage of development and are more able to logically differentiate between internal symptoms and external events (Piaget & Inhelder, 1969). With regard to the conceptualization of illness, Bibace and Walsh (1979; Bibace et al., 1994) propose two substages during this period of development, *contamination* and *internalization.* Children operating in the contamination stage view illness as being externally caused and transmitted through physical contact. The contaminating agent may range from germs or dirt to bad behavior. The child exhibits a greater sense of control over the illness by envisioning that its cure can be obtained by avoiding these agents. Whereas a child in the contagion stage may associate the cold air with becoming ill, it is not until the contamination stage that the child is able to verbalize a causal link that includes a more concrete explanation, for example, suggesting that the illness was caused by the cold air actually touching the child's skin.

In the internalization stage, children associate illness with having actually swallowed or inhaled external germs that subsequently affect their internal organs in some unclearly defined manner, e.g., believing that swallowing germs makes them cough. Healing is, therefore, believed to occur by ingesting medicine or by relying on the body's own healing power. With this level of conceptualization, children are likely to believe that they can avoid illness by keeping away from germs and also by engaging in health-promoting behaviors to boost the body's healing power (Bibace & Walsh, 1979). From an intervention perspective, this greater sense of control and understanding suggests that children can have an increased role in their own care. This may be especially relevant in the case of diabetic children needing to adhere to dietary restrictions.

Psychosocial development in later childhood continues to involve peer relationships, including learning how to work cooperatively with others. Children also are developing a sense of mastery and pride in their accomplishments. Clearly, these important developmental tasks can be thwarted by the repeated school absences and physical limitations experienced by children with a chronic illness (Stern, Norman, & Zevon, 1991, 1993). At this stage of development, usually by the age of 6 or 7 (corresponding to the acquisition of the cognitive concepts of conservation and reversibility), children have a clearer understanding that death is finite, a view that differs from earlier conceptualizations that associated death with sleep or temporary separation (Koocher & MacDonald, 1992). It is important for psychologists working with this age group to be sensitive to children's questions and concerns about death, especially when the children are in a hospital for their own treatment or for that of a family member.

Adolescence (12 to 18 years). Piaget (Piaget & Inhelder, 1969) posits that many, but not all, adolescents enter a stage of formal operations. This level of cognitive development is characterized by abstract thinking, such as the ability to infer biological processes from unobservable phenomenon and the ability to simultaneously consider different possible outcomes of any one event, including an illness. Two developmental substages in the conceptualization of illness correspond with the formal operations stage, *physiological* and *psychophysiological* (Bibace & Walsh, 1979; Bibace et al., 1994).

During the physiological substage, adolescents' descriptions of physical illness focus on the malfunctioning of internal organs that mediate the relationship between external causal agents and perceived symptoms of illness. For example, adolescents may now understand that cancer cells destroy healthy organ tissue and this leads to the experience of pain and related symptoms. At the psychophysiological stage, adolescents incorporate a psychological component as a contributing factor to their concept of illness. They can now recognize the potential impact of thoughts and feelings upon body functioning, although they may still believe that only physiologically-based interventions will produce healing.

Psychosocially, adolescents are in the process of developing a sense of personal identity and control over multiple domains in their lives, including family and peer relationships and issues related to their sexual and vocational development. Noteworthy here for its implications for intervention is that with higher levels of cognitive development comes a greater sense of internal locus of control. Clearly, interventions targeting this age group might be facilitated by tapping into adolescents' developing psychosocial resources and by encouraging them to become more involved in their own treatment. Aside from these general suggestions, it is important to keep in mind that the developmental period of adolescence is generally viewed as being comprised of several distinct substages, each associated with different tasks and challenges. Addressing the complexities inherent to this stage of development is, however, beyond the scope of this chapter.

The Development of Coping

Although a stage model is used to understand how children conceptualize illness, professionals working with pediatric patients must be aware that children and adolescents vary greatly in their cognitive, social, emotional, and biological functioning, making this population significantly more diverse than adults (Compas, Worsham, & Ey, 1992). Another area of wide variation, and one of central concern for psychologists working within a health setting, is how well children cope with or adapt to their illness. Because children learn how to cope with various stressors over the course of their childhood, it can be expected that they will react to medical stressors differently than adults, and what is regarded as normative for adults may not be normative for children. Therefore, it is important for practitioners working within this arena to be familiar with the general literature on the developmental nature of children's coping processes.

Coping is generally viewed as a process in which active problem-solving and emotion-focused efforts are used by individuals to manage stress. Effective coping has increasingly been described as those efforts aimed at either cognitively restructuring the way a situation is viewed or generating behavioral alternatives for problem-solving (Compas et al., 1992; Van Slyck, Stern, & Zak-Place, 1996). Greater resilience and competence, and hence better adjustment, have been associated with the use of more active, problem-based coping strategies. Such efforts, however, clearly vary as a function of a child's developmental level as well as the degree to which the child perceives he or she can control the situational stressor. Research examining the developmental changes and stabilities in problem- and emotion-focused coping has generally found that the use of both major strategies of coping increases with age, although the evidence is more consistent for problem- as opposed to emotion-based coping (see Compas et al., 1992).

Compas and colleagues (1992) argue that problem-focused and emotion-based strategies emerge at different points in development, with problem-based strategies appearing at an earlier point in most children's development. For example, the literature suggests that a child's capacity to generate multiple solutions to a problem, an essential component of problem-solving, begins to emerge when the child is around 4 or 5 years of age. These authors suggest that children may readily acquire these problem-based strategies through modeling of overt adult behaviors. In contrast, emotion-based strategies for dealing with stressful situations may be more difficult for a child to learn through direct observation. It should be emphasized, however, that, although emotion-based strategies may not develop until later childhood and adolescence, they are not necessarily more sophisticated. In fact, these forms of coping have consistently been associated with poorer outcomes and adjustment (McCrae & Costa, 1986; Stern & Zevon, 1990).

What emerges from examining the literature on coping with illness is that the research has evolved from focusing on assessing which factors characterize maladjustment at each developmental stage to addressing which factors are predictive of better or worse adaptation (Johnson, 1994). One line of research that illustrates this trend compared the ability of adolescents with cancer and healthy adolescents to resolve important developmental tasks such as career and self-image identity formation (Stern, Norman, & Zevon, 1991, 1993). The findings suggested that the ability to resolve these tasks varied as a function of age and health status and that areas of poorer as well as more adaptive functioning can be identified. Thus, in evaluating how well children and adolescents are managing health-related stressors, practitioners must identify coping strengths and weaknesses as well as the child's developmental level of functioning.

Clearly, an individual child's repertoire of available strategies to deal with any particular stressor will vary both as a function of the developmental sequence in which these skills are acquired and the environmental context in which these processes occur (Compas et al., 1992). Social support from the family is an important contextual factor in any child's ability to cope effectively with a medical stressor; unfortunately, this support can have both positive and negative effects on the child (e.g., Melamed, 1992; Quittner, 1992). For example, the effects of maternal support provided to children preparing for medical treatment has been found to differ as a function of several factors. Mothers' use of active, problem-focused strategies has been found to be associated with less distress and more positive coping outcomes for children undergoing surgery. In contrast, children with mothers who show more anxiety in response to their child undergoing various medical procedures have been found to be more anxious and to cope more poorly with these procedures (Melamed, 1992). Thus, to more accurately reflect the contextual and systemic framework from which a child health psychologist must work, the assessment of a child's ability to cope must also include an evaluation of how well the family is coping with the health-related stressor. This broadening of focus is a fundamental issue for child-based health psychologists and directly relates to issues of evaluation, assessment, and intervention.

Assessment

Psychological assessment lays the groundwork for making informed decisions regarding diagnosis, treatment, and evaluation of interventions. In medical settings, these important processes take place in a context where the working norms of the culture stress expediency and quantification (Roberts, 1986; Roberts & McNeal, 1995). Unfortunately, such an approach may inadvertently miss important emotional and subjective information that can expand the medical team's understanding of a case and their ability to administer treatment appropriately (Hamlett & Stabler, 1995). For example, when a child's fears are interfering with his or her compliance with medical protocol, obtaining psychosocial information may help the medical team choose interventions that will not only deal with the patient's symptoms, but also decrease his or her fears and increase his or her compliance with treatment. With their developmental and psychosocial training, child health psychologists are uniquely qualified to provide this very critical perspective on assessment.

Assessment and evaluation of pediatric patients may be complicated by the difficulty inherent in getting complete information from children. Children's limited communication skills and understanding of illness present special challenges for evaluation and assessment. Yet, the ability to elicit information from children is clearly essential in order to obtain an accurate sense of how they perceive their symptoms, illness, and treatment (Mash & Terdal, 1990). Such communication would undoubtedly be enhanced by a knowledge of normative developmental processes, including children's concepts of illness and coping skills (Burbach & Peterson, 1986). Further, information obtained from children might be augmented by adults who can provide an accurate psychosocial history and contextual factors relevant to the child's illness. Parents, teachers, and other health care professionals may participate in interviews, complete parent or teacher forms of standardized assessments, and corroborate children's self-reports (Johnson, 1994; La Greca, 1990).

Mental health professionals must be especially aware of how sociocultural factors impact on assessment, diagnosis, and treatment interventions when working with minority and culturally diverse children, adolescents, and their families. Culturally diverse patients often have health-related beliefs and practices, including their perceptions of symptomatology and treatment, that differ from those of the majority culture (Canino & Spurlock, 1994). A lack of awareness of such cultural belief systems can result in erroneous diagnoses and misinformed treatment interventions. See chapter 15 for a full delineation of these issues.

In addition to informal methods of gathering information, such as unstructured interviews, many more formal approaches to assessment have been utilized in medical settings. These include traditional paper-and-pencil inventories, structured interviews, and behavioral observations. In using these strategies, mental health professionals must consider psychometric information such as reliability, validity, and norm groups. Many instruments have been designed and normed using healthy populations from the dominant culture or children referred to clinics primarily for mental health problems. Standard norms may, therefore, not apply to children and families from varied cultural backgrounds who are confronting medically-related stressors (La Greca, 1994). Several factors may influence the profile of responses given by a child with a physical illness, including age at disease onset, chronicity of disease, etiology and course of the illness, physical symptoms, visibility of the illness, and side effects from treatment or medication (Mash & Terdal, 1990).

Attempts have been made to develop psychometrically sound instruments to assess various aspects of specific illnesses. It is important to note, however, that each illness presents unique influences on children's development, behavior, and coping (Roberts, 1986). A brief summary of some important factors that cut across many illnesses and that pertain to critical issues of pain and adherence follow.

Pain Assessment

Pediatric pain has been conceptualized as falling into four categories (Varni, 1983):

1. pain associated with physical injuries or traumas (e.g., fractures)

2. pain not associated with a well-defined disease or injury (e.g., recurrent abdominal pain or headaches)
3. pain associated with medical and dental procedures (e.g., bone marrow aspirations or surgery)
4. pain associated with chronic diseases, such as cancer or arthritis

The accurate assessment of pain in all of these domains is critical for several reasons. Pain can signal changes in one's medical condition that can alert medical personnel to the need for further intervention. For example, acute pain in a child with hemophilia can serve as a warning for the onset of a new bleeding episode. Many treatment procedures induce pain, which can trigger anticipatory anxiety in children and subsequently impact their behavior and compliance with prescribed treatment regimens. Clearly such potential responses to treatments such as chemotherapy or insulin injection warrant careful assessment and utilization of preventive strategies. Finally, chronic pain calls for continual assessment because of its association with depression, school absences, and inactivity, all of which have been shown to interfere with a child's psychosocial development (Varni, Blount, Waldron, & Smith, 1995).

One myth about pain that does not hold true is that children are unable to communicate how they feel (Varni et al., 1995). In a review of child health assessment methods and instruments, Dahlquist (1990) concluded that children as young as 5 are able to use different colors to communicate qualitative aspects of their pain experiences. Semi-structured interviews, questionnaires with an open-ended format, drawings, and projective instruments may be used to elicit this information. Many children associate the color red with higher intensity of pain, although some children have been found to associate other dark colors such as green or black with the same level of high-intensity pain. These findings suggest that it is imperative for the child health psychologist to understand the child's subjective scale of pain intensity before attempting to interpret the results.

The Varni/Thompson Pediatric Pain Questionnaire (Varni, Thompson, & Hanson, 1987) is one example of a widely used, comprehensive, multidimensional approach to the assessment of both acute and chronic pain. The instrument is particularly noteworthy because of its sensitivity to children's cognitive developmental stage. It has forms suitable for assessing children's, adolescents', and parents' perceptions of pain (Varni et al., 1995). The pediatric version utilizes visual analog scales and body outlines to assess the sensory and affective components of pain. This approach is consistent with a young child's level of understanding of illness. Moreover, numerical (e.g., Likert) as well as visual analog scales have been reported to be useful in the assessment of pain with children aged 8 and above (Dahlquist, 1990). The adolescent form elicits information that incorporates adolescents' increasing understanding of the impact of psychosocial factors upon their experience of pain. The parent form has components similar to those of the pediatric and adolescent forms to allow for corroboration of the patient's self-reported information by an adult.

Adherence Assessment

Another important ongoing issue in the health care arena is adherence to pre-scribed treatment regimens. Although adherence to medical protocol has life or death implications for individuals with illnesses such as diabetes and hemophilia, there is mounting evidence to suggest that a significant propor-tion of children and adolescents do not adhere to prescribed medical regi-mens (La Greca & Schuman, 1995). Assessing adherence becomes critical in evaluating the effectiveness of a given treatment protocol. This information may suggest a need to change the protocol or intervene directly to increase a patient's adherence.

La Greca and Schuman (1995) categorized factors purported to predict adherence into five major domains:

1. child's developmental status (e.g., age, cognitive maturity, and psy-chosocial development)
2. individual patient characteristics (e.g., coping ability and resources, and biological functioning)
3. family factors (e.g., parental support, family conflict, and parental problem-solving skills)
4. medical system factors (e.g., quality of communication regarding the treatment regimen)
5. disease and regimen considerations (e.g., chronicity, complexity, and immediacy of effects)

Several issues that are subsumed in the categories specified here, but that are especially important when assessing adherence in pediatric patients, include (Johnson, 1994):

1. the child and family's understanding of the illness and the importance of treatment

2. their ability to complete the tasks assigned by the physician
3. the degree to which the medical procedures interfere with the family's lifestyle
4. the amount of support available to the child and family

These important issues must be considered when designing and evaluating treatment protocols that families are expected to follow. Such assessment may be facilitated by the ability of health care providers to communicate effectively with children and their families. This line of communication is critical and is an area where counseling psychologists can serve as educational consultants in the medical setting.

Evaluation of adherence is further complicated by variations in the way the construct is defined. One approach considers the prescribed medical regimen as a whole and categorizes patients as either "adherent" or "nonadherent" depending on whether the entire protocol is followed. This approach to assessment would seem to be most reasonable when compliance with the entire procedure is imperative for therapeutic gain. Another definition of adherence examines specific behaviors within the prescribed treatment and does not presume that compliance with one protocol component indicates compliance with another. This approach might be most appropriately used with complicated medical regimens that involve multiple tasks, such as those associated with many chronic illnesses, for example, diabetes or cystic fibrosis.

Measures of treatment adherence generally fall on a continuum ranging from direct to indirect assessment. Direct methods of assessment, such as blood assays and behavioral observation of the child performing the prescribed task, are most often used in short-term assessment protocols. Indirect approaches include pill counting, evaluation of therapeutic outcome, and ratings completed by physicians, parents, or patients (La Greca, 1990). Although the direct approaches are often considered more objective and reliable because they may be less subject to inherent biases of self-report, indirect methods can provide unique and equally valuable information. Structured 24-hour recall interviews are one example of an indirect assessment method with demonstrated reliability and validity in assessing adherence to diabetes management protocol (Johnson, Silverstein, Rosenbloom, Carter, & Cunningham, 1986). These instruments can also be used to elicit important contextual information. For instance, diabetic children needing to carefully control their diets might experience teasing from their peers that inhibits their motivation to adhere to the protocol. Eliciting such information would facilitate the design of appropriate treatment strategies that might include social skills and coping training to address these problems.

For ongoing assessment of adherence, self-monitoring, geared to the developmental level of the child and his or her medical needs, seems most appropriate. However, multiple measures must be used to obtain a complete assessment of adherence (Johnson, 1994; La Greca, 1990). Children's self-report should be cross-validated with behavioral observations and physiological indicators, as well as reports by parents, teachers, and health workers. Indeed, most successful interventions aimed at increasing adherence with complex treatment regimens involve the use of several interrelated strategies, including education, monitoring, and reinforcement. Moreover, to be successful, patients, and their families and other individuals important to the child, must be engaged in the treatment process (La Greca, 1990).

Intervention

Child health psychologists work in a variety of medically-based settings including hospitals, HMOs, outpatient pediatric clinics, and private pediatric group practices. Each setting provides the practitioner with unique challenges and specific presenting patient issues. However, there are key characteristics inherent to the practice of child health psychology that tend to cut across all work settings, including the need to take a pragmatic, flexible orientation in the delivery of short-term, cost-effective services. As a result of this orientation, the most frequently used intervention strategies tend to be crisis-oriented and behavioral in nature, although other theoretical orientations and treatments might in fact be more appropriate as well as more effective and expedient in working with certain children and their families (Roberts, 1986).

Regardless of the treatment strategy employed, the focus is on providing nonpsychiatric care to children coping with medically related stressors. In providing such services, all systems related to the child must be considered in the treatment plan to adequately address the child's presenting issues (Mullins, Gillman, & Harbeck, 1992; Rodrigue, 1994). Children must always be viewed within their ecological context, which includes examining the reciprocal impact of the child's illness on family members, peers, teachers, schools, and community. Clearly, the level of system involvement will vary depending on the child's age and stage of cognitive development. A multi-faceted assessment approach is therefore essential for understanding the complex network of systems in which a child is involved. Similarly, intervention strategies may be most effective when they target multiple levels of these interlocking systems. One empirically validated program provides ongoing clinical care for children diagnosed with cancer by intervening at several contextual levels affected by the child's illness (e.g., family, peers, and school; Varni, Katz, Colegrove, & Dolgin, 1993). Findings from this as well as other programs suggest that psychosocial services should be provided across all phases of chronic illness and that treatment protocol should vary as a function of the salient issues present at each stage of the illness (Powers, Vannatta, Noll, Cool, & Stehbens, 1995).

The complexity and breadth of issues that child health psychologists may confront make defining treatment strategies in a succinct manner difficult at best (La Greca & Varni, 1993). Helping children adjust to chronic illness, deal more effectively with pain and stress, and increase adherence to medical protocols are prevalent areas for intervention (Rodrigue, 1994). Treatment strategies used to address these vary greatly as a function of type and etiology of illness or medical problem, prognosis of treatment, as well as child age and developmental stage. Some common interventions that may be employed in working with children are highlighted below. Treatment modalities include individual, family, or group interventions that target the pediatric patient, the family, and the medical staff, although other groups such as school personnel may also be involved. These modes of treatment can be implemented simultaneously as components of a multifaceted approach to intervention.

Individual

Psychological interventions with medically ill children are generally aimed at reducing pain and stress and encouraging adaptive coping. Treatment strategies may range from broad-based interventions such as supportive counseling to more symptom-focused strategies that target behavior modification. Supportive counseling typically involves one-to-one contact between a child and mental health professional in order to develop a trusting alliance, provide empathy and acceptance, and allow for ventilation of feelings and concerns related to coping with a medically-related stressor. Drawings, journals, and therapeutic play can be utilized to facilitate emotional expression within an empathic environment. Play modalities such as games or puppet role-plays may be especially relevant in working with younger children to facilitate communication and to elicit their feelings and fears as well as to help them acquire coping strategies to deal more effectively with distressing medical procedures (Hart, Mather, Slack, & Powell, 1992).

Preparation for surgery and cancer treatment procedures constitute two distressing medical situations that have been the subject of both clinical and empirical inquiry. Most professionals working with pediatric patients now believe that preparing children for medical procedures is important, although the level of preparation may vary (Peterson & Harbeck, 1988). One well-documented example of coping and stress inoculation training uses a film-modeling technique as a way of preparing children for surgery. The best known example of this technique is a 7-minute film entitled "Ethan Has an Operation" that depicts a child's experience from admission to and discharge from the hospital (Melamed & Siegel, 1975). This technique has been found to be consistently effective in reducing anxiety in children, even with those as young as 4 years old. Pinto and Hollandsworth (1984) have also found that this type of film-modeling decreases parental anxiety about child surgery.

In dealing with pediatric cancer, patients often undergo a variety of painful and anxiety-provoking medical procedures, including bone marrow aspirations and lumbar punctures. Effective strategies for working with these patients include, but are not limited to, distraction techniques and hypnosis (Hilgard & LeBaron, 1982; Kellerman, Zeltzer, Ellenberg, & Dash, 1983), biofeedback, relaxation and imagery techniques to reduce anticipatory nausea, and the provision of information (Stroebel, 1982). In using educational interventions, the level and type of information disseminated to children must be carefully considered so that they are congruent with a child's primary coping style, that is, whether the child tends to repress or is especially vigilant to stressful information (Peterson & Harbeck, 1988; Stern, Ross, & Bielass, 1991). Hypnotherapy has been shown to be an especially effective treatment approach in reducing children's pain and emotional distress associated with medical procedures (Kellerman et al., 1983; Smith, Barabasz, & Barabasz, 1996; Zeltzer & LeBaron, 1982). It has been argued that children are likely to respond well to hypnosis because they use imagination and fantasy more easily than adults (Olness & Gardner, 1988).

As an example, hypnotherapy was effective in treating a 9-year-old girl with acute lymphocytic leukemia. Amanda had undergone eight bone marrow aspirations over the course of one year. During these procedures, she became exceedingly anxious, combative, screamed and yelled, and occasionally required physical restraint. Amanda's pediatrician became concerned after being informed by her family that she had attempted to run away from home in order to avoid her next scheduled appointment. Amanda was subsequently referred to a pediatric psychologist who recommended hypnotherapy as a course of treatment. An imagery-based hypnotic induction technique was utilized to help Amanda achieve a state of relaxation. Several hypnotic pain control methods were then taught to Amanda as outlined by Olness and Gardner (1988). These included:

1. *direct suggestions*—"Imagine injecting an anesthesia into your back. Notice the change in the feeling as the area becomes numb."
2. *distancing suggestions*—"Imagine putting all the discomfort of the spinal tap into the little finger of your right hand. Now let it float away."
3. *suggestions for feelings antithetical to the pain*—"Think of the funniest movie you ever saw."
4. *distraction techniques*—instructing Amanda to defocus on the pain by engaging in a discussion on a topic of interest to her or focusing on the IV rather than the spinal tap.
5. *directing attention to the pain itself*—helping Amanda to develop and then shift from pain imagery to relief imagery.

Amanda then selected the methods with which she felt most comfortable and audiotapes were made for home practice. Amanda practiced these hypnotic pain control methods at home privately as well as with coaching by the therapist or her parents. Hypnotic pain control techniques enabled Amanda to enhance her sense of mastery in actively addressing her feelings of fear, anxiety, helplessness, and powerlessness related to the treatment of her leukemia. Amanda tolerated her subsequent bone marrow aspirations with less reported pain and with far less agitation.

Family

Treatment involving the family is essential when working with children and is especially important with close-knit families, such as those often found among culturally diverse groups (Canino & Spurlock, 1994). Family therapy can be employed to assist family members with validating, normalizing, and coping with feelings associated with a threatening diagnosis or lengthy hospitalization of a child or sibling. Interventions may also focus on providing families with information about the potential psychological impact of having acute or chronic illnesses. This information will vary according to the age, developmental level, and cultural background of the child.

For example, adolescent noncompliance with daily tasks required for diabetes management has been documented as both a medical issue and a concern for parents (Peterson & Harbeck, 1988). Parents may respond to this situation by increasing their scrutiny of the adolescent's behavior to a point where parents attempt to take full responsibility for maintaining treatment compliance. Adolescents are unlikely to respond favorably to such parental actions, and parent-child conflicts may ensue that ultimately compromise the child's health. Psychological intervention at the family level can help the family reframe the situation by viewing the adolescent's responses within a normal developmental context, that is, understanding that the highly structured routine necessary in diabetic care is at odds with the adolescent's needs for individuation, independence, and autonomy. Family-based interventions that focus on communication training, conflict resolution, and education have been recommended for use with this population (Drotar, 1997; Peterson & Harbeck, 1988; Wysocki, 1993).

A related role of child health psychologists is in providing education and support to family members of prematurely born infants. A series of studies has shown that when a child is born prematurely, parental reactions and treatment of the infant may be inaccurately based on their expectations of vulnerability for the child (Stern & Karraker, 1990, 1992). These inaccurate expectations and overprotective parental reactions have been demonstrated to negatively impact the child's cognitive and social development. Education-based intervention strategies aimed at increasing understanding and fostering more appropriate expectations have been shown to mitigate the development of the vulnerable child syndrome (Stern & Karraker, 1990, 1992). A related approach to working with parents of prematurely born infants who are at-risk for later psychological and cognitive deficits is interaction coaching (Field, 1992), whereby parents acquire information about dealing with their infant through a combination of information dissemination and observing and modeling of a professional's behaviors. This type of interaction coaching could also be conducted within a group format.

Group

Group interventions can be effective for providing education and support services to medically ill children and their families. For example, as part of a multifamily support group treatment, parents of adolescents with diabetes participated in a simulated treatment protocol which included having them give self-injections of saline, take blood glucose tests, and regulate their diet. Parents' participation was related to increased family empathy regarding their children's adherence to medical protocol and decreased family conflict about the illness (Satin, La Greca, Zigo, & Skyler, 1989). Peterson and Harbeck (1988) also describe group therapy programs to help children gain an understanding of diabetic control and self-care issues.

Another area in which group strategies have been found to be useful is in helping siblings of children with cancer or other life-threatening illnesses deal with their emotional and behavioral responses to the stressful situation impacting their family (Stern & Newland, 1994). Such group experiences can provide an important function in helping to normalize the experiences of medically ill children, especially for those at an age where peer contact is critical. Summer camp programs for chronically ill children are good examples of such services and provide children with normalizing peer experiences as well as provision of specific information about their illness.

Consultation

Three major models of pediatric psychological consultation have been identified: independent functions, indirect service, and collaborative (Roberts, 1986). The *independent functions model* operates when psychological services are primarily provided in a noncollaborative fashion. The referring physician and child health psychologist do not maintain an ongoing dialogue about the case, although they may exchange some information about patients and their functioning at the outset and termination of the consulting relationship. One example of such a role would be when an adolescent with cancer is referred by a physician for psychological evaluation regarding depressive symptomatology. The *indirect service model* operates when psychologists working in a medical setting serve as mediators between patients and their families and the complex medical system so that optimal treatments may be designed (Hamlett & Stabler, 1995). In this case, the focus of service is often on medical staff requesting information rather than on direct patient care, for example, providing stress management group support for health care professionals dealing with burnout issues. The *collaborative model* operates when the psychologist is included as an integral member in a team that provides patient services. It has been suggested that this approach to consultation results in more comprehensive assessment and highly coordinated care for the patient; however, in actual practice it is less commonly used than other models (Mullins et al., 1992).

Working within the indirect model, a consultant might intervene with health care providers to mitigate stereotypes that affect how these providers interact with patients and their families. Recent research has suggested that health care providers hold negative expectations for children identified as vulnerable, including infants born prematurely and children identified as in remission from cancer (e.g., Kohrman & Diamond, 1986; Stern & Carmel, 1995; Stern, Ross, & Bielass, 1991). Despite the fact that health care providers believe that their personal values about a patient do not interfere with their treatment of that patient, biases do exist which influence the provider's behavior and relate to the level of patient satisfaction. In the case of the infant born prematurely, the initial and often most influential information concerning the characteristics of and appropriate expectations for a premature infant comes from health care professionals. Paradoxically, research indicates that mothers report not receiving such information from health care providers whereas physicians consistently report providing such information (Stern & Karraker, 1992). An important role played by child health psychologists is educating health care providers about the operation of stereotypes and how to clearly communicate with parents regarding realistic expectations for their infants' development.

Chronic pain syndromes, which often include physical distress, functional disability, and the use of maladaptive coping strategies, may best be treated using a collaborative team model in which physicians, psychologists, and other health care providers coordinate interventions that focus on different aspects of patient care. For instance, 14-year-old Cory was referred by his pediatrician for increased pain complaints, anxiety, escalating use of narcotic pain medication, and sleep difficulties. He had been diagnosed with spinal muscular atrophy at 20 months old and had used a wheelchair since the age of four. At about the time Cory entered ninth grade at a new high school, he underwent surgery for spinal fusion. His presenting symptoms were noted approximately seven months after these events.

In this case, Cory's pediatrician carefully managed the medical aspects of his physical condition and associated pain symptoms. In close alliance with the pediatrician, the psychologist developed a treatment plan focused on teaching Cory cognitive-behavioral self-regulation strategies to help him reduce his pain and psychological distress and improve his sleep. Cory was taught to utilize deep breathing, meditative imagery, soothing cognitive self-statements ("my mind is calm and quiet"; "relax, I can cope with this"), and progressive muscle relaxation to achieve a state of lowered stress and arousal. Audiotapes were made of these techniques for Cory to practice at bedtime to improve his sleep and to practice throughout the day to decrease his anxiety, pain, and tension.

During the course of treatment, it became clear that Cory was also feeling quite overwhelmed with the stress of adjusting to high school. Thus, in addition to teaching Cory these self-regulation techniques for pain management, weekly supportive therapy was undertaken. The purpose of these supportive therapeutic contacts was to provide a safe, nonjudgmental environment in which Cory could address his feelings, fears, and developmental issues related to this particular life transition. Following several weeks of supportive psychotherapy, as well as learning and practicing pain management techniques, Cory expressed considerable pain relief, decreased anxiety, and improved sleep. Comfortable and more confident in his sense of mastery with these pain management strategies, Cory also reduced his narcotic medication use by two-thirds over the two months following intervention.

Recently, another approach to consultation has been proposed that involves multiple levels of intervention (Mullins et al., 1992; Rodrigue, 1994). One such multilevel intervention strategy involves children with cancer, their parents, teachers, and peers in a school reintegration program (Varni et al., 1993). In this program, the primary target is the patient, who is taught interpersonal problem-solving skills and coping strategies to deal with specific stressors that are likely to be encountered upon returning to school after diagnosis and hospitalization (e.g., teasing, name-calling). As part of this program of intervention, parents are trained to rehearse and engage in role plays with their children to reinforce the learning of social skills. Prior to the child returning to school, the child health psychologist coordinates educational discussions with teachers and classmates as a way of increasing understanding and acceptance as well as facilitating communication about the child's illness. This multilevel approach to consultation has been shown to decrease children's stress when they return to school and to provide them with interpersonal skills that prepare them to cope with new stressors as they arise (Varni et al., 1993).

Salient Issues and Controversies

Psychologists working in health care settings face several professional issues that are common when working within a complex medically dominated organization. These include, but are not limited to, turf issues, differences in jargon, and differences in the way problems are conceptualized (Roberts, 1986). In addition to these cross-cutting concerns, child health psychologists face issues that are unique to working with children. They play multiple roles as members of interdisciplinary health care teams, mental health clinicians, and advocates for children and families in their medical and psychological treatment. As previously stressed, dealing with children necessitates the involvement of families and other social networks pertaining to the child and requires a thorough knowledge of developmental issues.

Making ethical and legal decisions within these multiple roles and systems becomes especially complex when working with children. For example, psychologists must consider a child's capacity to make competent decisions, while also recognizing parents' legal responsibility to provide consent for treatment (Rae, Worchel, & Brunnquell, 1995). Child health psychologists must grapple with a variety of ethical and legal considerations, such as bioethics (decisions pertaining to medical treatment), consent, and confidentiality.

Many medical decisions involve balancing potential risks against benefits of treatment and the patient's right to self-determination. Psychologists may play a role in helping patients and their caregivers cope with difficult decisions regarding the child's care, including withholding or withdrawing life-sustaining treatment. One such struggle might be when parents decide whether to maintain the life of their infant born extremely premature when the quality of that life may be severely compromised. Another example might involve balancing the potential benefits of childhood cancer treatments with the invasiveness, debilitating nature, and long-lasting physical and psychosocial effects of such treatment. Psychologists can help parents and patients deal with these decisions by assessing the child's current and potential social, emotional, and cognitive functioning (Johnson, 1991). These decisions must also involve consideration of the family's cultural and religious background and beliefs.

Parents are legally responsible for consenting to treatment for their children, but psychologists are ethically bound to obtain children's assent for treatment (Rae et al., 1995). "Assent" also serves to increase the child's sense of control and motivation for treatment and has been found to be related to better overall psychological health (Nitschke, Wunder, Sexauer, & Humphrey, 1977). Similar to issues of consent, limits of confidentiality arise when the patient is a minor because parents (or legal guardians) have a legal right to be informed about information disclosed by their child during treatment. Therefore, discussions about the nature and limits of confidentiality must include the degree to which information will be made available to each family member, as well as to other medical personnel, for example, information pertaining to drug use and sexuality. As with assent, such a discussion must be congruent with both the patient's cognitive developmental level and cultural background. Competent management of assent and confidentiality issues requires that therapists and medical providers negotiate with patient and family members as to what information will be shared in the interest of optimal patient care. A full delineation of these issues are discussed in chapter 3.

Summary

Professionals working with children in a medical setting are presented with a unique set of challenges. To address these challenges, child health psychologists must have a strong working knowledge of cognitive, emotional, and psychosocial developmental processes and how these factors affect children's understanding of illness and their ability to cope with medical stressors. Psychologists must additionally consider systemic factors that affect children's functioning, including those factors related to family and school environments. These developmental and systemic factors must be considered in planning methods for assessment and intervention. A variety of approaches have been found to be effective in working with children dealing with medical stressors. With their training as scientist/practitioners and their focus on normative development, counseling psychologists are particularly suited for working within the child health arena. They may contribute to the knowledge base of the field through clinical intervention and/or by engaging in clinically relevant, basic, and applied research activities.

Suggested Resources

The Pediatric Psychologist: Issues in Professional Development and Practice (Peterson & Harbeck, 1988) provides an introduction and overview of pediatric/child health psychology. The authors present a cogent, yet eminently readable discussion of professional issues, research, and practice relevant to the field. The historical roots, current status, and challenges for the future of the field are highlighted. *Pediatric Psychology: Psychological Interventions and Strategies for Pediatric Problems* (Roberts, 1986) is an additional source of information for those interested in a more thorough examination of professional issues.

Handbook of Pediatric Psychology (Roberts, 1995) is an excellent resource that provides an extraordinary amount of useful as well as scholarly information. Chapters cover a wide range of topics, issues, and considerations relevant for clinical practitioners and research investigators. Chapters are written by eminent scholars in their respective fields and generally discuss professional issues in child health psychology in the prevention and treatment of physical, developmental, behavioral, and emotional problems related to children and adolescents' health concerns. Specifically, the chapters cover such topics as child health assessment, pain management, adjustment to chronic illness, prevention of injuries and disease, diabetes, leukemia, brain injuries, cardiovascular disease, prematurity, obesity, sleep disturbances, and much more.

A counseling psychologist interested in working in child health psychology should also be familiar with the stress and coping literature. *Stress and Coping in Child Health,* edited by La Greca, Seigel, Wallender, and Walker (1992), gives a solid foundation of the current thinking and research on this topic within the child health arena. Both individual and family factors in coping with acute and chronic health stressors are considered.

Readers interested in the most current research in the field should also refer to the *Journal of Pediatric Psychology,* the official journal of the Society of Pediatric Psychology. This journal publishes articles relating to theory, research, and professional practice in the interdisciplinary field of pediatric psychology. A wide variety of topics are explored related to the relationship between the psychological and physical well-being of children and adolescents. The journal also features special issues devoted to such topics as child health assessment, chronic illness, failure to thrive, pediatric AIDS, and family issues in intervention.

Discussion Questions

1. What factors should be considered in understanding a child's manner of organizing and responding to a medically-related stressor?
2. What individual and contextual variables need to be taken into account in evaluating how well a pediatric patient is coping with and/or adapting to a chronic illness?
3. What would you consider to be the most important considerations in facilitating an effective collaborative relationship between medical and psychological staff in a pediatric AIDS clinic?
4. Based on Bibace and Walsh's model of how children conceptualize illness, how might you develop a cognitive-behavioral intervention for a 6-year-old child with a fear of injections? A 15-year-old adolescent with chronic headaches?

References

Altmaier, E. M. (1990). Research and practice roles for counseling psychologists in health care settings. *The Counseling Psychologist, 19,* 342–364.

Bibace, R., Schmidt, L. R., & Walsh, M. E. (1994). Children's perceptions of illness. In G. N. Penny, P. Bennett, & M. Herbert (Eds.), *Health psychology: A lifespan perspective* (pp. 13–30). Langhorne, PA: Harwood Academic.

Bibace, R., & Walsh, M. E. (1979). Developmental stages in children's conceptions of illness. In G. C. Stone, F. Cohen, & N. E. Adler (Eds.), *Health psychology* (pp. 285–301). San Francisco: Jossey-Bass.

Burbach, D. J., & Peterson, L. (1986). Children's concepts of physical illness: A review and critique of the cognitive-developmental literature. *Health Psychology, 5,* 307–325.

Canino, I. A. & Spurlock, J. (1994). *Culturally diverse children and adolescents: Assessment, diagnosis, and treatment.* New York: Guilford.

Compas, B. E., Worsham, N. L., & Ey, S. (1992). Conceptual and developmental issues in children's coping with stress. In A. La Greca, L. J. Seigel, J. L. Wallander, & C. E. Walker (Eds.), *Stress and coping in child health* (pp. 7–24). New York: Guilford.

Dahlquist, L. M. (1990). Obtaining child reports in health care settings. In A. M. La Greca (Ed.), *Through the eyes of the child: Obtaining self-reports from children and adolescents* (pp. 395–439). Boston: Allyn & Bacon.

Drotar, D. (1997). Relating parent and family functioning to the psychological adjustment of children with chronic health conditions: What have we learned? What do we need to know? *Journal of Pediatric Psychology, 22,* 149–165.

Field, T. M. (1992). Interventions in early infancy. *Infant Mental Health Journal, 13,* 329–336.

Hamlett, K. W., & Stabler, B. (1995). The developmental progress of pediatric psychology consultation. In M. C. Roberts (Ed.), *Handbook of pediatric psychology* (2nd ed., pp. 39–54). New York: Guilford.

Hart, R., Mather, P. L., Slack, J. F., & Powell, M. A. (1992). *Therapeutic play activities for hospitalized children.* St. Louis: Mosby Year Book.

Hilgard, J. R., & LeBaron, S. (1982). Relief of anxiety and pain in children and adolescents with cancer: Quantitative measures and clinical observations. *International Journal of Clinical and Experimental Hypnosis, 4,* 417–442.

Johnson, S. B. (1991). The psychological impact of risk screening for chronic and life-threatening childhood illness. In J. H. Johnson, & S. B. Johnson (Eds.), *Advances in child health psychology* (pp. 345–352). Gainesville, FL: University of Florida.

Johnson, S. B. (1994). Chronic illness in children. In G. N. Penny, P. Bennett, & M. Herbert (Eds.), *Health psychology: A lifespan perspective* (pp. 31–50). Langhorne, PA: Harwood Academic.

Johnson, S. B., Silverstein, J., Rosenbloom, A. L., Carter, R., & Cunningham, W. (1986). Assessing daily management in childhood diabetes. *Health Psychology, 5,* 545–564.

Kellerman, J., Zeltzer, L., Ellenberg, L., & Dash, J. (1983). Hypnosis for the reduction of acute pain and anxiety associated with medical procedures. *Journal of Adolescent Health Care, 4,* 85–90.

Kohrman, A., & Diamond, L. (1986). Institutional and professional attitutdes: Dilemmas for the chronically ill child. *Topics in Early Childhood and Special Education, 5,* 82–91.

Koocher, G. P., & MacDonald, B. L. (1992). Preventive intervention and family coping with a child's life-threatening or terminal illness. In T. J. Akamatsu, M. A. Stephens, S. E. Hobfoll, & J. H. Crowther (Eds.), *Family health psychology* (pp. 67–86). Washington, DC: Hemisphere.

La Greca, A. M. (1990). Issues in adherence with pediatric regimens. *Journal of Pediatric Psychology, 15,* 423–436.

La Greca, A. M. (1994). Assessment in pediatric psychology: What's a researcher to do? *Journal of Pediatric Psychology, 19,* 283–290.

La Greca, A. M., & Schuman, W. B. (1995). Adherence to prescribed medical regimens. In M. C. Roberts (Ed.), *Handbook of pediatric psychology* (2nd ed., pp. 55–83). New York: Guilford.

La Greca, A. M., Seigel, L. J., Wallander, J. L., & Walker, C. E. (Eds.). (1992). *Stress and coping in child health.* New York: Guilford.

La Greca, A. M., & Varni, J. W. (1993). Interventions in pediatric psychology: A look toward the future. *Journal of Pediatric Psychology, 18,* 667–679.

Mash, E. J., & Terdal, L. G. (1990). Assessment strategies in clinical behavioral pediatrics. In A. M. Gross, & R. S. Drabman (Eds.), *Handbook of clinical behavioral pediatrics* (pp. 49–79). New York: Plenum.

McCrae, R. R., & Costa, P. T., Jr. (1986). Personality, coping and coping effectiveness in an adult sample. *Journal of Personality, 54,* 385–405.

Melamed, B. (1992). Family factors predicting children's reactions to anesthesia induction. In A. La Greca, L. J. Seigel, J. L. Wallander, & C. E. Walker (Eds.), *Stress and coping in child health* (pp. 140–156). New York: Guilford.

Melamed, B. G., & Seigel, L. (1975). Reduction of anxiety in children facing hospitalization and surgery by use of filmed modeling. *Journal of Consulting and Clinical Psychology, 43,* 511–521.

Mullins, L. L., Gillman, J., & Harbeck, C. (1992). Multiple-level interventions in pediatric psychology settings: A behavioral-systems perspective. In A. La Greca, L. J. Seigel, J. L. Wallander, & C. E. Walker (Eds.), *Stress and coping in child health* (pp. 377–399). New York: Guilford.

Nitschke, R., Wunder, S. Sexauer, C. L., & Humphrey, G. B. (1977). The final-stage conference: The patient's decision on research drugs in pediatric oncology. *Journal of Pediatric Psychology, 2,* 58–64.

Olness, K., & Gardner, G. (1988). *Hypnosis and hypnotherapy with children* (2nd ed.). New York: Grune & Stratton.

Peterson, L., & Harbeck, C. (1988). *The pediatric psychologist: Issues in professional development and practice.* Champaign, IL: Research.

Piaget, J., & Inhelder, B. (1969). *The psychology of the child.* NY: Basic.

Pinto, R. P., & Hollandsworth, J. G. (1984). Using videotape modeling to prepare children psychologically for surgery: Influence of parents and costs and benefits of providing preparation services. *Health Psychology, 8,* 79–95.

Powers, S. W., Vannatta, K., Noll, R. B., Cool, V. A., & Stehbens, J. A. (1995). Leukemia and other childhood cancers. In M. C. Roberts (Ed.), *Handbook of pediatric psychology* (2nd ed., pp. 310–326). New York: Guilford.

Quittner, A. L. (1992). Reexamining research on stress and social support: The importance of contextual factors. In A. La Greca, L. J. Seigel, J. L. Wallander, & C. E. Walker (Eds.), *Stress and coping in child health* (pp. 85–115). New York: Guilford.

Rae, W. A., Worchel, F. F., & Brunnquell, D. (1995). Ethical and legal issues in pediatric psychology. In M. C. Roberts (Ed.), *Handbook of pediatric psychology* (2nd ed., pp. 19–36). New York: Guilford.

Roberts, M. C. (1986). *Pediatric psychology: Psychological interventions and strategies for pediatric problems.* New York: Pergamon.

Roberts, M. C. (Ed.). (1995). *Handbook of pediatric psychology* (2nd ed.). New York: Guilford.

Roberts, M. C., & McNeal, R. E. (1995). Historical and conceptual foundations of pediatric psychology. In M. C. Roberts (Ed.), *Handbook of pediatric psychology* (2nd ed., pp. 3–18). New York: Guilford.

Rodrigue, J. R. (1994). Beyond the individual child: Innovative systems approaches to service delivery in pediatric psychology. *Journal of Consulting and Clinical Psychology, 23,* 32–39.

Satin, W., La Greca, A. M., Zigo, M. A., & Skyler, J. S. (1989). Diabetes in adolescence: Effects of multifamily group intervention and parent simulation of diabetes. *Journal of Pediatric Psychology, 14,* 259–275.

Smith, J. T., Barabasz, A., & Barabasz, M. (1996). Comparison of hypnosis and distraction in severely ill children undergoing painful medical procedures. *Journal of Counseling Psychology, 43,* 187–195.

Stern, M., & Carmel, S. (1995, March). *The prematurity stereotype in Israeli health care providers: A cross-cultural comparison.* Paper presented at the meeting of the Society for Research in Child Development, Indianapolis, IN.

Stern, M., & Karraker, K. (1990). The prematurity stereotype: Empirical evidence and implications for practice. *Infant Mental Health Journal, 11,* 3–11.

Stern, M., & Karraker, K. (1992). Modifying the prematurity stereotype in mothers of premature infants and ill full-term infants. *Journal of Clinical Child Psychology, 21,* 76–83.

Stern, M., & Newland, L. (1994). Working with children: Providing a framework for the roles of counseling psychologists. *The Counseling Psychologist, 22,* 402–435.

Stern, M., Norman, S., & Zevon, M. (1991). The career development of adolescent cancer patients: A comparative analysis. *Journal of Counseling Psychology, 38,* 431–439.

Stern, M., Norman, S., & Zevon, M. (1993). Adolescents with cancer: Self-image and social support as indices of adaptation. *Journal of Adolescent Research, 8,* 124–142.

Stern, M., Ross, S., & Bielass, M. (1991). Impact of health status label on medical students' expectations for children's coping style and choice of approach strategy. *Journal of Social and Clinical Psychology, 10,* 91–101.

Stern, M., & Zevon, M. (1990). Stress, coping, and family environment: The adolescent's response to naturally occurring stressors. *Journal of Adolescent Research, 5,* 290–305.

Stroebel, C. F. (1982). *QR: The quieting reflex.* New York: Putnam.

Van Slyck, M., Stern, M., & Zak-Place, J. (1996). Promoting optimal adolescent development through conflict resolution education training and practice: An innovative approach for counseling psychologists. *The Counseling Psychologist, 24,* 433–461.

Varni, J. W. (1983). *Clinical behavioral pediatrics: An interdisciplinary biobehavioral approach.* Elmsford, NY: Pergamon.

Varni, J. W., Blount, R. L., Waldron, S. A., & Smith, A. J. (1995). Management of pain and distress. In M. C. Roberts (Ed.), *Handbook of pediatric psychology* (2nd ed., pp. 105–123). New York: Guilford.

Varni, J. W., Katz, E. R., Colegrove, R., & Dolgin, M. (1993). The impact of social skills training on the adjustment of children with newly diagnosed cancer. *Journal of Pediatric Psychology, 18,* 751–767.

Varni, J. W., Thompson, K. L., & Hanson, V. (1987). The Varni/Thompson pediatric pain questionnaire. I. Chronic musculoskeletal pain in juvenile rheumatoid arthritis. *Pain, 28,* 27–38.

Wysocki, T. (1993). Associations among teen-parent relationships, metabolic control, and adjustment to diabetes in adolescents. *Journal of Pediatric Psychology, 18,* 441–452.

Zeltzer, L., & LeBaron, S. (1982). Hypnosis and nonhypnotic techniques for reduction of pain and anxiety during painful procedures in children and adolescents with cancer. *Journal of Pediatrics, 101,* 1032–1035.

13

Older Adults and Geriatrics

Sue C. Jacobs
Mary Jean Formati

Many of the patients whom counseling psychologists and other mental health providers encounter in health care settings are elderly. Older adults use medical services more than younger adults (U.S. Senate Special Committee on Aging, 1991) and are much more likely to take their mental health problems to a medical provider than to a mental health provider (Koenig & Blazer, 1990).

It is crucial that mental health providers working with older adults in medical settings understand that the psychosocial and medical problems are both complex and interactive. While psychologists have the necessary assessment and intervention skills to work with adults with mental health problems, most have not been adequately trained to work with older medical patients (Haley, 1996).

In order to adequately assess and intervene with older patients, health care providers need to recognize the possible interaction of psychological and physical factors and the evolution of these factors with age. Failure to do so could mean decline in patient function or quality of life—perhaps even death. For example, research suggests that depression following myocardial infarction increases the risk of reinfarction (Frasure-Smith, Lespérance, & Talajic, 1995). This highlights the importance of assessing and treating depression in patients who have had a heart attack. For instance, a provider could fail to provide a life-saving treatment to a 75-year-old woman if the provider misdiagnosed and treated her sadness, inactivity, and fatique after a heart attack as a grief response to loss and/or anticipatory loss of health rather than as clinical depression.

Just as most mental health providers lack adequate training for working with older adults, so do most medical providers. Primary care physicians, the gatekeepers and main medical providers for most older patients, often do not recognize, treat, or make necessary referrals for their older patients who present with such problems as depression (Haley, 1996). Although physicians trained in geriatric medicine, an internal medicine subspecialty, emphasize attention to psychosocial issues as part of the comprehensive assessment and management of elderly patients, most older adults do not have access to these specialists or to geriatric assessment teams (interdisciplinary teams with specialists from medical and psychosocial professions).

In the absence of a geriatric assessment team, treatment of older adults in medical settings should be interdisciplinary and involve a clinical geropsychologist. A clinical geropsychologist is a licensed psychologist from either counseling psychology, rehabilitation psychology, clinical neuropsychology, community psychology, or clinical psychology who engages in psychological practice with older adults. This subspecialty emerged in 1987 when psychologists were included in Medicare. The goal of the subspecialty is to apply the knowledge and techniques of adult development, aging, and psychology to help older adults "maintain well-being, overcome problems, and achieve maximum potential in later life" (Lichtenberg et al., 1996, p. 1). The American Psychological Association Interdivisional Task Force is developing qualifications for practice in clinical or applied geropsychology, which may include training recommendations at three levels: general exposure to aging, generalist training in clinical geropsychology, and specialist training in clinical geropsychology (Lichtenberg et al., 1996). Since interdisciplinary care is not available for most older adults, psychologists need to obtain adequate training and find other professionals with whom to consult and refer.

This chapter focuses on those concerns most salient for mental health providers working with older adults in health care settings. The importance of the mind-body connection and of providers recognizing the increasingly complex interplay of psychological, physiological, social, cultural, pharmacological, and belief systems in older adults is emphasized. Also considered are issues of assessment, diagnosis and treatment, consultation and referral, and work with other professionals in this context. Controversies affecting the provision of psychological services for older medical patients are noted at the end of the chapter.

The Older Adult Population

Adults over the age of 65 make up the largest group of health care users in the United States. This trend is expected to increase, creating an even greater need for adequately trained providers. Life expectancy in the United States has risen dramatically from 48 years in 1900 to 75.5 years in 1991; the relative percentage of elderly in the population has also risen markedly (U.S. Bureau of Census, 1992).

Quality of Life

Perhaps more important than length of life is quality of life. Counseling psychologists can contribute to the primary health promotion and disease prevention objectives for older adults by facilitating behaviors that increase the years of healthy life and decrease the years of dependence on others. Regular exercise, health screens, and social support are essential to the health and independence of older adults. By understanding the factors that lead to decreased functioning and dependence, mental health providers can help identify patients at risk for problems and provide interventions to reduce risk. For example, the risks for osteoporosis, cancer, and heart disease can possibly be reduced by changes in behavior, such as adherence to regular weight-bearing exercise, following a healthy diet, and taking hormone replacement therapy. The quality of life for many older adults who suffer from urinary incontinence could possibly be improved by providing information on effective and available treatments (U.S. Department of Health and Human Services, 1990). In addition, simple interventions like telephone reminders can increase the rate of medical appointments kept by older adults and thus increase prevention behaviors (American Psychological Association, 1993).

Heterogeneity

More perhaps than for other segments of the population, it is important that psychologists recognize that older people are a heterogeneous group.

Gender and ethnic differences are important in older adulthood, especially differences in cultural expectations, life expectancy, economic resources, and support systems. Life expectancy for women is almost 80 years, while that for men is only 73 (Zarit & Knight, 1996). This means that most of the oldest-old—those over age 80—are women, many of whom suffer from chronic illnesses.

With advanced age, differences among people and how they age increase. For example, one 76-year-old may run a marathon, work part-time, and begin a second marriage, while another may reside in a nursing home, have multiple medical problems, receive a variety of medications, and be depressed and dependent on others.

Coping and Adjustment Issues

Older adults are likely to experience more losses than younger adults, especially losses of health, roles, relationships, income, and function. In general, however, the sources of stress for older adults are the same as for younger adults, with health-related stressful events being the most common. Deaths of friends, peers, and spouses are frequent. The loss of friends and relatives tends to be more difficult for women, while the loss of a spouse appears more traumatic for men (Fiske & Chiriboga, 1990; Pearlin & Skaff, 1995). Changes in living situations or the community may be perceived as threats to safety and security. Chronic stressors may include illness, role strains (e.g., an adult alcoholic child), or difficulties related to diminished functioning. Older adults have a lifetime of strengths and coping skills to draw upon as they confront multiple stresses, losses, and/or medical problems. As with younger adults, they vary with respect to what is perceived as stressful and how they cope.

Mental Health Problems

That older adults are not a homogenous group is also evident in the diversity of psychological and adjustment problems that come to the attention of mental health providers and in the variety of service settings in which older adults are seen. As noted earlier, older people are more likely to go to a medical provider for mental health problems than to a mental health provider. They receive psychological services in a variety of community settings, such as outpatient clinics, HMOs, day hospitals, inpatient and partial psychiatric and medical hospitalization settings, nursing home/extended care settings, and rehabilitation clinics, or they may receive in-home care. It is estimated that over half of older patients treated for physical disorders in hospitals, medical clinics, or nursing homes also have at least one mental health problem that is not recognized or treated. Common mental health problems among older medical outpatients include depression, anxiety, sleep disorders, alcohol-related disorders, and sexual dysfunction. Further, older patients vary a great deal in functional ability and degree of impairment. Patients may range from physically frail and/or cognitively impaired nursing home residents to functionally capable patients in an outpatient HMO.

Besides needing services for psychological problems such as anxiety, depression, or chronic mental illness, older adults often require mental health services related to special issues of later life. These issues include recurrences of earlier life problems, new problems such as unintentional abuse or misuse of prescription medicines, alcohol abuse, homelessness, sleep disorders, or problems coping with loss of function and transitions such as retirement, widowhood, and/or moving from one's home. Older adults may seek help for chronic pain, decisions about medical treatment or living arrangements, or coming to terms with terminal illness and death.

Older adults, especially white males over age 80, are at high risk for suicide, accounting for about 25 percent of the total suicides in the United States (Blazer, 1991). Over 70 percent of elderly male suicide victims have seen a primary care physician within a month of suicide. These physicians typically do not recognize the risk of suicide, which likely stems from depression, reaction to illness, social isolation, and/or recent loss (American Psychological Association, 1993).

Older adults also face an increased risk of cognitive impairment. Nearly 30 percent of those over age 85 have some form of dementia, commonly caused by Alzheimer's or cerebrovascular disease. Older patients with progressive dementias often have coexisting symptoms, such as depression, anxiety, paranoia, or behavioral problems.

Normal Aging

Older adults today are better educated and healthier than previous generations. With the aging of the baby boomers, this trend is likely to accelerate (Zarit & Knight, 1996). A growing number of older adults are likely to be psychologically-minded and want counseling, "healthy lifestyles" programs, or other preventive interventions. Aging and the deterioration of body and mind do not automatically go together. Senescence is accompanied by a gradual decline in bodily functioning. The belief that old age must be accompanied by profound changes in cognitive ability and/or physical functioning is a myth, as most elderly remain active until the end of their lives. Azar (1996), for example, found that some forms of memory improve with age, while other memory functions, which require a quick response time, decline as the central nervous system slows.

Comorbidity of Psychological and Medical Problems

Unlike their younger counterparts, 85 percent of older adults are affected by at least one chronic medical condition, such as hypertension, heart disease, arthritis, or hearing impairments (U.S. Senate Special Committee on Aging, 1991). Chronic medical problems, including the three leading causes of death for older adults—heart disease, cancer, and stroke—often result in functional impairment or disability. For example, among noninstitutionalized Americans, 11.4 percent over age 65 and 34.5 percent over age 85 have difficulty with one or more activities of daily living (U.S. Senate Special Committee on Aging, 1991).

The older the individual, the more likely he or she is to have multiple medical conditions. With increasing chronic medical conditions and increasing functional impairment, there is also an increase in mental health problems, including anxiety and depression (American Psychological Association, 1993). In a 1993 review, Blazer suggested that almost 40 percent of older medical inpatients are significantly depressed, while only 3 percent of adults over age 65 in community (noninstitutionalized) samples are estimated to suffer from major depression (Friedhoff, 1994). However, in a more recent review by Zeiss, Lewinsohn, and Rohde (in press), the authors suggested that disease only predicts depression if it affects functional status, that older adults' loss of ability to engage in usual patterns of living is a significant risk factor for depression, and that greater functional impairment increases this risk.

With advancing age, each bodily system increasingly affects other physical and psychological systems and functioning. Biological, psychosocial, medical, pharmacological, environmental, and spiritual factors become more interdependent. This can at times seem like what Haley (1996) referred to as a vicious circle. For example, a history of depression may increase the risk of myocardial infarction (Pratt et al., 1996), may be a consequence of a heart attack or stroke, and/or may also affect prognosis or recovery (Frasure-Smith et al., 1995). Or, medication given for insomnia in order to decrease depression may cause delirium, disorientation, or a fall, resulting in a hip fracture, which in turn may result in increased functional impairment and depression. Comorbidity of medical and psychological problems in the oldest-old is high, necessitating a team approach to care or at least continual consultation with other health care professionals.

Diagnostic and Assessment Considerations

Assessments are best when they are interdisciplinary, comprehensive, and tailored to the specific needs of the individual, his or her family, and other caregivers (Zarit & Knight, 1996). A thorough assessment takes into account how problems interrelate and the role that medications, functional impairments, cognitive or sensory decline, physical disease, family, social support, beliefs, and resources play in behavioral or psychological problems. Psychologists conduct several types of assessments as part of this interdisciplinary process or, more often, independently on a consultation basis to other health care providers. Assessment may encompass physical, cognitive, emotional, behavioral, social, functional, nutritional, cultural, and environmental domains, as well as unique characteristics of the individual. What is of major importance, however, is the ability to distinguish between normal aging and disease process (Rowe & Kahn, 1987). Changes in sensory abilities and biological functioning occur gradually as one ages and affect sight, hearing, memory, response time, concentration, and energy levels. For example, metabolic slowing changes an individual's ability to tolerate, utilize, and eliminate medications. Psychologists must be knowledgeable about the possible contributions of disease, functional impairment, and medications to psychological or cognitive problems, in order to know when and how to refer for further evaluation.

Sources of Information

While many older patients are the primary source of assessment information, it is advisable to consult with other sources if the patient has cognitive, sensory, or physical limitations. To fully assess what is contributing to or maintaining a patient's problem, information should be gathered from as many relevant sources as possible and necessary, including relatives, friends, physicians, nursing staff, and social agencies.

To illustrate the importance of interdisciplinary assessment and the use of multiple sources of information, consider the following case. A 68-year-old man was brought to a hospital clinic by his daughter for treatment of possible depression and substance abuse. A Native American, he had spent his life on his Northern Plains reservation, until three months prior to assessment when his wife died and he joined his daughter in a large city. During the intake interview, the man was found to be clinically depressed, drinking four to five beers per day, and on multiple medications—the names of which he could not remember. He had been diagnosed with diabetes, had a myocardial infarction nine months before, and retired within the past two years. He reported eating only one or two meals per day, usually cereal, because he was not hungry and could not see well enough most days to cook or reheat prepared food. When asked about meals with his daughter, he reported that his dentures do not fit and "it hurts to chew." He got minimal exercise, lived with his daughter, and had no other current ties to his community or family.

It is highly unlikely that one professional would have the knowledge or skill to deal with all of the possible factors contributing to this man's problems. It would be more helpful to put together a team consisting of, besides the psychologist, a geriatrician, an internist, a cardiologist, an endocrinologist, a pharmacist, a dentist, an ophthamologist, a nutritionist, a specialist in geriatric psychiatry, a case manager, a social worker, an exercise specialist or physical therapist, someone from the clergy, and his daughter or others who understand his traditions, including perhaps his tribe's healer. Such a comprehensive team approach could assist in fully meeting this man's complex needs.

Assessment of older medical patients should always include questions regarding recent or past medical problems, trauma or injuries suffered throughout the life span, exposure to toxins, and substance or alcohol abuse. It is important to obtain a list of current and past prescription and nonprescription medications. A social and cultural history also needs to be gathered and should include information on education, employment and financial status, current living situation, social supports (family, friends and spouse), religious affiliation, social activities, ethnicity and cultural background, family history, and a list of current or past pleasurable activities. The individual's ability to maintain daily activities in a variety of settings must be assessed. Assessment of individual strengths and deficits is necessary not only for proper diagnosis, treatment planning, and implementation but also for continued evaluation of patient goals and expectations. Kaszniak (1996) provides an overview of various comprehensive interview protocols developed for use with older adults and their families, as well as professional caregiver reports or checklists.

Types of Assessment

Often several forms of psychological assessment are necessary. Self-report measures, cognitive and neuropsychological testing, direct behavioral observation, and psychophysiological techniques can add valuable information to the clinical interview. Cognitive and neuropsychological testing assesses the nature and possible bases of an older adult's cognitive or behavioral problems or functional impairment. Psychologists working with older adults should be able to conduct a mental status examination or neuropsychological screening evaluation, such as Folstein's Mini-Mental State (Folstein, Folstein, & McHugh, 1975), and interpret it. For information on assessing dementias and cognitive function in older adults, see Storandt and VandenBos (1994) and Kaszniak (1996), along with chapter 10 in this text.

As discussed earlier, mental health providers are often called upon to assess the ability of an older adult to function and independently take care of him- or herself in a variety of environments. Functional abilities include activities of daily living (ADLs; such activities as grooming, eating, toileting, and mobility) and instrumental activities of daily living (IADLs; i.e., activities and skills necessary to survive in the community, such as communication, household chores, shopping, and health maintenance). Kemp and Mitchell (1992) provide a comprehensive review of ADL and IADL assessments for older adults.

For psychologists working with older adults in hospitals, rehabilitation, or nursing homes, behavioral assessments and treatment are almost indispensable. Behavioral analysis is useful for assessing the older patient's strengths and weaknesses and targeting areas to strengthen adaptive behavior. A functional assessment of behavior is often helpful for problem areas such as noncompliance with treatment or medications. Examining the behaviors that surround noncompliance by doing a functional assessment to determine the causes of reduced adherence to recommended treatment is a first step in changing the unwanted behavior. The patient's lack of understanding, a too complex regimen, or simple human error are just a few of many possible reasons that may be found with a functional assessment.

Instruments that measure anxiety or depression symptoms or personality traits need either to be either designed for use with older clients or to have known psychometric properties relative to older adults. Kaszniak's (1996) chapter is a good starting place for techniques and instruments for the psychological assessment of older adults.

Special Considerations

As previously noted, knowledge of the normal aging process is especially important for mental health providers working with older adults. Psychologists need to be able to differentiate normal changes from cognitive and psychological changes caused by medication, nutritional changes, functional impairment, and disease processes.

Exploring and understanding the possible effects or interactions of medical conditions and medications is a chief concern in assessment of older adults. Around 86 percent of older adults have chronic conditions for which ongoing pharmacological treatment is necessary, and approximately 34 percent of them take three or more prescription medications; it is not uncommon for patients with multiple chronic conditions to take eight or more medications at once (APA, 1993). Such use of multiple medications dramatically increases the likelihood of drug interactions, which, in turn, cause new symptoms. Medication side effects are seven times more likely to occur in older adults than in younger adults (Andresen, 1995).

Further complicating the issue is that older adults may not comprehend the proper use of medications, may not be able to afford them, and/or may not comply regularly with treatments. More than 25 percent of admissions to emergency rooms of individuals over age 65 were due to drug-related reactions (Andresen, 1995). Although psychologists working with older adults may not be completely conversant with the side effects and interactions of various medications, they can and need to learn about particularly problematic drugs. A number of commonly prescribed medications can contribute to delirium, depression, anxiety, mania, or other psychological problems. Sources for understanding drug interactions in older adults are Andresen (1995) and Schwartz (1994).

In addition to medications and disease processes, normal age-related changes can affect the assessment of geriatric patients. Changes in vision, hearing, and sensorimotor capability, and physical limitations such as arthritis are commonplace in older adults. By the age of 65 almost one-half of adults experience vision loss to 20/70 or less. The same is true for auditory ability, with loss being detected in about 50 percent of those over age 75. Diminished hearing and vision can lead to errors in communication and information processing, thus contributing to invalid testing protocols or misinterpretation of assessment results. It is helpful to remind patients to bring correctional devices, such as eyeglasses and hearing aids, to the assessment appointment. Change in speed of information processing also impacts validity and reliability across the assessment process. Older adults process material more slowly than younger adults and many testing procedures have timed components. Fatigue and pain are other factors to consider that can bias results and the implementation of treatment plans.

The likelihood of comorbidity of one or more medical and mental disorders creates diagnostic difficulties. The effects of normal aging can be confused with some of the symptoms of depression or mild dementia. Older adults often report loss of energy, changes in eating or sleeping patterns, or loss of sexual interest. Age-related changes in psychopathology are not well researched, although there is some indication that older adults may manifest a disorder differently from younger populations (Gurland, 1987). It is important to remember that, with advancing age, a change in one system is more likely to affect other systems within the individual.

Delirium, common after the age of 60 (Conn, 1991), can be the result of medical conditions, changes in body metabolism, or medication effects. This treatable condition often goes unrecognized by medical teams and can have potentially deleterious effects if left unaddressed. Dementia is also of increasing concern in older adults; approximately one-quarter of those presenting with delirium have a preexisting dementia (Conn, 1991). The ability to identify both disorders and to differentiate between them is crucial.

The psychologist working with older medical patients must incorporate many sources of information in assessment, diagnosis, and treatment planning. It should never be assumed that others are trained to ask the same questions or incorporate findings into a comprehensive body of information that reflects the patient's level of functioning. The expertise of various professionals is necessary for a comprehensive assessment of the older patient; an interdisciplinary approach is preferred. In the absence of a geriatic team, it is necessary to learn how to best draw on the information and expertise available from other professionals and relevant sources.

Interventions

For the most part, the assessment and therapeutic skills that mental health clinicians use with adult clients apply to work with older patients as well. The main differences occur in the process of psychotherapy (e.g., pacing, goals, and issues of treatment) and in implications of conducting treatment in different settings (Zarit & Knight, 1996). For an empirically-based overview of interventions with older adults, their familes, and caregivers in different settings and from different theoretical perspectives, we recommend Zarit and Knight (1996).

Adapting Treatment for Older Patients

Counseling psychologists and other clinicians need to modify their therapeutic approaches with older patients, taking into account age-related changes in hearing, vision, and information processing, as well as physical or functional limitations such as those caused by chronic pain or fatigue. This may translate into conducting therapy at a slower pace, with shorter sessions, or with breaks. Age-related hearing loss means that lower pitches are heard better than higher pitches; therefore the provider needs to position him- or herself directly in front of the patient and speak clearly and slowly with a low voice pitch. For patients with mild memory problems it is helpful to write notes. A well-lit room with direct lighting available for written material or chalkboards and large-print reading material are helpful for many adults with visual deficits. When providing information or teaching skills, it is important to provide demonstrations and present material in multiple formats—verbally and visually. Providers need to remember to say it, write it, and show or demonstrate it. The patient should then say and demonstrate the skill. Finally, end the session with written or audiotaped reminders.

Other specific interventions, such as relaxation training, may need to be adapted to physical limitations. If, for example, a patient with chronic obstructive pulmonary disorder is unable do rhythmic breathing or finds it uncomfortable to focus on breathing, techniques that elicit the relaxation response without a focus on breathing may be used. Among others, these include meditation, progressive muscle relaxation, repetitive exercise, or repetitive prayer. For a physically impaired patient unable to use progressive muscle relaxation because the tensing and relaxing of certain muscle groups causes pain, alternative techniques might include body scan relaxation, imagery, or gentle yoga stretching.

Mental health providers also need to be aware of their own attitudes and feelings toward older patients, both positive and negative, so they do not interfere with adequate assessment or effective treatment. If there is a great age difference between the patient and the psychologist, this should be addressed. It is also important to have some awareness of and sensitivity to the patient's specific attitudes and beliefs. For example, many older woman believe that public exercise is not proper and so do not want to walk around the hospital or go to cardiac rehabilitation following cardiac surgery, which could ultimately hamper their recovery. A common dysfunctional attitude among older adults is that they are too old to learn or change. Because such beliefs may be harmful to the patient's physical or mental health, it is therapeutic to challenge the logic of these beliefs to reduce the frequency of their occurrence. Since many older adults frequently use the coping style of changing the meaning of a situation, this process may be used to change the meaning of a belief, such as it not being proper to exercise in public. The mental health provider, through a cognitive-behavioral approach, could suggest that the patient change the meaning of exercise to something more acceptable, like walking and visiting in the mall.

Special Concerns with Older Medical Patients

Working with older medical patients involves adapting psychotherapy to the setting and to different presenting issues. Since there is little research on therapy with older adults in medical settings, the following comments are based on clinical literature and experience. A change for many psychologists starts with the initial contact. The patient will immediately need a rationale for psychological evaluation and treatment (Haley, 1996). If concerned about medical problems, the patient will likely feel those concerns are minimized or discounted if the provider begins with questions regarding psychological functioning. It is useful to explain that when older people develop medical problems, they may also develop psychological problems, problems in memory or thinking, or limitations in activities they used to enjoy. Throughout, it is important to normalize the patient's concerns. For example, when assessing anxiety with a cardiac patient, the clinician may note that it is common for patients who have been on heart monitors to be fearful and anxious and even to think they are having palpitations for days or weeks after they are out of the cardiac care unit. It is important to ask about health problems, not simply to gain rapport, but also to gather vital information about the client's knowledge and compliance.

Psychologists should not assume that an older patient's medical problems and disabilities mean acceptance of a poor life quality or depression. One goal may be to help the patient learn to live with his or her limitations and find other enjoyable life activities. This highlights the importance of close collaboration with physicians in order to determine what is realistic given the patient's medical condition.

In addition, providers may need to change their perspective or role. Often psychologists see patients only briefly on a consultation basis in the patient's room, which limits confidentiality because there is another patient in the next bed. Further, someone else may carry out the intervention. For example, a nurse may teach the patient a relaxation technique or an aide may get the patient to reminisce about pleasant events. Psychotherapy can include collaboration with family members and/or other health care providers. Treatments may involve the staff in a nursing home or the family of a home-bound patient rather than be directly with the patient. Interventions vary from having the staff of a day treatment program implement a behavioral program to increase the frequency with which the patient interacts with others to having an Alzheimer's patient's spouse participate in a caregiver's support group.

Mental health providers in medical settings may need to help older patients face their own death and help their families and loved ones face it. Often older adults accept their death before their spouses or other relatives. This can be especially stressful if the patient says he or she is ready to let go and die while the relatives are not and want extraordinary measures taken to keep their loved one alive. Family counseling including the dying patient is appropriate at this time to enable individuals to share their feelings, say their good-byes, and accept the death. Families that wish to play an active role in the death, being with their loved one or guiding them in meditation or prayer, often seek suggestions from mental health providers.

Following the death, spouses may need to be encouraged to join a bereavement group. Gallagher-Thompson, Futterman, Farberow, Thompson, and Peterson (1993) advocate this for men because they have increased mortality rates following their spouse's death. Bereavement groups or other ways to enrich social networks are important to older men who have lost their confidante and the person responsible for their social life. Grief work for older adults involves both accepting the loss and finding a new life without the deceased.

Death is a common occurrence in nursing homes or medical units of hospitals. If a patient dies suddenly or unexpectedly, it can be traumatic for the provider and other patients as well as for family and friends. Providers need to be open to processing how the death of a nursing home patient affects other patients, other caregivers, and themselves, all of whom need to grieve. The boundaries of therapy change when working with older adults in these settings. While it would be inappropriate to hold hands in traditional therapy, it may be extremely comforting to hold the hand of older patients who are in pain or frightened. It would also be appropriate to share your grief at the loss of their loved one with the family.

Counseling psychologists can also play a role in developing psychoeducational programs for maintaining and enhancing the health of older adults. Wellness programs focus on helping older adults acquire the skills and knowledge to cope with transitions, losses, and/or medical symptoms. These groups can be for older adults only and organized around a specific transition, such as retirement; they can be open to all adults with common medical problems, such as chronic pain or cancer; or they can include individuals with varied medical symptoms. Within a group, patients become aware of physical and mental stress and learn techniques for reducing symptoms caused or exaccerbated by stress and for enhancing health and well-being. Techniques taught include meditation, cognitive restructuring, exercise, nutrition, and knowledge about particular medical conditions.

Other programs that may be offered are bereavement groups or life review or reminiscence therapy groups. Reminiscence therapy, as well as relaxation techniques, has also been used with older adults to reduce anxiety prior to surgery. Programs for caregivers and respite care programs have been found to reduce caregiver distress and thus possibly maintain the caregiver's health (Knight, Lutzky, & Macofsky-Urban, 1993). Psychologists can also play a role in starting up and training peer leaders of self-help groups, such as those for cancer patients or caregivers of patients with Alzheimer's disease.

Psychological Treatments for Common Problems

In a comprehensive review of the efficacy of psychotherapy with older adults, Gallagher-Thompson and Thompson (1995) note several types of psychotherapy that have been demonstrated to be effective. These include brief forms of cognitive, behavioral, personal construct, control mastery, and psychodynamic therapies as well as various cognitive-behavioral, psychodynamic, and psychoeducational group treatments. Recent meta-analyses of 17 controlled empirical studies of psychotherapy with older adults suggest that these therapies are reliably more effective than no treatment for depression (Scogin & McElreath, 1994). Research has also indicated the effectiveness of behavioral or psychotherapeutic treatments for other common problems faced by some older adults. Several comprehensive reviews provide further details about these therapies and their empirical basis (Carstensen & Edelstein, 1987; Zarit & Knight, 1996).

Controversies

Because older adults are such a diverse group and because the problems they present to the health care system include so many interacting and complex factors involving different professions, controversies abound. Two problems in particular, (a) the issue of how to train providers and which providers are most appropriate to deliver services, and (b) the future role for counseling psychologists in providing care to older adult medical patients, are highlighted below.

As discussed in this chapter, most physicians and psychologists are inadequately trained to meet the prevention, assessment, and treatment needs of older adults. Interdisciplinary geriatric assessment teams are rare. For mental health care providers working with older adults, a major question is how to integrate information relevant to psychological functioning and aging with the physician's knowledge. The primary care physician is often the gatekeeper to older adults getting other services; however, he or she often does not have the training to recognize the risk factors for problems such as depression in older adults. There are several contradictory solutions proposed to this problem:

- Increase the training of physicians to recognize these problems and refer.
- Integrate mental health care providers with psychological and aging knowledge into primary care practices.
- Increase psychologists' knowledge of geriatric medicine.

Another question clinical geropsychologists must grapple with is what the future role of psychologists will or should be in providing care to older medical patients. This question arises from different directions. One is the changing health care system. Managed care demands empirical data to demonstrate the necessity of involving psychologists in the health and mental health care of older adults. A challenge will be to empirically demonstrate how and why we need to be part of the "team." Another direction is the need to increase adequate assessment and care of older patients. In order to meet the increased service demand, it is suggested that psychologists working with older adults will give very little direct patient care but will have increased roles as consultants, trainers, supervisors, team facilitators, and team builders. An added future challenge will be the giving away or teaching of psychological assessment and intervention skills to the public and other professions, both to increase older adult self-care and to ensure the adequate care of older medical patients.

There are a number of other issues that counseling psychologists working with older medical patients should note. Ageism, the term coined by Robert Butler (1987) for a "process of systematic stereotyping and discrimination against people because they are old, just as racism and sexism accomplish this for skin color and gender" (p. 22), may influence how older adults view themselves, how younger people view them, and how health care providers treat them. Younger adults often see older adults as different and separate from themselves; this can be seen in medical residents' references to being on the "vegetable" rotation. Ageism has also shaped our theories and treatments; once-accepted myths of aging include the theory of disengagement, sexlessness, and senility.

The mental health provider must be aware of the issues surrounding living wills, "do not resuscitate" orders, advanced directives, physician-assisted suicide, and rationing of health care. A good background source for socio-legal, medical-ethical, and political perspectives interacting with clinical geropsychology on these issues is Smith (1996).

Summary

Counseling psychologists and other mental health care providers in health care settings face a number of challenges in the prevention, assessment, and treatment of older patients. The first is understanding normal aging and some of the various biopsychosocial factors that can render diagnosis and treatment of the problems of the oldest-old extraordinarily complex. The second is recognizing the necessity of involving many players and finding a way to communicate with them about the patient, which is especially difficult in the absence of a team. The third is adapting a wide range of interventions to meet the needs of the patient and including the caregivers, family, or nursing home staff in these interventions. The final challenge involves learning and building on the patient's own unique strengths.

Suggested Resources

For an overview of psychology's possible contributions to older adults and productive aging, see *Vitality for Life: Psychological Research for Productive Aging* (APA, 1993). For further information on the United States health goals for older adults, consult *Healthy People 2000: National Health Promotion and Disease Prevention Objectives* (U.S. Department of Health and Human Services, 1990). To keep current with general issues of aging, older adult health and mental health, contact the National Institutes of Aging (NIA); a good place to start is their homepage on the worldwide Web (http://www.nih.gov/nia/).

For an overview of clinically effective, empirically-based interventions with older adults, their families, and caregivers in different settings and from different theoretical perspectives, we recommend *A Guide to Psychotherapy and Aging: Effective Clinical Interventions in a Life-Stage Context* (Zarit & Knight, 1996). This volume includes chapters on the use of behavioral, cognitive-behavioral, interpersonal, modern psychoanalytic, and family therapy with older adults as well as addressing ethical considerations, interventions with caregivers, work in nursing homes and the medical context of psychotherapy with older adults. Kaszniak's (1996) chapter in this volume provides an excellent review and further references for techniques and instruments for the psychological assessment of older adults. Specific information on assessing dementias and cognitive function in older adults can also be found in Storandt and VandenBos (1994). Kemp and Mitchell (1992) review ADL and IADL assessments for older adults.

It is very important that mental health providers working with older adults in medical settings have some understanding of normal aging and the impact of multiple medical problems and medications. The chapter by Haley (1996) provides some further references on geriatric teams and geriatric medicine. Beginning sources for understanding drug interactions in older adults are Andresen (1995) and Schwartz (1994).

Counseling psychologists and other applied psychologists interested in working with older adults should consult the draft report of the American Psychological Association (APA) Interdivisional Task Force on qualifications for practice in clinical and applied geropsychology (Lichtenberg et al., 1996) for further information on training and practice issues in clinical geropsychology. Since training and credentialing issues are rapidly changing, contact is advised with such groups as Section 2 (clinical geropsychology; counseling psychologists also belong to this section) of APA Division 12 (clinical psychology; contact http://www.apa.org/about/division.html#d12), the Aging Special Interest Group in APA Division 38 (health psychology; contact by e-mail "Dr. Alex Zautra" <Alex.Zautra@asu.edu>), APA Division 20 (http://www.iog.wayne.edu/APADiv20/apadiv20.htm), the newly formed APA Committee on Aging, the Association for the Advancement of Behavior Therapy Aging and Behavior Therapy Special Interest Group (http://server.psyc.vt.edu/aabt/), and the Gerontological Society of America (GSA; http://www.geron.org/). The worldwide Web homepages of NIA, GSA, and Division 20 of APA are also particularly useful for keeping current on issues and pointing to sources of information on normal aging and geriatric medicine.

Discussion Questions

1. What type of specialized training, if any, is necessary to work with older adults in medical settings? What changes may be needed to meet the possible changing roles of clinical geropsychologists in medical settings?
2. Why is there a need for comprehensive geriatric assessment teams? Discuss possible advantages and disadvantages to this team approach.
3. How might a counseling psychologist integrate his or her services with other health care professionals in settings where there is not a geriatric team?
4. What is ageism? How can it impact the work of counseling psychologists in health care settings?

References

American Psychological Association, Science Directorate. (1993). *Vitality for life: Psychological research for productive aging.* Reston, VA: American Psychological Association.

Andresen, G. (1995). *Caring for people with Alzheimer's disease: A training manual for direct care providers.* Baltimore, MD: Health Care Professionals.

Azar, B. (1996). Some forms of memory improve with age. *The APA Monitor, 27*(11), 27.

Blazer, D. (1991). Suicide risk factors in the elderly: An epidemiological study. *Journal of Geriatric Psychiatry, 29,* 175–189.

Blazer, D. G. (1993). *Depression in late life* (2nd ed.). St. Louis, MO: Mosby.

Butler, R. N. (1987). Ageism. In G. L. Maddox (Ed.), The encyclopedia of aging (pp. 22–23). New York: Springer.

Carstensen, L. L., & Edelstein, B. A. (1987). *Handbook of clinical gerontology.* Elmsford, NY: Pergamon.

Conn, D. (1991). Delirium and other organic mental disorders. In J. Sadavoy, L. W. Lazarus, & L. F. Jarvik (Eds.), *Comprehensive review of geriatric psychiatry* (pp. 331–336). Washington, DC: American Psychiatric Press.

Fiske, M., & Chiriboga, D. A. (1990). *Change and continuity in adult life.* San Francisco: Jossey-Bass.

Folstein, M. F., Folstein, S., & McHugh, P. R. (1975). Mini-mental dtate: A practical method for grading the cognitive state of patients for the clinician. *Journal of Psychiatric Research, 12,* 189–198.

Frasure-Smith, N., Lespérance, F., & Talajic, M. (1995). Depression and 18-month prognosis after myocardial infarction. *Circulation, 91,* 999–1005.

Friedhoff, A. J. (1994). Consensus panel report. In L. S. Schneider, C. F. Reynolds, B. D. Lebowitz, & A. J. Friedhoff (Eds.), *Diagnosis and treatment of depression in late life: Results of the NIH Consensus Development Conference.* Washington, DC: American Psychiatric Press.

Gallagher-Thompson, D., Futterman, A., Farberow, N., Thompson, L. W., & Peterson, J. (1993). The impact of spousal bereaveement on older widows and widowers. In M. S. Stroebe (Ed.), *Handbook of bereavement: Theory, reasearch, and intevention.* New York: Cambridge University.

Gallagher-Thompson, D., & Thompson, L. W. (1995). Psychotherapy with older adults in theory and practice. In B. Bonger, & L. Beutler (Eds.), *Comprehensive textbook of psychotherapy* (pp. 357–359). New York: Oxford University.

Gurland, B. (1987). Psychopathology. In G. L. Maddox (Ed.), *The encyclopedia of aging* (pp. 549–550). New York: Springer.

Haley, W. E. (1996). The medical context of psychotherapy with the elderly. In S. H. Zarit, & B. G. Knight (Eds.), *A guide to psychotherapy and aging: Effective clinical interventions in a life-stage context* (pp. 221–239). Washington, DC: American Psychological Association.

Kaszniak, A. W. (1996). Techniques and instruments for assessment of the elderly. In S. H. Zarit, & B. G. Knight (Eds.), *A guide to psychotherapy and aging: Effective clinical interventions in a life-stage context* (pp. 163–219). Washington, DC: American Psychological Association.

Kemp, B. J., & Mitchell, J. M. (1992). Functional assessment in geriatric mental health. In J. E. Birren, R. B. Sloan, & G. D. Cohen (Eds.), *Handbook of mental health and aging* (2nd ed., pp. 671–697). San Diego, CA: Academic.

Knight, B. G., Lutzky, S. M., & Macofsky-Urban, F. (1993). A meta-analytic review of interventions for caregiver distress: Recommendations for future research. *The Gerontologist, 33,* 240–249.

Koenig, H. G., & Blazer, D. G., II. (1990). Depression and other affective disorders. In C. K. Cassel, D. E. Riesenberg, L. B. Sorensen, & J. R. Walsh (Eds.), *Geriatric medicine* (2nd ed., pp. 473–490). New York: Springer-Verlag.

Lichtenberg, P. A., Duffy, M., Edelstein, B., Gallagher-Thompson, D., Gatz, M., Hartman-Stein, P., Hinrichsen, G., LaRue, A., Niederehe, G., Taylor, G., & Teri, L. (1996). *Draft report of the APA interdivisional task force on qualifications for practice in clinical and applied geropsychology: Draft #4.* Unpublished manuscript.

National Institutes of Health Consensus Panel (1992). Diagnosis and treatment of depression in late life. J*ournal of American Medical Association, 268,* 1018–1024.

Pearlin, L. I., & Skaff, M. M. (1995). Stressors and adaptation in late life. In M. Gatz (Ed.), *Emerging issues in mental health and aging* (pp. 97–103). Washington, DC: American Psychological Association.

Pratt, L. A., Ford, D. E., Crum, R. M., Armenian, H. K., Gallo, J. J., & Eaton, W. W. (1996). Depression, psychotropic medication, and risk of myocardial infarction: Prospective data from the Baltimore ECA follow-up. *Circulation, 94*(12), 3123–3129.

Rowe, J. W., & Kahn, R. L. (1987). Human aging: Usual and successful. *Science, 237,* 143–149.

Schwartz, J. B. (1994). Clinical pharmacology. In W. R. Hazzard, E. L. Bierman, J. P. Blass, W. H. Ettinger, & J. B. Halter (Eds.), *Principles of geriatric medicine and gerontology* (3rd ed., pp. 259–275). New York: McGraw-Hill.

Scogin, F., & McElreath, L. (1994). Efficacy of psychosocial treatments for geriatric depression: A quantitative review. Journal of Clinical and Consulting *Psychology, 62,* 69–74.

Smith, G. P., II. (1996). *Legal and healthcare ethics for the elderly.* Washington, DC: Taylor & Francis.

Storandt, M., & VandenBos, G. R. (Eds.). (1994). *Neuropsychological assessment of dementia and depression in older adults.* Washington, DC: American Psychological Association.

U.S. Bureau of Census. (1992). Sixty-five plus in America. *Current population reports: Special studies* (series No. P23–178). Washington, DC: U.S. Government Printing Office.

U.S. Department of Health and Human Services, Public Health Service.(1990). *Healthy people 2000: National health promotion and disease prevention objectives.* Washington, DC: Author.

U.S. Senate Special Committee on Aging, American Association of Retired Persons, Federal Council on Aging, and U.S. Administration on Aging. (1991). *Aging America: Trends and projections.* Washington, DC: Department of Health and Human Services.

Zarit, S. H., & Knight, B. G. (1996). Introduction: Psychotherapy and aging: Multiple strategies, psositive outcomes. In S. H. Zarit, & B. G. Knight (Eds.), *A guide to psychotherapy and aging: Effective clinical interventions in a life-stage context* (pp. 1–13). Washington, DC: American Psychological Association.

Zeiss, A. M., Lewinsohn, P. M., & Rohde, P. (in press). Functional impairment, physical disease, and depression in older adults. In P. Kato, & T. Mann (Eds.), *Health psychology of special populations.* New York: Plenum.

14

Women's Health Issues: A Focus on Infertility, Gynecological Cancer, and Menopause

Sharon E. Robinson Kurpius
Susan E. Maresh

No one would be surprised at the statement that women are biologically different from men. However, addressing women's health issues from a multidisciplinary perspective in an organized fashion is very new to the health care community. Previously, issues such as how being a woman affects the disease process, how the disease process affects women, and why certain diseases primarily affect women have been ignored. Although gender-based health differences exist from conception to death, medical research informing health care professionals on these differences has been absent or fragmented.

Concerns over the gender disparity in our medical knowledge base were documented in a 1985 report of the Public Health Service Task Force on Women's Health Issues (United States Public Health Services, 1985). This report's recommendations led the National Institute of Health (NIH,1986) to publish a policy statement in their *Guide for Grants and Contracts* urging the inclusion of women in clinical studies. Four years later the United States General Accounting Office (GAO; 1990) issued a report stating that the NIH policy had been virtually ignored. The GAO report provided the catalyst to unify the efforts of Congress, the NIH, the medical, health, and scientific communities, and the public at large in far-reaching reforms that would lead to substantial changes in health research. For example, the NIH mandated that no research application be funded unless women (and minorities) were adequately represented and established the Office of Research on Women's Health (NIH, 1990). The Director of NIH spearheaded the launch of the Women's Health Initiative, the most comprehensive study of women's health in history (Healy, 1991). As is evident from this brief historical overview, focusing specifically on women's health issues is a very recent phenomenon.

Traditionally, scientific research using male-only populations was based on the idea that the research would not be obscured by the effects of hormonal influences on physiological processes. Pregnancy, lactation, and menopause were viewed as interfering with accurate knowledge of the course of a disease and its response to treatment (Sherman, 1993). It has now been demonstrated, however, that the endocrine status of women can confound medical diagnoses and alter the impact of interventions. The reliance on the male model has resulted in limited information on specific indications and contraindications for treatment of women. This is especially poignant when one considers that women are more likely than men to take both prescription and over-the-counter drugs and are more frequent users of medical health services (Rodin & Ickovics, 1990). According to the American Medical Association (AMA) Council on Ethical and Judicial Affairs (1991), the gender disparities in research efforts have left health care providers with insufficient knowledge for relevant preventive strategies, diagnostic procedures, and safe and efficacious interventions.

A recent report (Tobin, Wassertheil-Smoller, & Wexler, 1987) on gender disparities illustrates some of the consequences of insufficient research and a weak medical knowledge base. This report noted that even though cardiovascular disease is the number one killer of women, men are at least six times more likely than women to be referred for cardiac catherization, even after controlling for age and disease severity. Although the risk of lung cancer is similar between women and men with similar smoking usage, there is a 50 percent greater chance that cytologic studies of sputum to diagnose lung cancer will be ordered for men than for women (AMA, 1991). Disparities also exist in receiving a transplant. Women aged 46 to 60 undergoing renal dialysis are 50 percent less likely to receive a kidney transplant than are men the same age (AMA, 1991).

Counseling health psychologists are in a position to help female patients and their medical care providers. In addition to helping women evaluate treatment options in light of their lifestyles and life choices, they can help the medical team to view and treat female patients in light of their womanhood. In order to serve as an advocate, assist in health decision making, and facilitate adaptive coping strategies, the counseling health psychologist must be able to integrate knowledge about women's unique physiology, about psychological concerns, and about various medical concerns. For example, without the knowledge of common medical concerns of women, such as hypothyroidism, a health psychologist may treat a patient for depressive symptomatology for a considerable time without decreasing her depression, since in actuality the patient might be experiencing a thyroid disorder, not clinical depression (Vliet, 1995). To avoid such an instance, the patient should be referred to her physician in order to rule out potential physiological causes for the depression.

In addition to incorrectly diagnosing a woman's concern as a psychological condition, other significant reasons exist for becoming knowledgeable about women's psychophysiology. Lifestyle factors can directly affect disease onset, duration, and outcomes that, in turn, affect morbidity and mortality. For example, a common misperception is that osteoporosis is only relevant to women of advanced age. However, women have 20 percent less bone mineral resources than men, and the turnover of bone loss occurs twice as rapidly for women. Bone mass turnover begins around age 35. By the time women are age 50 they can already be deficient if they are not taking a calcium supplement and vitamin D (Bilezikian, 1995). In addition, both smoking and heavy consumption of carbonated drinks negatively affect calcium absorption, which results in more bone mass turnover. Although women live longer than men, the complications from diseases like osteoporosis diminish the quality of those years. About 20 percent of women die from hip fracture complications within three months of the fracture, and over 50 percent never walk independently again (Vliet, 1995). It is important for psychologists to know the lifestyle risk factors for osteoporosis (Kaltenborn, 1992) to be competent when working with patients with this concern.

Without specific biopsychosocial knowledge about areas specific to women's health, the counseling health psychologist will be mediocre at best in helping the medical team and female patients in addressing health issues. While the topic of this chapter is women's health issues, there are too many to cover them all. Therefore, three of the most pressing issues will be addressed—infertility, gynecological cancers, and women's midlife health concerns related to menopause.

Infertility

The vast majority of women assume that if they decide to have children, they will just get pregnant as expected. However, statistics now indicate that one in six couples will experience infertility (Menning, 1980), and of those who seek medical intervention, only 50 percent will be successful in their attempt to conceive (Daniluk, 1996).

Historically, women have been blamed for not conceiving. Indeed, famous for his many wives, Henry VIII systematically "did away with" most of them for their failure to conceive or for not conceiving a male child. Up until the 1970s, when medical practitioners were able to identify physical causes for infertility, the woman was blamed for having emotional problems that were interfering with her conception (Burns, 1987). Only in the last 25 years has the man in the relationship been routinely included in any clinical workup investigating potential causes of infertility (Leiblum, 1988). Today we know that there is a known physical cause for 90 percent of the couples trying to conceive, with 40 percent of the causal factors related to the man, 40 percent to the woman, and 20 percent shared (Menning, 1988). According to Leiblum, factors implicated in infertility include:

1. more liberal attitudes toward sexual behaviors that have resulted in a drastic increase in genital infections (genital inflammatory disease, PID) that damage fallopian tubes, ovaries, and uterus
2. greater exposure to environmental toxins
3. use of contraceptive procedures that may damage the reproductive tract
4. increased age at time of attempted conception

Diagnosing infertility, generally defined as having attempted unsuccessfully for one year to conceive, is a complex process often involving multiple medical tests and procedures, which result in considerable emotional strain on the couple. Medical interventions may include surgery such as laparoscopy that requires a general anesthesia, hormonal regimes with physical and psychological side effects, and daily recording of basal temperature (Leiblum, 1988). This daily recording is a constant reminder for the couple that they have failed to conceive and often interferes with their sexual spontaneity. In addition to the costliness of these medical procedures, they invade the core of the couple's most private life together.

It is essential to understand factors influencing infertility. However, since the focus of this discussion is women's health issues, only biospychosocial factors related to women's infertility will be discussed. The primary physiological factors include "(a) obstructed or damaged fallopian tubes; (b) failure by the ovary to produce a viable ovum(s); (c) cervical abnormalities that prevent the penetration of sperm; and (d) inability of the uterus to accept or maintain the conceptus" (Leiblum, 1988, p. 118). It should be evident from this list that mental health professionals working with patients who have been unable to conceive need a thorough understanding of female reproductive anatomy and the psychophysiological aspects of reproduction and conception.

Emotional factors may also be related to infertility in a small proportion of cases. It has been assumed that stress impacts fertility through hypothalamic-pituitary-gonadal relations; however, research has failed to demonstrate this relationship except in cases of extreme environmental stress (Leiblum, 1988). Further, while depression has been clinically linked to infertility, the role of depression in decreasing the release of follicle-stimulating hormone (FSH) and luteinizing hormone (LH) has not been empirically supported. Finally, although psychosexual problems have been theoretically linked to infertility, it is difficult to say whether sexual problems are a cause or effect of infertility. Sex on demand, when the woman's basal temperature is ideal, is less than romantic and can cause sexual dysfunction. Women may experience vaginismus, involuntary contraction of vaginal muscles, when anxiety about failure to conceive is high and the time for intercourse is determined by body temperature rather than mood. Women may also experience a sense of urgency that interferes with their ability to enjoy sex and achieve orgasm. All of these may have serious emotional consequences for the couple and the woman, and thus impede the ability to become pregnant.

Fertility is a chronic crisis—it recurs month after month (Conway & Valentine, 1988). Women who consistently fail to achieve pregnancy are on an emotional roller coaster, vacillating between hope and despair. Feeling helpless, powerless, and a lack of control, they question their fundamental beliefs about themselves, their bodies, and their partners (Berg & Wilson, 1991; Daniluk, 1988). It is not surprising that they feel angry and cheated and envy others who are pregnant or have children (Conway & Valentine, 1988). This anger may be turned against the medical establishment, against themselves for being "flawed," against friends and family, against God, or against their partner (Covington, 1988). If the woman has delayed her attempts to get pregnant due to other priorities such as a career or has had an abortion earlier in her life, she may experience guilt and self- blame (Covington, 1988). Depression is common among women experiencing the challenges of infertility. For some this depression is brief and cyclical, associated with each month's failure to conceive, while for others depression may become a part of their daily lives (Mahlstedt, 1985).

One of the strongest emotions is a profound sense of loss. This loss includes the loss of being pregnant, actually giving birth, being able to breast-feed, and having a child to raise and to carry on one's life. While these losses may be invisible to others, they are very real to the woman and her partner. Like other losses in life, they need to be grieved. Since the loss due to infertility is one of potential rather than of a person or a tangible object, others may not understand the depth of the pain being felt (Forrest & Gilbert, 1992). Since there is no closure for this type of loss, couples must find ways to deal with a grief that "is not recognized or validated by society" (Forrest & Gilbert, 1992, p. 47).

At some point, if conception has not occurred, the couple must decide to end attempts to achieve pregnancy (Matthews & Matthews, 1986). In the process of finding acceptance of and adaptation to infertility (Fleming & Burry, 1988), the multitude of experienced feelings such as anger, guilt, loss, and isolation needs to be revisited and integrated until they no long hold deep pain for the woman. Infertility may also result in the loss of the partner relationship if the emotional and physical drain of infertility becomes too heavy.

Although the empirical literature is relatively sparse on working with the psychosocial concerns related to infertility, there are some excellent writings available. For example, Leiblum (1988) talks about four areas of intervention:

1. cognitive attributions related to blame, hostility, and guilt
2. sexual problems, with the goal of treating actual sexual dysfunctions, and encouraging the couple who has lost the joy of sex to abandon the demand component and resume spontaneous sex
3. marital relations in which the infertility has caused distress, poor communication, and a loss of intimacy
4. psychological problems related to the ceaseless pursuit of pregnancy

Interventions might include:

- thought-stopping for negative or self-defeating thoughts
- cognitive restructuring
- imagery and relaxation training
- appropriate confrontation

Coping is an ever-present demanding process. The individuals must cope not only with medical aspects but also with consequent psychological effects of infertility.

Whether the medical practitioner refers the patient for psychological services or whether the patient is self-referred, the role of the counseling health psychologist is significant. The patient may lack the knowledge necessary to understand the normal emotional reactions to the prolonged crisis of infertility; therefore, the mental health professional needs to provide this type of psychoeducational information. In addition, she may need more support than her partner, family, or friends are providing. She and her partner may need help in determining which medical interventions are acceptable to them. For example, using a donor sperm may be acceptable to both of them, to one partner but not the other, or to neither. It is also possible that the couple's priorities differ, in that one is willing to endure the costs of continued medical interventions (often varying between $2,000 and $5,000 per procedure), while the other believes that they cannot afford to continue since these procedures often are not reimbursable by insurance coverage (Forrest & Gilbert, 1992). The following case exemplifies the diverse and difficult decisions facing couples who are experiencing infertility.

A 33-year-old female patient and her 39-year-old husband were referred to a psychologist by her gynecologist. The woman had been attempting to get pregnant for over a year and had become quite distraught about the failure to achieve pregnancy. The husband stated that he had a son by a previous marriage and that he didn't have any particular desire to have another child. However, since it meant so much to his wife, he was willing to try. They had undergone extensive medical tests and were now trying to decide whether the wife should take a fertility drug or have in vitro fertilization. Although the physician had explained the medical complications (multiple births, premature delivery, greater risk to mother during pregnancy) of using fertility drugs and the chances of not conceiving during in vitro fertilization, the psychologist had been asked to work with them on making a final decision. During therapy, the psychologist helped the couple examine how the consequences of each decision would influence their relationship and their individual lives. The woman talked about her parents' disappointment over not having a grandchild and her envy of her friends who already have their children. The psychologist assisted them in uncovering and discussing the losses of not achieving pregnancy; their anger at each other, the medical system, and others; and the emotion turmoil they had been experiencing in their attempts to conceive. In discussing the pros and cons of each medical procedure, the couple was able to make a decision that was acceptable to both of them.

As this case demonstrates, infertility is complex and multidimensional. It requires counseling health psychologists to understand both the physiological and psychological aspects of infertility and the breadth of medical interventions possible. By working closely with the medical health providers, the counseling health psychologist can assist patients through the life crisis of infertility, help to resolve resulting emotional consequences, help with appropriate decision-making, and assist with marital and sexual difficulties.

Gynecological Cancer

Cancer is surpassed only by heart disease as the leading cause of death in America (McGinnis, 1994). Until recently, a diagnosis of cancer was considered synonymous with a death sentence. Even the word *cancer* can be frightening and has been used as a metaphor for any insidious condition that slowly erodes and destroys—for example, "the cancer of our society" (Holland, 1990a, p. 4). In 1975, Ingelfinger coined the term "cancerophobia" to describe the tremendous fear American society had/has about receiving a diagnosis of cancer (Holland, 1990b, p. 13). This fear often causes individuals to delay seeing a physician if they suspect that they might have cancer. This delay frequently results in serious health risks. For example, Eddy and Eddy (1984) found that between one-fourth and three-fourths of cancer patients delay more than three months, which decreases their chances for long-term survival by 10–20 percent. Perhaps having more accurate information about cancer could decrease both fears and delaying behaviors.

Educating the public about cancer and possible early detection first began in the 1890s in Europe; a gynecologist, Winter, wrote pamphlets urging women to be informed about the danger signals of cancer (Holland, 1990b). The American Cancer Society (ACS) was founded in 1913 during a time when surgery first was being successfully used to remove some cancers. A 1912 issue of the *Ladies Home Journal* told its readers, "Be careful of persistent sores and irritations, external and internal. Be watchful of yourself, without undue worry. At the first suspicious symptoms go to a good physician and demand the truth. . . . The risk is not in surgery, but in delayed surgery" (Fact Book, ACS, cited in Holland, 1990a, p. 4). If one examines similar magazines today, the same message is still being given—Watch for signs and see your physician immediately! Now, however, the messages are much more explicit and are being given through a variety of media. Television documentaries, sitcoms, and dramas are all offering programs focusing on cancer, particularly breast cancer. It is not unusual to find brochures and pictures posted in women's bathrooms describing how to conduct a breast self-exam. The media has assumed an active role in informing women about breast cancer.

Although breast cancer is the leading gynecological cancer among women, there are other gynecological cancers about which women need to be concerned. These include cervical, endometrial, vaginal, ovarian, and fallopian tube cancers. These cancers and breast cancer are the focus of the following discussion.

Breast Cancer

One in eight women will be diagnosed with breast cancer (ACS, 1997). The probably of having breast cancer increases exponentially as one gets older. For example, at age 25, one in 21,411 women will be diagnosed with breast cancer; at age 35, one in 622; at age 45, one in 96; and by age 55, one in 34 will be diagnosed with breast cancer (ACS, 1996). While 76.8 percent of women with new diagnoses of cancer are over the age of 50, breast cancer is the leading cause of death for women between the ages of 15 and 54 (ACS, 1997). Although white women are more likely to develop breast cancer than African American women, African American women are more likely to die of the breast cancer (ACS, 1997).

The five-year survival rate for women with localized (carcinoma in situ) breast cancer has improved from 79 percent in 1940 to 96 percent today, while the prognosis for women whose cancer has invaded nearby tissue (invasive carcinoma) is less optimistic, with a 75 percent five-year survival rate. Noninvasive cancers constitute 15–20 percent of all breast cancers (National Cancer Institute [NCI], 1997), and if detected early, survival rate is greatly increased. While the survival rate beyond five years is increasing for other cancers, for breast cancer it is decreasing. Of women diagnosed with breast cancer, regardless of stage, the average survival rates are approximately 84 percent 5 years after diagnosis, 67 percent at 10 years, and 56 percent at 15 years (ACS, 1997). There are primarily two types of breast cancer—ductal carcinoma, the most prevalent type, and lobular carcinoma. Ductal carcinoma is found in the milk ducts of the breast, while lobular car-cinoma is found throughout the lobes of the breast and is usually bilateral (found in both breasts). Most women (80 percent) find the first signs of breast cancer themselves. When a lump is confirmed by a physician's exam-ination, a mammography, and perhaps an ultrasound, and a localized needle biopsy are typically performed to help determine whether the lump is malig-nant or benign. The traditional medical intervention for breast cancer has been mastectomy, which results in a combined local and distant recurrence rate of 1–2 percent (NCI, 1997). However, in recent years, breast-conserva-tion therapy (e.g., lumpectomy) for early-stage breast cancer has been shown to be just as effective as mastectomy in treating the disease. Jacobson and colleagues (1995) reported results from a 10-year study comparing these two medical procedures for women with Stage I and II breast cancer. Lumpectomy (also called excisional biopsy) with radiation was as effective as mastectomy with respect to local and distant recurrence rates. Ten-year survival rates were 69 percent for mastectomy and 72 percent for lumpecto-my with radiation.

There are four stages of breast cancer (NCI, 1997), with each stage hav-ing various treatment options and prognoses.

Stage I breast cancer indicates that the cancer

(a) is no larger than 2 centimeters and
(b) has not spread (in situ) outside the breast.

Stage II indicates that the cancer

(a) is no larger than 2 centimeters but has spread (invasive) to the lymph nodes under the arm,
(b) is between 2 and 5 centimeters and may or may not have spread to the lymph nodes under the arm, or
(c) is larger than 5 centimeters but has not spread to the lymph nodes under the arm.

Stage III is divided into two stages:

(a) Stage IIIA cancer is more than 5 centimeters and has spread to lymph nodes under the arm,
(b) Stage IIIB cancer has spread to the tissue near the breast (skin or chest wall, ribs, or muscles) or to lymph nodes inside the chest wall along the breast bone.

Stage IV indicates that the cancer

(a) has spread to other organs in the body, most often the bones, lungs, liver, or brain, or

(b) has spread locally to the skin and lymph nodes inside the neck, near the collarbone.

In addition to knowing the stages of cancer, the mental health professional working with patients who have breast cancer needs to be aware of medical vocabulary, treatments available, and related recurrence rates. For example, the primary types of treatment (NCI, 1997) include surgery (removing the cancer in an operation), radiation therapy (using high dose X-rays to shrink and kill the cancer cells), chemotherapy (taking drugs orally or intraveneously to kill cancer cells), and hormone therapy (using hormones to stop cancer cells from growing). Tamoxifen is a hormone typically given to early stage breast cancer patients with no lymph node involvement. In contrast, estrogen, another hormone, has been linked to cancer, and since some breast cancers have estrogen receptors, which facilitate cancer growth, administering estrogen would be counterproductive. Estrogen therapy also increases the risk of cervical cancer.

Bone marrow transplant is a relatively new treatment for cancer. The patient's own bone marrow is harvested and frozen. The patient is then given high dosages of chemotherapy with or without radiation to kill the cancer, and as a result the immune system is destroyed. Finally, as a reverse procedure, the bone marrow is given back to the patient via transfusion (Antman, 1996). Stem cell transplants, similar to bone marrow transplants, involve the harvesting of stem cells (immature cells from which blood cells develop) from the blood, freezing and treating them, and then transplanting them back into the patient (NCI, 1997).

Each of these therapies offers potential risks and benefits that must be carefully considered by the patient. Basic knowledge of potential treatments is essential for the counseling health psychologist to communicate effectively and helpfully.

Other Gynecological Cancers

A body of knowledge is also required for working with women who have been diagnosed with other gynecological cancers, which include cancers of the cervix, endometrium, ovary, fallopian tube, and vagina. Following breast cancer, cervix cancer is the most prevalent gynecological cancer. The mortality rate for cervical cancer has steadily declined over the past 50 years primarily due to the increased use of PAP smears (Mettlin & Murphy, 1982). Risk factors for cervical cancer include several sexual partners, giving birth to numerous children, poor medical care postpartum, unhappiness and depression, marital disruption, and inadequate hygienic self care (DiSaia & Creasman, 1984). Women with herpes virus type-2 are also more prone to cervical cancer (Levy, Ewing, & Lippman, 1988).

Vaginal cancer is relatively rare, comprising only 1–2 percent of all cancers, and is typically diagnosed in women over the age of 62. The primary predisposing condition is previous treatment for cancer of the cervix (Levy et al., 1988). Endometrial cancer is among the most curable cancers if it is diagnosed early; it has been linked to estrogen, as has breast cancer. Obesity is also a prevalent risk factor. The preferred treatment for endrometial cancer is surgery with radiation.

Ovarian and fallopian tube cancers are insidious cancers in that they are difficult to detect. They have silent growth patterns so that most patients present with advanced disease (Levy et al., 1988). The prognosis is usually poor, with ovarian cancer the most fatal of the gynecological cancers. About 60 percent of ovarian cancers appear between the ages of 40 and 60, although the prevalence rate is low, about 15 to 17 per 100,000 (Levy et al., 1988). Risk for ovarian cancer is highest for women who have delayed childbearing or who have not had children. Hormones have been linked to both ovarian and fallopian cancers.

Emotional Reactions to Gynecological Cancer

Many patients who have breast or gynecological cancer struggle with issues of body-image and sense of femininity (Shover, 1991). The fear of cancer and of losing a breast can result in depression, anticipatory grief, anxiety, anger, decreased sexual desire, and feelings of helplessness. It can also negatively affect the marital relationship. Women who take a more active role in their treatment, who make lifestyle changes through exercise, diet, relaxation, and leisure time, and who express their emotions report having a better quality of life and tend to cope better with their disease (Royak-Schaler, 1992).

The counseling health psychologist can offer individual therapy to these patients or work with them in educational or support groups (Wenzel,

Robinson, & Blake, 1995). Self-help groups such as Reach-for-Recovery or Bosom Buddies are excellent sources of support from those experiencing similar health concerns. Counseling health psychologists can also work with the patient and her spouse to explore how the cancer is influencing their lives and how they can grow together as a result of this health crisis (Robinson, 1994; Robinson & Stiefel, 1985). In addition, we have the skills to help patients cope with the side effects of chemotherapy and other medications through strategies such as relaxation and guided imagery. Helping patients make lifestyle changes is one of the mainstays of our profession, and the knowledge base for facilitating these changes can be readily applied to patients coping with cancer.

Although research has failed to support the "cancer-prone personality" that was once thought to increase one's chance of developing cancer, we now know that those who do best are not acquiescent, unaggressive patients. Rather, a long course of illness and better immune functioning has been associated with a more combative, angry stance toward the disease and often toward the medical practitioners (Levy, Herberman, Maluish, Schlien, & Lippman, 1985). Counseling psychologists can help patients express this anger in a way that will help them fight their disease, be it breast or another gynecological cancer. Women have been socialized to accept and follow the lead of those in authority. If this means that they do not ask questions, challenge diagnoses, and ask for second opinions, they may need to be taught assertive behaviors to help them deal with the cancer and with health care professionals. Women need to be active partners in their treatment and decision making.

Counseling health psychologists have an essential role to play in working with women with gynecological cancer:

1. Support the patient during the stressful time when she is waiting for the results of any biopsy, then help her and her loved ones to accept her diagnosis.
2. Assist in her coping with medical regimens.
3. Facilitate interaction with other care providers such as nutritionists and physical therapists.
4. Help in planning aftercare and adjusting her lifestyle to prevent recurrence if possible.

Psychological intervention can be important at each phase of the process—from the point at which cancer is a possibility through medical treatment and follow-up.

Midlife Health Concerns Related to Menopause

Due to medical advances, hygiene practices, and better nutrition, a woman of 55 can expect to live to an average of 84 years in most industrialized countries (Sherwin, 1994). At the turn of the century, women were fortunate if they celebrated their 48th birthday, and most did not live long enough to experience menopause. Now over 1.3 million women experience menopause each year, at a median age of 50. These numbers will dramatically increase as more women of the babyboomer generation enter into midlife. By the year 2000, more than 21 million women will become menopausal (U.S. Department of Commerce, Bureau of Census, 1989). Women and their health care providers must be prepared to address the health decisions of a huge segment of our population during a transition that may begin as early as age 35 and that can have long-term physiological and psychological consequences.

Approximately 24 percent of all health care visits in 1989 were made by women over 44 years of age (U.S. Department of Commerce, Bureau of Census, 1989). These visits were often for symptoms attributable, at least in part, to ovarian hormone shifts related to menopause. However, what is critical is that women and their physicians are frequently not aware of these biological connections to health concerns (Vliet, 1991). Too frequently, the link between hormonal shifts and health concerns is not addressed by health care providers, resulting in women's dissatisfaction with health care providers. For example, Bart and Grossman (1976) found that 45 percent of a sample of midlife women were dissatisfied with the attitudes of their physicians and found them unhelpful. With approximately 40 million women currently over the age of 50 and millions more experiencing premenopausal symptoms, women are beginning to challenge the medical profession's silence surrounding the subject of menopause (Rebar, 1994).

Although the vast majority of women will now live long enough to experience menopause, most know very little about what to expect before, during, and after menopause. In addition, their physicians often fail to discuss the broad spectrum of possible symptoms. The North American Menopause Society assessed where women receive most of their information on menopause and found that popular magazines are the primary source. They also revealed that when physicians do address the subject of menopause, the discussion is not likely to cover women's more pressing concerns (Randall, 1993). While women most frequently cited osteoporosis (33 percent), emotional well-being (28 percent), and heart disease (27 percent) as their most serious health concerns, only about half said that their physicians discussed emotional symptoms or heart disease. Physicians were more likely to discuss short-term physical problems such as hot flashes.

Physiological Changes during Menopause

The focus of medical commentary has traditionally been on the behavioral aspects of the menopausal transition and has minimized the bothersome nature of recognized physiological changes. For example, estrogen levels affect endocrine-related midlife symptoms displayed through other target organs, including the brain, vulva, vagina, bladder and urethra, uterus, skin and mucous membranes, vocal chords, cardiovascular system, skeleton, and breasts (Stuenkel, 1989). The majority of the physical effects from declining hormonal levels can be grouped into vasomotor, urogenital, cardiovascular, and skeletal categories. According to Campbell and Whitehead (1977), specific physical changes in these four categories include:

- symptoms of dyspareunia (difficult or painful intercourse)
- vaginitis (inflammation and atrophy of the vagina)
- dry hair or loss of hair
- hirsutism of the face
- voice changes
- atherosclerosis
- angina
- heart disease
- osteoporosis
- drooping breasts

In addition to these symptoms, 80 percent of the women studied by Anderson, Hamburger, Liu, and Rebar (1987) reported a wide variety of physical complaints, including:

- hot flashes
- muscle and joint pain
- headaches
- increased weight
- light headedness
- increased appetite
- dizziness

- constipation
- numbness or tingling

Another 60–70 percent reported emotional or psychological symptoms upsetting enough to cause them to seek help. The most common of these reported symptoms include:

- irritability
- fatigue
- tension
- nervousness
- depression
- lack of concentration
- short temper
- lack of motivation
- early awakening
- insomnia
- sexual problems
- loss of memory

Not only are the midlife years for women marked by unparalleled hormonal changes, but women are also more frequently treated for depressive disorders during this time period. Approximately 40 percent of the first episodes of depressive illness in women occur between the ages of 40 and 60. Further, evidence from hospital admissions, records of suicide attempts, community studies, and histories of prescriptions for antidepressants suggests an excess of depression in women compared to men.

Fluctuating ovarian hormonal levels may be responsible for this higher incidence of depression. The occurrence of affective disorders at times of dramatic hormonal changes like pregnancy and menopause have led health care providers to believe that the rate of hormonal shifts may be more important than the absolute hormonal level itself. This notion of changes in reproductive endocrine levels affecting neurotransmitter regulation and affective disturbances during the midlife years was first described by Fothergill in 1776 (in Wilbush, 1979). Now, research reported over 200 years later has shown that the depressive symptoms present premenstrually, postpartum, and during menopause are responsive to estrogen therapy (Magos, Brincet, & Studd, 1986).

In clarifying the relevant etiological issues surrounding menopause, researchers have examined how ovarian function changes with age. From a biological perspective, it is commonly reported that menopause occurs due to the elimination of follicles from the ovary that lead to an anovulatatory state (cessation of ovulation). The timing of menopause is determined by the original size of the fixed store of follicles present at birth and by the rate of follicle depletion, the determining factor in female reproductive aging (Gosden & Faddy, 1994).

Although the role of follicle depletion is important, neural and neuroendocrine changes play an even more important etiological role in the decline of the regular reproductive cycles. The integrity of the hypothalamic supra chiasmatic nucleus, the master oscillator regulating most circadian rhythms, is altered during aging and is responsible for diverse hormonal and neurotransmitter changes. The identification of the role of the hypothalamus, which regulates temperature, sleep, and mood, is important to understanding commonly experienced menopausal symptoms (Wise et al., 1994).

The effects of aging on the hypothalamus also include decreased progesterone and estrogen cyclic production and increased plasma levels of androgens relative to the reduction in estrogen values (Utian, 1987). These hormonal alterations during the menopausal process affect neurochemical functioning related to affective disorders. For example, among the most significant neurophysiological mechanisms of estrogen is its ability to increase the rate of degradation of monoamine oxidase (MAO), which catabolizes serotonin. A deficiency of serotonin is thought to be one casual factor in depression. Estrogen is also a precursor for choline acetyl transferase (CAT), needed to synthesize acetylcholine. A deficiency of brain acetylcholine concentrations is a hallmark of Alzheimer's disease (McEwen & Woolley, 1994).

Another major hormonal change experienced by many women in midlife is a shift in their androgen levels. The androgen testosterone has been shown to be an important endocrine determinant of sexual interest, sexual responsiveness, and coital frequency (Sherwin, Gelfand, & Brenner, 1985). Physicians are now beginning to offer androgen supplements to menopausal women to assist in sexual dysfunction.

In contrast to the antidepressant effects of estrogen on various brain mechanisms, the other primary female sex hormone, progesterone, has powerful sedating and anesthetic properties. Administering large doses of progesterone induces dizziness, drowsiness, and even deep sleep. While estrogen decreases MAO activity in the amygdala, hypothalamus, and limbic area, resulting in an increased availability of mood-elevating neurotransmitters, progesterone increases MAO activity, resulting in lower concentrations of brain serotonin. Lower levels of serotonin may predispose women to dysphoric moods, anxiety phenomena, and depression (Sherwin, 1996). Neurophysiological actions of estrogen, progesterone, and testosterone have also been shown to occur in the emotional and sexual centers of the brain.

Having a basic understanding of the psychophysiology of menopause enables mental health professionals to make more accurate psychological diagnoses to help the midlife patient understand the biological changes she is experiencing and to refer back to the physician when necessary.

Hormone Replacement Therapy

A critical and complex decision to be made by most menopausal women is whether to take hormone replacement therapy (HRT), particularly if they have become prematurely menopausal as a result of surgeries such as hysterectomies and oophorectomy. Considerable controversy exists regarding the management of menopause. Philosophically, there are two medical views. One defines menopause in more biological terms based upon changing endocrine function that requires medical intervention, that is, HRT. The opposing view is that menopause is a natural event needing no medical intervention. These diverse positions can confuse women and compromise their ability to make an informed decision. Further, technological, pharmacological, and research advances have resulted in a variety of therapeutic options from which women can chose.

The decision-making process about HRT requires a substantial input from women to facilitate favorable outcomes and treatment compliance. The base risk rates for commonly experienced problems such as vasomotor, urogenital, skeletal, or psychological symptoms are reported to be approximately 80 percent. In addition, each year 390,000 women die from coronary heart disease and 50,000 from osteoporosis. Personal risk factors such as age, race, exercise habits, calcium intake, and family history also need to be explored. A self-analysis of personal values helps women to rate how they would feel about each potential health risk. Taking all of these factors into consideration, a woman can decide on the appropriateness of HRT.

It does little good to make a decision regarding HRT use only to discontinue treatment, however. Extensive research now supports the use of HRT for women experiencing common climacteric complaints and in the prevention of postmenopausal bone loss and death from coronary heart disease. Regardless of the reported effectiveness of HRT, reported compliance rates are very low. Of the 22 percent of women who initially start HRT, 60 percent discontinue it after 1 year, and 20–30 percent never have their prescriptions filled (Vliet, 1995).

A woman's beliefs about menopause need to be explored in order to help her make the best decision regarding HRT. Some women, believing that nature knows best, may attempt to "tough it out" or seek alternative natural remedies such as food supplements or meditation. Other women may be concerned about the long-term effects of HRT, based upon a fear of cancer. Some women mistakenly think that HRT will repair some of the damage of aging and will help them regain a more youthful appearance. Fear of heart disease or bone fractures may motivate others to use HRT. It is essential to help patients debating the use of HRT to examine their beliefs about it. By explicitly examining these, women are more likely to choose better individualized care options and increase their ability to comply with it. This process is especially critical for health care issues that have a life-threatening component and may need years of compliance to alter occurrence or severity.

Interventions

Counseling health psychologists can help women understand the relationship between their biological and psychological experiences and help them make informed treatment decisions. In addition, we are in an ideal position to provide psychosocial interventions to address the health concerns and difficulties of women in midlife.

Considerable confusion surrounds the midlife years, and women have been expected to suffer silently during this poorly understood life stage. Not only do women lose their primary reproductive function and their role as mothers, but they are portrayed in the media as being moody and in need of medication to return to a more youthful appearance. Unfortunately, the lack of normative data on menopausal changes has led both women and physicians to misdiagnose normal events as pathological.

Counseling health psychologists can provide patients with current information about the physiological, psychological, and sociological aspects of menopause through community-based workshops and classes. In order to be proactive about their health, women need to know generally what to expect before, after, and during menopause. Mental health professionals can also work with physicians to help them provide this type of information to their patients.

Psychotherapy can provide an empathic environment for support as well as an ideal setting for discussing accurate information related to menopause. Women can be taught to become resistant to negative external stereotypes and encouraged to develop their own image of midlife as a phase of new opportunities for personal growth or redefined roles. Cognitive reframing strategies can be used to counter negative stereotypes about body image and attractiveness perpetuated in this culture's obsession with youth. Counseling health psychologists can teach women protective and resilient coping skills such as renewed purpose in life, healthy self-esteem, active decision-making, internal locus of control, increased self-efficacy, and assertiveness training. Other women who may experience a sense of loss for their procreative lives can be helped to mourn this change and move forward to another role in which their experience is valued. Discussions of career planning, job training, financial and estate planning, college programs, and volunteer opportunities can provide a new revitalized focus for women in midlife who may feel that they have lost their usefulness.

A number of treatment modalities can address these relevant issues for midlife women. Individual therapy may be a place for an examination of severe health-related symptoms or a safe place for a grieving experience. Support groups can help women cope with physical symptoms, such as hot flashes, or serve to address the difficulties of re-entering college, divorce, caregiving to elderly parents, financial strain, or chronic pain. The group format counters the sense of being alone and provides therapeutic empathy. Counseling health psychologists may also organize a multidisciplinary team from medical centers to offer workshops to the community about such topics as heart disease, osteoporosis, and hormone replacement therapy. This major transition for women will be facilitated by health psychologists' leading the way for the acceptability of aging processes and their interaction with physical, psychological, social, and sexual factors. By striving to accurately and sensitively communicate information about these changes, we will impact quality-of-life issues for many women, which may begin as early as age 35 and continue until their eighties.

Summary

Counseling health psychologists have a wide variety of roles to play in working with women experiencing health concerns. In addition to the interventions suggested, having a conceptual model to direct interventions is essential. Several conceptual models have been developed that may assist counseling health psychologists working with women making other medical decisions. While traditional models have emphasized an authoritarian approach headed by physicians, current models emphasize patient-centered rights and responsibilities as well as a highly interactive process of communication. Gambone and Reiter's (1991) PREPARED model facilitates information regarding:

1. the procedure or the course of action being considered
2. the reason for the procedure
3. the expectation for benefits
4. the likelihood of meeting the expectation
5. the alternatives or other procedures and options
6. the risks or potential harmful outcomes of the procedure
7. the expenses or all direct and indirect costs
8. the decision which involves a fully informed patient choice

By advocating the use of such a model, a health psychologist may enhance in patients a sense of greater control of their own health behaviors and of their illness. By involving patients in decision-making, a number of improved health outcomes have been reported, including:

• faster recoveries
• improved treatment effectiveness
• fewer related health complaints
• compliance to treatment

Suggested Resources

In the general area of women's health, the *Handbook of Behavioral Medicine for Women,* edited by Blechman and Brownell (1988), is particularly informative. It covers a diversity of topics essential to understanding and working with women having health problems. The chapters by Levy, Ewing, and Lippman on gynecological and breast cancer and by Leiblum on infertility are particularly helpful.

The reader is also referred to the special 1992 issue of the *Journal of Mental Health Counseling,* edited by Robinson and Roth, which focuses on women's health issues. The article by Forrest and Gilbert, "Infertility: An Unanticipated and Prolonged Life Crisis," provides an excellent overview of the issues faced by women experiencing infertility and the role of the mental health professional.

The Handbook on Psychooncology, by Holland and Rowland (1990), is an excellent resource for not only gynecologic cancers but also for discussions of biopsychosocial factors in a wide variety of cancers.

For both physiological and psychological information about women in midlife experiencing menopause, the reader is referred to *Screaming To Be Heard: Hormonal Connections Women Suspect . . . and Doctors Ignore* (Vliet, 1995).

In addition, readers should consult the "Update on Women's Health Issues" published monthly by the Committee on Women's Health of the APA Division on Health Psychology for reports of the most recently published research on psychosocial aspect of women's health. The newly founded journal, *Women's Health: Research on Gender, Behavior, and Policy,* and the established *Women and Health* journal are also excellent resources for information on factors influencing women's health.

The Internet also has a variety of Web sites to explore for women's health issues. Some of the most useful include:

- www.twu.edu/hs/hs/decide/decide1.htm (Women's Health Decision Guide)
- nhic-nt.health.org (National Health Information Center)
- www.nysernet.org/breast/Default.html (Breast Cancer)
- www.haverford.edu/biuology/wmbweb/biblio.html (Annotated Bibliography of Women's Health)

Discussion Questions

1. What are the potential losses associated with infertility? How do these affect the psychological well-being of the patient?
2. What are the major psychosocial issues to be targeted in interventions with women who are experiencing infertility?
3. When working with patients trying to make a decision about medical interventions related to her breast cancer, what psychosocial considerations need to be discussed?

4. If they live long enough, all women will experience menopause. What biopsychosocial changes can a woman expect to experience during this life phase?

References

American Cancer Society (1997). *Cancer facts and figures, 1997.* Atlanta, GA: Author.

American Cancer Society (1996). *Cancer facts and figures, 1996.* Atlanta, GA: Author.

American Cancer Society (1980). *Fact Book for the Medical and Related Professions.* New York: Author.

American Medical Association, Council on Ethical and Judicial Affairs. (1991). Gender disparities in clinical decision making. *Journal of the American Medical Association, 266,* 559.

Anderson, B., Hamburger, S., Liu, J., & Rebar, R. (1987). Characteristics of menopausal women seeking assistance. *American Journal of Obstetrics and Gynecology, 156,* 428–433.

Antman, K. (1996, September). When are bone marrow transplants considered? *Science American,* 124–125.

Bart, P., & Grossman, M. (1976). *Menopause. Women and Health, 1,* 3–11.

Berg, B. J., & Wilson, J. F. (1991). Psychiatric morbidity in the infertile population: A reconceptualization. *Fertility and Sterility, 53,* 1–8.

Bilezikian, J. (1995). Osteoporosis: Why calcium is important. *Journal of Women's Health, 4,* 483–494.

Blechman, E. A., & Brownell, K. D. (1988). *Handbook of behavioral medicine for women.* Elmsford, NY: Pergamon.

Burns, L. H. (1987). Infertility as boundary ambiguity: One theoretical perspective. *Family Process, 26,* 359–372.

Campbell, S., & Whitehead, M. (1977). Estrogen therapy and the menopausal syndrome. *Clinical Obstetrics and Gynecology, 4,* 31–47.

Conway, P., & Valentine, D. (1988). Reproductive losses and grieving. *Journal of Social Work and Human Sexuality, 6,* 43–64.

Covington, S. N. (1988). Psychosocial evaluation of the infertile couple: Implications for social work practice. *Journal of Social Work and Human Sexuality, 6,* 21–36.

Daniluk, J. D. (1988). Infertility: Intrapersonal and interpersonal impact. *Fertility and Sterility, 49,* 982–990.

Daniluk, J. C. (1996). When treatment fails: The transition to biological childlessness for infertile women. *Woman and Therapy, 19,* 81–98.

DiSaia, P. J., & Creasman, W. T. (1984). *Clinical gynecologic oncology.* St. Louis, MO: Mosby.

Eddy, D. M., & Eddy, J. F. (1984). Delay factors in detection of cancer. *Proceedings of the American Cancer Society, Fourth National Conference on Human Values and Cancer* (pp. 32–40). New York: American Cancer Society.

Fleming, J., & Burry, K. (1988). Coping with infertility. *Journal of Social Work and Human Sexuality, 6,* 37–41.

Forrest, L., & Gilbert, M. S. (1992). Infertility: An unanticipated and prolonged life crisis. *Journal of Mental Health Counseling, 14,* 42–58.

Gambone, J., & Reiter, R. (1991). Quality improvement in healthcare. *Current Problems in Obstetrics Gynecology and Fertility, 14,* 151–175.

Gosden, R., & Faddy, M. (1994). Ovarian aging, follicular depletion, and steroidogenesis. *Experimental Gerontology, 29,* 265–274.

Healy, B. (1991). Women's health, public welfare. *Journal of the American Medical Association, 266,* 566.

Holland, J. C. (1990a). Historical overview. In J. C. Holland, & J. H. Rowland (Eds.), *Handbook of psychooncology* (pp. 3–12). New York: Oxford.

Holland, J. C. (1990b). Fears and abnormal reactions to cancer in physically healthy individuals. In J. C. Holland, & J. H. Rowland (Eds.), *Handbook of psychoocology* (pp. 13–23). New York: Oxford.

Holland, J. C., & Rowland, J. H. (Eds.) (1990). *Handbook of psychooncology.* New York: Oxford.

Ingelfinger, F. J. (1975). Cancer! Alarm! Cancer! [Editorial]. *New England Journal of Medicine, 293,* 1319–1320.

Jacobson, J. A., Danforth, D. N., Cowan, K. H., d'Angelo, R., Steinberg, S. M., Pierce, L., Lippman, M. C., Lichter, A. S., Glatstein, E., & Okunieff, P. (1995). Ten-year results of a comparison of conservation with mastectomy in the treatment of stage I and II breast cancer. *New England Journal of Medicine, 332,* 907–952.

Kaltenborn, K. (1992). Perspectives on osteoporosis. *Clinical Obstetrics and Gynecology, 35,* 901–912.

Leiblum, S. R. (1988). Infertility. In E. A. Blechman, & K. D. Brownell (Eds.), *Handbook of behavioral medicine for women* (pp. 116–125). Elmsford, NY: Pergammon.

Levy, S. M., Ewing, L. J., & Lippman, M. E. (1988). Gynecologic cancers. In E. A. Blechman, & K. D. Brownell (Eds.), *Handbook of behavioral medicine for women* (pp. 126–139). Elmsford, NY: Pergammon.

Levy, S. M., Herberman, R. B., Maluish, A. M., Schlien, B., & Lippman, M. E. (1985). Prognostic risk assessment in primary breast cancer by behavioral and immunological parameters. *Health Psychology, 4,* 99–113.

Magos, A., Brincet, M., & Studd, J. (1986). Treatment of the premenstrual syndrome by subcutaneous oestradiol implants and cyclical oral norethisterone: A placebo-controlled study. *British Medical Journal, 1,* 1629.

Mahlstedt, P. P. (1985). The psychological component of infertility. *Fertility and Sterility, 43,* 335–346.

Matthews, R., & Matthews, A. M. (1986). Infertility and involuntary childlessness: The transition to nonparenthood. *Journal of Marriage and the Family, 48,* 641–649.

McEwen, B., & Woolley, C. (1994). Estradiol and progesterone regulate neuronal structure and synaptic connectivity in adult as well as developing brain. *Experimental Gerontology, 29,* 431–436.

McGinnis, M. (1994). The role of behavioral research in national health policy. In S. Blumenthal, K. Matthews, & S. Weiss (Eds.), *New research frontiers in behavioral medicine: Proceedings of the national conference.* Washington DC: NIH.

Menning, B. E. (1980). The emotional needs of infertile couples. *Fertility and Sterility, 34,* 313–319.

Menning, B. E. (1988). *Infertility: A guide for the childless couple* (2nd ed.). Englewood Cliffs, NJ: Prentice Hall.

Mettlin, C., & Murphy, G. (1982). *Issues in cancer screening and communications.* New York: Alan R. Liss.

National Cancer Institute (1997, January). *PDQ state of the art: Cancer treatment information.* Washington, DC: Author.

National Institutes of Health (1986, November 28). *Guide to Grants and Contracts, Vol. 15.* Washington, DC: Author.

National Institutes of Health (1990, August 24). *Guide to Grants and Contracts, Vol. 19.* Washington, DC: Author.

Randall, T. (1993). Women need more and better information on menopause from their physicians. *Journal of the American Medical Association, 270,* 1664.

Rebar, R. (1994). Unanswered questions in hormonal replacement therapy. *Experimental Gerontology, 29,* 447–461.

Robinson, S. E. (1994). Chronic disease: Characteristics and sychosocial interventions. *Directions in Rehabilitation Counseling, 9,* 1–11.

Robinson, S. E., & Stiefel, S. (1985). Familiar techniques with new applications: Counseling cancer patients. *Journal of Counseling and Development, 64,* 81–83.

Rodin, J., & Ickovics, J. (1990). Women's health: Review and research agenda as we approach the 21st century. *American Psychologist, 45,* 1018.

Royak-Schaler, R. (1992). Psychological process in breast cancer: A review of selected research. *Journal of Psychosocial Oncology, 9,* 71–89.

Sherman, S. (1993). Gender, health, and responsible research. *Clinics in Geriatric Medicine, 9,* 261–269.

Sherwin, B. (1994). Sex hormones and psychological functioning in postmenopausal women. *Experimental Gerontology, 29,* 423–430.

Sherwin, B. (1996). Hormones, mood, and cognitive functioning in postmenopausal women. *Obstetrics and Gynecology, 87,* 20S–26S.

Sherwin, B., Gelfand, M., & Brenner, W. (1985). Androgen enhances sexual motivation in females: A prospective, cross-over study of sex steroid administration in the surgical menopause. *Psychosomatic Medicine, 47,* 339–351.

Shover, L. R. (1991). The impact of breast cancer on sexuality, body image, and intimate relationships. Cancer, 41, 112–120.

Stuenkel, C. (1989). Menopause and estrogen replacement therapy. *Psychiatric Clinics of North America, 12,* 133–153.

Tobin, J., Wassertheil-Smoller, S., & Wexler, J. (1987). Sex bias in considering coronary bypass surgery. *Annals of Internal Medicine, 107,* 19.

United States Department of Commerce, Bureau of Census. (1989). *Projections of the population of the United States by age, sex, and race: 1988-2080* (Current Population Reports, Series P-25, No. 1018). Washington DC: U.S. Government Printing Office.

United States General Accounting Office. (1990). *National Institutes of Health: Problems in implementing policy on women in study populations (Statement of Mark V. Nadel).* Washington, DC: Author.

United States Public Health Service (1985). *Women's health: Report of the Public Health Service Task Force on Women's Health Issues, Vol. 2.* Washington DC: U.S. Department of Health and Human Services.

Utian, W. (1987). Overview on menopause. *American Journal of Obstetrics and Gynecology, 156,* 1280–1283.

Vliet, E. (1991). New perspectives on the relationship of hormone changes to affective disorders in the periminopause. *NAACOG's Clinical Issues, 2,* Philadelphia, PA: Lippincott.

Vliet, E. (1995). *Screaming to be heard: Hormonal connections women suspect . . . and doctors ignore.* New York: M. Evans.

Wenzel, L., Robinson, S. E., & Blake, D. D. (1995). The effects of problem-focused group counseling for early-stage gynecological cancer patients. *Journal of Mental Health Counseling, 17,* 81–93.

Wilbush, J. (1979). La menespausic—the birth of a syndrome. *Maturitas, 1,* 145–151.

Wise, P., Scarbrough, K., Lloyd, J., Cal, A., Harney, J., Chin, S., Hinkle, D., & McShane, T. (1994). Neuroendocrine concomitants of reproductive aging. *Experimental Gerontology, 29,* 275–283.

15

Addressing the Needs of Diverse Racial/Ethnic Populations

Ester Ruiz Rodriguez

As the population in the United States continues to grow, shifts are occurring that will have consequences for how health care providers practice. The population trend toward aging continues, and by the year 2000, 13 percent of the population will be over the age of 65 (Spencer, 1989). Women will comprise the major source of new entrants into the work force and the number of children under the age of 5 will decline (Kutscher, 1990). All racial/ethnic groups are increasing in numbers, with Latinos growing the fastest, and White Americans comprising a smaller proportion of the total (Chapa & Valencia, 1993; Spencer, 1989). With these changes in the ethnic composition of the United States population, understanding the diverse nature of this country becomes increasingly important when considering health promotion, disease prevention and intervention, and impact on health care planning.

New knowledge in the psychobiological aspects of health have increased our awareness of the relationship between psychological distress and the body's neuroendocrine and immune systems (McBride & Austin, 1996), as well as the importance of psychosocial and sociocultural factors in healing. Such factors provide both psychological and physiological feedback, which reinforces the human organism's homeostatic mechanisms (Schwartz, 1984). Providing appropriate, culturally relevant services to racial/ethnic groups has been a concern for some years (Sanchez, Demmler, & Davis,

1990) and is now deemed a necessity. Faculty have been charged with an ethical responsibility "to promote their students' understanding of gender, race, ethnicity, culture, and class issues in psychological theory, research, and practice" (McGovern, Furumoto, Halpern, Kimble, & McKeachie, 1991, p. 602).

This chapter will begin with a focus on issues key to understanding the health needs of racial/ethnic groups. Issues germane to all racial/ethnic groups will first be addressed. Issues such as acculturation, racial/ethnic identity, discrimination, socioeconomic level, language, and migration history may contribute significantly to the psychosociocultural development of racial/ethnic individuals and their interactions with the U.S. health culture. The second part of this chapter is devoted to issues specific to particular racial/ethnic groups. Within each of the broad racial/ethnic groups, various subgroups exist, each with its own specific history, value orientations, and identity. Further complexity is added to the heterogeneity within each racial/ethnic group when genetic endowments are considered. There are both black and non-black Latinos. Non-black Latinos are closely related genetically to American Indians, and Alaska Natives may more closely resemble Asians than American Indians in their genetic endowment. Generalizations when discussing racial/ethnic groups can quickly descend into oversimplications if the heterogeneity within each major group is forgotten. Finally, the last section in this chapter will address implications for practice.

Key Issues and Concepts

Subjective Culture and Worldview of the United States Health Care System

Subjective culture as reformulated by Triandis and colleagues (1980) refers to social norms, roles, beliefs, and values that are shared from one generation to another. The transmission of subjective culture among racial/ethnic groups has been likened to a psychic language (Rodriguez, 1994), where attitudes and beliefs are transmitted without conscious awareness and may account for a group's attitude or position with regard to the dominant mainstream culture. This transmission of a group's position occurs even when the events initially leading to the group's position transpired many years before.

For example, a defensive posture continues to exist within the African American population with regards to slavery. This posture continues, even though slavery has been abolished for many years. Somehow this defensive posture has survival value, is communicated from one generation to the next, and has become part of the group's subjective culture. Subjective culture becomes part of one's worldview. Worldview includes those values, beliefs, and attitudes that organize and shape perceptions, expectations, and consequently, behavior (Ibrahim, 1991).

The subjective culture of the United States' health system has tended to be organ and disease specific. For many years the health culture has embraced a definition that incorporates dysfunction, either at the cellular or structural level, as the main explanation for disease. Such mechanistic, linear explanations have not tolerated explanations outside of this paradigm. In the recent past, any explanations, methodologies, or research involving alternative causalities were viewed as suspect and research in these areas typically went unfunded. Individuals seeking help from the health system were expected to adjust to the system's paradigm. Failure of clients to accommodate the United States' health culture has frequently been labeled as "patient noncompliance."

It is now recognized that not all cultural groups share the health culture's explanation for the causation of disease. In part, this recognition has been facilitated by the New Age movement, with its emphasis on holistic and alternative methods. Alternative causalities, assessment methods, and treatments abound in several cultural groups, in particular racial/ethnic groups. The significance of these alternative orientations increases as more attention is directed toward how cultural perceptions direct the meaning attributed to being ill, which is separate from the health culture's notion of the objective progression of a disease (Kleinman, 1987). When an individual subscribes to alternative views of disease causation, the likelihood is high that alternative views will also be held regarding what constitutes appropriate treatment and what is expected from the health provider (Kleinman, 1980; McGoldrick, Pearce, & Giordano, 1996). Failure to understand an individual's point of view, worldview, or subjective culture, contributes to mismatches in understanding (Ibrahim, 1991; Triandis, 1994). This applies whether the issue is medical or psychological. Health providers need to weave the client's conceptualization of his or her distress into the diagnosis and treatment plan. Failure to do so prevents a client from following what appears to the provider as the logical conclusion regarding appropriate treatment. Failure of the client to reach this same conclusion contributes to an unwillingness or resistance in complying with the provider's recommendations. As perceptions of disease, stress, conflict, and behavioral disorders are dependent on cultural context (Rodriguez, 1996), a client who does not understand or agree with recommended solutions may place less importance on these solutions. The provider, however, may unjustifiably view this as noncompliance or nonadherence.

Attention to clients' cultural meanings and conceptualization of their concerns is frequently considered a basic skill for health providers; however, this skill is not always practiced, especially when providers are pressed for time. Attending to cultural context results in a collaborative relationship with the client. Collaboration is basic, especially in this day of managed care, for uniting with the client toward health and forming a strong therapeutic relationship. Attention to cultural context also assists the health provider in understanding culture-bound phenomena that the client may subscribe to, such as "ataque de nervios" in Latino populations or "thin or low" blood in African American groups (Kleinman, 1980; Worley, 1997). Furthermore, in some racial/ethnic groups, the family's conceptualization of the presenting concern can be an important tool in understanding the client's experience and, consequently, can provide a framework within which explanations may be given and readily understood by the patient.

Acculturation

The importance of acculturation for particular groups has been well documented throughout the psychosocial and medical literature (Balcazar, Castro, & Krull, 1995; Berry, 1980; Mendoza & Martinez, 1981; Neff, Hoppe & Perea, 1987; Smart & Smart, 1994; Sodowsky, Lai, & Plake, 1991; Szapocznik & Kurtines, 1980). Acculturation refers to the process of accommodation that occurs as individuals experience and interact with new cultural environments (Mendoza & Martinez). It is a multifaceted process in which alternative accommodation options may be subscribed to, such as marginalization (lack of identification with either ethnic or majority group), segregation (forced separation), separation (withdrawal from society), assimilation (surrendering ethnic and assuming the majority identity), or integration (maintaining ethnic and incorporating majority identity) (Berry & Kim, 1988; Sodowsky et al., 1991). The stress and demands experienced as part of the adaptive process to the United States culture and lifestyles are commonly referred to as acculturative stress (Berry & Kim, 1988; Smart & Smart, 1994; Williams & Berry, 1991).

Different health conditions have been associated with different levels of acculturation. For example, less acculturated Mexican American men drink significantly more (Neff et al., 1987), less acculturated elderly are more prone to depression (Zamanian et al., 1992), and immigrants are susceptible to acculturative stress (Smart & Smart, 1994; Sodowsky et al., 1991). Furthermore, among Latino adolescents, depression and suicidal ideation are positively correlated with acculturative stress, while family support and positive expectations for the future are negatively correlated with acculturative stress (Hovey & King, 1996).

Multiple factors are correlated with acculturation, including age, gender, migration history, socioeconomic status (Rogler, 1994), higher education (Negy & Woods, 1992), generation in the United States (Sodowsky et al., 1991), and residence in rural or urban environments (Castro & Gutierres, 1997). This multiplicity of factors emphasizes the importance of soliciting sufficient information to allow health care providers to make accurate assessments regarding the acculturation level of their clients. Such assessments allow providers to adequately assess potential vulnerabilities to stress and other health conditions and have implications for evaluation, intervention, treatment, and training. Although several acculturation scales have been developed, inventories cannot replace the information elicited by good interviewers.

Racial/Ethnic Identity and Discrimination

Acculturation and racial/ethnic identity, although complexly related, are different concepts. Acculturation refers to the process of accommodating into a culture, while racial/ethnic identity refers to identification with a racial or ethnic group based on characteristics of that group. Past cultural traditions, sociopolitical history, sociological factors, and psychological factors arising out of early socialization influences are determinants of racial/ethnic identity. Racial/ethnic identity encompasses the extent to which an individual values his or her origins, engages in ethnic behaviors, possesses information about that behavior, and places importance on that knowledge (Rosenthal & Feldman, 1992).

Tjafel (1981) has postulated that racial/ethnic identity is a component of social identity, and thus a part of an individual's self-concept associated to group belongingness and the value and emotional importance attached to this belongingness. Thus, a racial/ethnic individual's self-esteem and worth are highly influenced by his or her perception of who he or she is as a racial/ethnic person. This influence is pervasive and permeates one's relationships with self, others, and societal systems. Ethnic identity is mostly based on an individual's experiences. According to Ho (1987) and Carter (1995), the reality of people of color in the United States is that they will experience racism. Racial discrimination and prejudice temper an individual's perceptions and expectations. As racial/ethnic persons incorporate perceptions of the dominant system, they will need to develop strategies for dealing with discrimination and prejudice. Racial/ethnic parents bear the burden of building their own and their children's self-esteem within their own culture and within a prejudiced society, yet socializing them into this same society in such a manner that they can function effectively (Julian, McKenry, & McKelvey, 1994). It is imperative that health professionals recognize that the guardedness or vigilance that racial/ethnic clients may present has had survival value for them. Health providers, especially health psychologists, should attempt to understand how this guardedness developed and not label this defensiveness as unwarranted or pathological without a clear understanding of the racial/ethnic client's perspective and experiences. Provider understanding of this dynamic is especially important, since psychosociocultural factors influence health, consequently, racial/ethnic identity may have a direct bearing on an individual's health.

Socioeconomic Level

Low income has a devastating effect on health. Morbidity and mortality, especially with chronic diseases, increases as income decreases. According to the National Center for Health Statistics (1990), poor children are especially vulnerable to low birth weights, infections, debilitating conditions, growth retardation, and other developmental limitations. This vulnerability continues into adulthood. The death rates for the poor are twice that of people with incomes above the poverty level (Amler & Dull, 1987). The incidence of cancer increases and survival rates decrease as income decreases (Amler & Dull, 1987; U. S. Department of Health and Human Services [USDHHS], 1985). Heart disease is 25 percent higher in the low income population (National Heart, Lung, and Blood Institute, 1990), and traumatic injury and accidents are strongly related to low income (National Center for Children in Poverty, 1990). In addition, higher rates of obesity, hypertension, and diabetes are directly linked to low socioeconomic status (Public Health Service, 1988). The economically disadvantaged also are more susceptible to psychosocial and psychophysiologic stress reactions (Louis Harris Associates, 1985).

Higher rates of teenaged pregnancies occur in deprived areas (Figueira-McDonough, 1996), where poor housing and family instability dominate. According to Wilson (1987), the high rates of joblessness among poor racial/ethnic men makes marriage economically unfeasible. For poor females there are also structural barriers to using contraceptives. First, obtaining effective contraceptives requires a clinic or doctor visit, which requires that the female acquire money, transportation, and parental consent (Chilman, 1988). Secondly, she must deal with inconvenient hours.

An additional issue related to poverty is violent crime. In the last three decades there has been a 300 percent increase in teenage homicides and rates of violent crime, especially in poor, urban areas. Violent crime increases as household income decreases. Homicides account for the highest rates of death in African American youth (Devereaux & Pickens, 1996) and also figure prominently in the death rate of Latino males between the ages of 20 and 24 (Smith, Mercy, & Rosenberg, 1986). Several structural sources have been identified that contribute strongly to gang development and violence: poverty, unemployment, weak family socialization, and lack of social capital (Decker & Winkle, 1996).

Most of the poor in the United States are not racial/ethnic people. In numbers there are more poor White people than other racial/ethnic groups; however, a higher percentage of racial/ethnic people are poor (Moccia & Mason, 1986), which serves to confuse ethnicity with poverty in our beliefs, attitudes, policies, and practices toward racial/ethnic populations.

Factors essential for sound physical and psychological health are reduced by poverty; these factors include adequate nutrition, shelter, health care, clothing, transportation, education, and employment. The effects of poverty are superimposed on race/ethnicity and contribute to inadequate social and physical environments, inadequate information and knowledge, increased risk-promoting lifestyles, attitudes, and behaviors, and diminished access to health care (Freeman, 1994), all of which lead to decreased quality of life and lower survival rates in racial/ethnic groups.

Educational level is highly correlated with socioeconomic status and has implications for occupational outcomes (Aponte, Rivers, & Wohl, 1995).

With the exception of the Asian/Pacific Islander group, racial/ethnic individuals are more likely than Whites to not have finished high school or attended college. Less education tends to trap racial/ethnic individuals in low-paying jobs, which are physically taxing, have inflexible work hours, and provide limited benefits.

Health providers have an ethical and moral responsibility to be aware of how a client's socioeconomic level affects the client's everyday life, especially with regard to priorities. For instance, resolving one's codependent tendencies may not be as relevant as finding someone to share expenses so that your children can eat. One's partner may be abusive but still provide a second income. When resources are scarce, it is unlikely that money will be devoted to self-help literature or activities that incur cost. Health providers need to be versatile enough that they can suggest creative solutions that are couched within the sociocultural context of the client, solutions that incorporate activities in which the client already participates. Examples include utilizing the family as support for Latino clients, the church for African American clients, or medicine men/women for Native Americans.

In addition, health providers must come to terms with their biases about the poor. Are people poor because they deserve it? Do people choose to stay in poverty? Affirmative responses to these questions indicate that the provider will most likely: (a) negate the role of environmental factors in enabling poverty in the United States, (b) ignore the effects of poverty, and (c) neglect to consider how socioeconomic level will affect treatment. A negative response may indicate a provider who is willing to grapple with upstream solutions to poverty, which entail looking at environmental factors that enable poverty. Understanding poverty entails working within economic and political policies that influence people to stay poor (Butterfield, 1990; Crawford, 1990) and affect racial/ethnic groups the most. There is a differential vulnerability connected with poverty. The mental health and well-being of people in the lower socioeconomic groups are more adversely affected by negative or stressful life events than that of those in higher socioeconomic groups.

Language

Language is the means used to think about ideas, share experiences, and validate perceptions with others. Spoken language is important in understanding the denotative or generalized meaning of a word and the connotative or more personal interpretation of a word (Arnold & Boggs, 1995). For health providers the connotative meaning may at times be more important. Language is punctuated by culture, ethnicity, religion, geography, age, or occupation. For example, youths tend to imbue words with connotative meanings different from what their parents generally associate with those words. Similarly, many occupations have their own professional or occupational jargon with specific word connotations.

Espin (1987) espouses that bilingual individuals may compartmentalize feelings by maintaining independence between the two language systems. Webster (1996), in her study on American Indians and alcohol treatment systems, discovered that her participants would switch from English to their native language when expressing particularly affect-laden information. Language-switching is not an infrequent occurrence when working with individuals whose primary language is other than English. Since racial/ethnic individuals function simultaneously in two systems—the immediate nurturing environment and the larger societal system (Norton, 1983)—health providers need to be sensitive to and listen for specific connotative meanings that may arise from culturally distinct environments. In addition, encoding experiences with affective meaning in the primary language is not uncommon (Espin, 1987; Gibson, 1983; Russell, 1988), and requesting that affect-laden material be related in the primary language and then translated for the provider may yield information important for the therapeutic relationship and subsequently for the treatment process. Being sensitive to differences in expression in one language versus the other can provide avenues of opportunity for understanding the client better. A health provider may also ask a client what a certain word or phrase is in the primary language and then use that word/phrase to better ground the client in the experience of the moment. Similarly, requesting translation of the words to songs in the client's primary language that the client listens to repeatedly may the help mental health provider break through an impasse or increase his or her understanding of the client's experience.

In health care, clients need to understand diagnoses, treatment options and regimens, as well as medication effects and side effects. Provider instructions cannot be followed if the client fails to understand what was requested. Likewise, patients cannot ask questions if language barriers exist between the provider and the client. When a translator must be utilized, the translator must not only possess a parallel vocabulary in English and the patient's primary language, but must also be able to convey medical information. Using the housekeeper or a child to translate does not guarantee that the message will be conveyed. For example, an individual may speak Spanish because his or her parents spoke Spanish at home. However, if this individual was educated only in English-speaking schools, his or her Spanish vocabulary may be limited to the mundane activities of daily living and he or she may be unable to adequately translate at the English equivalent level. In addition, children, although usually quite willing to translate for their parents, are also likely to censor what they perceive may be distressful to their parents.

Remaining cognizant of the intended receiver is important when using a translator: Is it the translator or the patient? If the intent is to communicate with the patient, then nonverbal and verbal expressions need to be directed toward the patient. The provider should be facing the patient, not the translator, and use a direct approach as if communicating in the same language so that the translation will be direct. For example, the provider should say, while facing the patient, "Do you . . ." rather than telling the translator, "Ask her if she . . ."

All translators need to be oriented to how you want to proceed. Do you want to talk for a while and then have the translation occur? Do you prefer to have each sentence translated as you go? It is important when using translators, as in interactions with all individuals, to be sensitive to cultural sanctions about what is culturally appropriate and permissible to discuss. In addition, the use of same gender, similar age translators, if possible, may be more productive. Being aware of and sensitive to cultures where being respectful is more important than seeking clarification will enhance the interaction. Traditional Asian or Latina women may nod their heads politely but not have comprehended what was stated. Asking for periodic back translations may ensure clarity and minimize misunderstandings. Misunderstandings are common when people speak the same language; they are even more likely when different languages are being spoken.

Different cautions are relevant when working with clients for whom English is a second language. The pace may be slower. The client needs time to translate English into his or her native language and then back again. Usually these clients understand more than they can express. To facilitate the communicative transaction, the provider should speak slowly and enunciate clearly, but not more loudly. Speaking English as a second language does not automatically imply that client has hearing difficulties. Also, providers should avoid slang, professional jargon, or medical terminology that may increase the client's anxiety and decrease understanding. As with all transactions involving health treatment, nonverbal behavior should be scrutinized for messages that may not be verbally expressed.

Migration History

The influences of migratory experiences are seldom considered in the provision of health services, and yet such experiences can have a profound effect on racial/ethnic individuals who may present for services. As an example, many American Indians move back and forth between the reservation and a metropolitan environment. Their economical sustenance may be derived in the city, but their emotional sustenance may come from the family and tribal support system on the reservation.

The reasons that immigrants seek entrance into the United States are varied and may affect their presenting demeanor and expectations for health services. Immigrants who come to the United States in search of the American Dream are different from immigrants who come as refugees. For one group the move was planned and voluntary, and the individual possessed control of the move. For the other group, the move was unplanned (few days to prepare) and involuntary, and control was forsaken in the service of survival. Refugees, many of whom have experienced persecution, may not know what has happened to loved ones left behind and upon entering the United States may be detained in detention centers for years (Sue & Sue, 1990; Williams & Berry, 1991). Voluntary immigrants may be anticipating a better future, but refugees have incurred many losses: loss of family members, country, traditions, livelihood. Regardless of the motivation for migration into the United States, a high probability exists that the United States' health care system is significantly different from their country of origin's health care system. Initial education regarding health care in the United States may be warranted and provide dividends in enhancing an immigrant's ability in accessing health care appropriately and becoming a health consumer.

Such factors will influence an immigrant's acculturation process and the level of acculturative stress experienced (Smart & Smart, 1994). For example, first-generation immigrants perceive significantly more prejudice, are more closely affiliated with their cultural groups, and are less likely to speak English (Sodowsky et al., 1991). Baptiste (1987) has commented that work with immigrants involves working with losses and grief about leaving the country of origin and reconciling unrealized expectations.

Migrant farmworkers in the United States present a different migratory history. Their highly mobile lifestyle subjects them to additional stresses related to unstable support systems, substandard housing, low wages, inaccessible health services, hazardous working conditions, and minimal opportunities to interact with the dominant culture and begin to acculturate. In addition, the ability of migrant workers' children to obtain educational opportunities that might enhance their ability to function better in society is severely limited by the peripatetic lifestyle (Hibbeln, 1996).

Racial/Ethnic Groups

Latinos

The Latino population, commonly referred to as Hispanic by government sources such as the U.S. Census Bureau, the media, health care institutions, and social and behavioral scientists (Marín & Marín, 1991), is rapidly increasing in size. This population increased by 53 percent between 1980 and 1990 and is projected to double again by 2010. Currently Latinos comprise 9 percent of the population, making them the second largest racial/ethnic group, and by 2050 they are expected to be the largest racial/ethnic group, comprising 21 percent of the total population. Over 70 percent of Latinos were born in the United States, and over 87 percent live in urban areas (National Coalition of Hispanic Health and Human Services Organizations [NCHHHSO], 1988).

In general, Latinos are a young population with a median age of less than 26, compared with an overall U.S. population median age of 34 (U.S. Bureau of Census, 1991). The youthfulness of this group is generally attributed to a high birth rate. There are several subgroups within this diverse group (Chapa & Valencia, 1993; NCHHHSC, 1988):

- 66 percent are Mexican Americans, with the greatest concentration in the western and southwestern United States.
- 12 percent are Puerto Ricans, mostly in the eastern coast states.
- 5 percent are Cuban Americans, mostly in Florida.
- The remainder are Central and South Americans, including Spanish-speaking immigrants from the Caribbean Islands.

Health Status

There is also variability in the health status within the Latino subgroups. Mexican Americans have low rates of cerebrovascular disease while Puerto Ricans have a high stroke rate. Cuban Americans have the highest prenatal care utilization rate while Mexican Americans have the lowest. The leading causes of death for the group overall are heart disease and cancer; however, these rates are lower than for non-Latino groups, including Whites (NCH-HHSO, 1988). Unintentional injuries, homicides, chronic liver disease, cirrhosis, and AIDS are higher for Latinos than for non-Latino populations; however, suicides, stroke, and chronic obstructive pulmonary disease are lower (NCHHHSO). In the southwest, Latino men aged 20 to 24 are four times more likely than White men the same age to die by homicide (Smith, Mercy, & Rosenberg, 1986). Likewise, the incidence of AIDS in the overall Latino population is five times higher than for non-Latino Whites. For Puerto Ricans, the rate is seven times higher (Selik, Castro, & Papaionnou, 1988). HIV transmission through intravenous drug use and heterosexual contact is eight times higher in Latinas than non-Latinas (Selik et al., 1988).

Heavy alcohol use, smoking, and drug use are problems. Mexican men are less frequent but higher quantity alcohol drinkers, especially among the less acculturated (Neff et al., 1987). Forty-three percent of Latino men smoke. Puerto Rican and Cuban American youth aged 12 to 17 have higher rates of cocaine use than non-Latino Whites or Blacks, while Mexican American men use marijuana more (NCHHHSO, 1988). Latinos consistently underutilize outpatient mental health services and represent about 5 percent of inpatient admission to psychiatric services (Cheung, 1991; Snowden & Cheung, 1990).

While several groups comprise the migrant farm worker group, Latinos comprise the largest number of this group. Migrant farmworkers have an infant mortality rate that is 25 percent greater than the overall population and a life expectancy of 49 years compared to the overall population life expectancy of 75 years (National Migrant Resource Program, 1990).

Acculturation

Padilla, Wagatsuma, and Lindholm (1985) have reported that each generation of Latinos experiences acculturative stress differently. In their research, first-generation and third-generation Mexican Americans experienced the most stress. While it is understandable that first-generation immigrants would experience acculturative stress—they have left their country of origin, with its values, customs, and language—it is harder to explain why Mexican Americans, born and raised in the United States, with parents born in the United States, and who speak English, experience acculturative stress. Hayes-Bautista (1994) provides a plausible explanation. He found that by the third generation whatever psychological and physiological immunity Latino immigrants possessed was lost. For example, immigrant Mexican women are notorious for not seeking prenatal care, yet have the lowest rates of low-birthweight infants and complications compared to all other racial/ethnic groups and Whites. However, by the third generation, smoking and drinking patterns have increased to approximate rates in the mainstream society (Black & Markides, 1993) and the rates of low-birthweight infants and depression in adults have increased as well (Golding, Karno, & Rutter, 1990). It would appear that in some ways acculturation is not always beneficial to Latino health.

On the other hand, several studies have refuted the notion that increasing acculturation increases vulnerability for Latinos.

- Fernandez and Sanchez (1993) reported that weak identification (low acculturation) is more likely to lead to acculturative stress. When low acculturation is accompanied by high ethnic identification, adjustment is hampered and stress increased.
- Moyerman and Forman (1992) reported that socioeconomic stress is a significant intervening variable in the acculturation and stress debate. Their results indicate that a higher socioeconomic level is correlated with greater increases in adjustment and acculturation. Likewise, a higher socioeconomic level is related to larger and more developed networks and greater acculturation.
- Griffith and Villavicencio (1985) reported that the number of extended family members was unrelated to level of acculturation; however, more acculturated participants reported more primary family members, friends, and neighbors in their social networks compared to the less acculturated participants.
- Keefe (1980) speculated that increased time in the United States enhances the probability of stability, the likelihood that primary kin will be sent for, and procreation will occur, thereby increasing the number of primary family members in the network.

One of the value orientations that seems to persist across the Latino subgroups is that of a strong sense of the importance of family, commonly referred to as familismo or familism. This central value is characterized by strong feelings of loyalty, unity, solidarity, commitment, and reciprocity (Marín & Marín, 1991). Within this value is a pervasive sense of family support. For Latinos the perceived effectiveness of one's support system is a better measure than actual access (Salgado de Snyder, 1987), emotional closeness is more important than physical closeness (Hovey & King, 1996), and a high level of perceived family support has been found to be the most stable dimension of familismo (Sabogal, Marín, Otero-Sabogal, VanOss Marín, & Perez-Stable, 1987). Lending support to the notion of familismo, the study by Marín, Marín, Perez-Stable, and Sabogal (1990) explored intentions to quit smoking with 263 Latinos and 150 non-Latino Whites. Cultural differences in attitudes were identified. Family-related consequences (such as harming the health of their children, providing a bad example to their children, or family criticism) and concerns about the smell (e.g., bad breath) were more likely to motivate Latinos to cease smoking, while concerns about the effects of withdrawing from tobacco were more salient to the non-Latino Whites.

When working with Latino clients then, health providers should remember the importance of the family and assess the client's perceived level of family support. In addition, exploration with the client as to whether and how to include family members in the treatment plan might prove beneficial in attaining the treatment goals. Including the spouse or adult children when discussing chronic disease management may enhance treatment outcomes.

Healing System

The folk healing system of Latinos is somewhat diversified by the major subgroups. Mexicans tend to resort to curanderismo, Puerto Ricans to espiritismo (spiritualism), and Cubans to santeria (Aponte et al., 1995). Each of these practices tends to prevail in areas of high concentration of the respective Latino subgroup. These healing systems are predicated on the belief that natural forces (air, moonbeams) and supernatural forces (God, other divine entities, or evil) can cause disease. Treatment is directed at restoring harmony and/or balance with the forces involved. It is not uncommon that variants of these systems will be used for the treatment of emotional/psychological conditions prior to or instead of Western mental health services. Both the Mexican and Puerto Rican systems incorporate the hot-cold theory of imbalance. Diseases are either hot or cold; therefore, you treat hot diseases with cold treatments, and cold diseases with hot treatments. Divine intervention is invoked in all three systems: for the Mexican curanderismo divine interventions originate from God, Puerto Rican espiritismo relies on the Holy Spirit, and Cuban santeria invokes orishas, gods who have become interwined with Christian saints. Each system has its own traditional healer who will diagnose and treat the illness utilizing such treatments as massage, structural manipulations, herbs, prayer rituals, and ceremonies.

It is difficult to estimate how widespread the use of traditional healing methods is in the Latino population. Some practices, such as the use of herbs, are so interwoven into the culture that they are rarely considered alternative medicine but are seen as cultural practices. For example, the use of teas such as yerba buena (spearmint) to treat stomach upsets and manzania (chamomile) to soothe and aid sleep are widespread. The following vignette illustrates the use of another tea in treating colic.

Ongoing colic in a newborn was frustrating a new Mexican American mother who was also a registered nurse. The pediatrician advised her that the child would eventually grow out of it, and she must hang in there as there was no effective treatment for colic. Her mother advised her to make a tea with several seeds of cumin, sweeten it, and feed it to the infant first thing in the morning for three days. She at first rejected this remedy, but then administered it since she was concerned with her infant's discomfort. She was pleasantly surprised at how well it worked, but never told the pediatrician. She was afraid he would question her nursing abilities for giving in to ethnic practices.

Utilization rates for curanderismo have been reported as high as 54 percent in Texas, 32 percent in Colorado, and 1–8 percent in California (Aponte et al., 1995). Widespread use of espiritismo and santeria are reported in areas where high concentrations of Puerto Ricans and Cubans reside, respectively; however, exact estimates are not available. The following vignette illustrates the pervasiveness of early cultural beliefs on disease causation and treatment.

A pregnant psychologist was preparing to leave the hospital after a visit with her traditional, Latino father. He cautioned her, "Be careful. The moon is full." Initially she was confused by this statement, until she recalled that moonrays from a full moon were believed to cause birth defects in the newborn if the pregnant mother was exposed to them. She reassured her father, while reminding herself that she didn't believe in that stuff anymore. However, upon facing the huge full moon, she recalled that metal deflects the harmful rays and decided, "It's better to be safe than sorry," and held her keys at the apex of her pregnant abdomen, "just in case."

African Americans

African Americans comprise approximately 12 percent of the United States population and constitute the largest racial/ethnic group. African Americans live in all regions of the United States; however, over 85 percent live in poor urban areas where 50 percent or more of the residents are African Americans (Norton, 1983; Spector, 1996). The poverty rate in this group is three times that of White Americans. The life expectancy for this group was 69.4 years in 1987 and is now lagging even further behind at 65.6 years (United States Bureau of Census, 1992b).

Health Status

African American males are two times more likely to die from strokes and have a higher nonfatal stroke prevalence (USDHHS, 1985). Their heart disease rates are similar to the overall population; however, when compared within income categories, the rates for African Americans are lower (USDHHS, 1990). Interestingly, sudden out-of-hospital cardiac arrests occur more in African American than White American patients, and initial resuscitation and survival to hospital discharge are poorer for African Americans (Cowie, Fahrenbruch, Cobb, & Hallstrom, 1993). The poorer outcomes are due to poorer levels of health, less bystander-initiated cardiopulmonary resuscitation, and differences in underlying cardiac disorders. Wenneker and Epstein (1989) and Goldberg, Hartz, Jacobsen, Krakauer, and Rimm (1992) have documented that White Americans receive several more cardiac assessments and treatments (coronary angiography, bypass, and angioplasty) than do African Americans.

Diabetes in African Americans is 33 percent higher than in White Americans and is especially prevalent in overweight African American females. More diabetic complications (cardiovascular disease, neuropathy, renal failure) occur as well (USDHHS, 1985). In addition, African American infants are twice as likely to die during their first year of life (USDHHS, 1985), and African American adolescents generally have lower levels of health, utilize health facilities less, and lack usual sources of both routine and sick health care (Lieu, Newacheck, & McManus, 1993).

Hypertension is more common among African Americans than in the total population (Subcommittee on Definition and Prevalence, 1985). They are 20 times more likely to suffer from hypertension than are White Americans in the same age group. In a study by Klag, Whelton, Coresh,

Grim, and Kuller (1991), hypertension was reported to correlate positively with the darkness of African Americans' skin and negatively with their socioeconomic level. Higher blood pressure is also related to darker skin and lower socioeconomic level. These findings were independent of age and body mass index and persisted irrespective of blood glucose concentration, serum urea nitrogen, serum uric nitrogen, serum uric acid, and urinary sodium and potassium levels (Klag et al., 1991). On a brighter note, Alexander and colleagues (1996) reported that African Americans who meditated twice a day lowered their blood pressure. These findings held regardless of activity level, stress level, obesity, and alcohol or salt consumption. Transcendental meditation yielded a higher drop in blood pressure than progressive muscle relaxation. Changes in exercise and diet did not contribute to a similar decrease in blood pressure.

Homicide is the leading cause of death for young African American men between the ages of 15 and 34. African American men in the 25–34 age group are seven times more likely to die from homicide than White men. African American women are four times more likely to die from homicide than White women (USDHHS, 1985).

African Americans as a whole are more likely to contract AIDS than any other group, with a risk three times greater than for White Americans. African American women are 10 to 15 times more likely to contract AIDS than White women, and African American children comprise 50 percent of all children with AIDS (Selik, Castro, Papaionnou, & Ruehler, 1989). This higher proportion of AIDS is due to intravenous drug use and heterosexual contact with subsequent transmission from mother to infant.

An issue affecting mostly persons of African descent is sickle cell disease. Sickle cell disease refers to a group of genetic disorders characterized by the presence of sickle hemoglobin, crescent- or sickle-shaped red blood cells. Typical symptoms include chronic anemia and acute and chronic tissue injury secondary to blockage of blood flow. All tissues are at risk for damage and the more common complications include painful episodes involving soft tissue and bones, acute chest syndrome, priapism, cerebral vascular accidents, and splenic and renal dysfunction. In sickle cell anemia, splenic dysfunction predisposes the infant to overwhelming infection.

By far the most common form of sickle cell disease is sickle cell anemia, where an individual inherits two ß-sickle genes. Other forms of the disease exist as well, including ß-thalassemia or other abnormal ß globin genes. Although sickle cell disease affects mostly persons of African descent

(Worley, 1997), it has also been found in persons of Mediterranean, Caribbean, South and Central American, and East Indian ancestry (Sickle Cell Disease Guideline Panel, 1993).

Sickle cell trait occurs when an individual has inherited both a normal ß globin and a ß-sickle globin gene. Persons with sickle cell trait produce mostly normal hemoglobin and their red blood cells do not sickle except under adverse circumstances. The sickle cell trait is an important consideration for couples deciding to have children, as they are at risk for having children with sickle cell disease.

Information on differences between the disease and the trait, risks of the child developing sickle cell anemia, morbidity and mortality information, and family planning options available to individuals with sickle cell disease or trait must be provided. In addition, the importance of health care maintenance, compliance with prophylactic penicillin regimens, and the need for prompt medical attention during acute illness must also be stressed. Additional counseling involves assisting the couple or individuals to make informed decisions. As with all genetic counseling, the health provider needs to be sensitive to the wide range of issues that can surface and how these issues affect marital and family planning decisions. Some of the issues that can surface include: feelings of grief, guilt, anxiety, or anger; personal, cultural, and religious values; attitudes regarding control; desire to have children; taking risks; and coping with adversity. The decisions made will affect the individuals for the rest of their lives.

African Americans are overrepresented in inpatient psychiatric admissions and residential care. This overrepresentation occurs at rates of 21 percent and 10.2 percent, respectively, and is significantly greater than would be predicted based on population statistics (Cheung, 1991). Access issues to outpatient psychiatric treatment and delay in seeking conventional outpatient care due to alternative help-seeking behaviors may partially account for the overrepresentation. Nonetheless, bias in providers' clinical judgement and diagnosis has been implicated (Snowden & Cheung, 1990).

Further bias is noted in a study conducted to ascertain if racial differences existed in the use of medical procedures in elderly Medicare patients. Escarce, Epstein, Colby, and Schwartz (1993) discovered pervasive racial differences:

1. Significantly more medical procedures and diagnostic tests performed by different specialties for different conditions were conducted on White elderly patients versus African American patients.

2. Elderly White Americans had an advantage in terms of access to higher technology or newer services.
3. Racial differences increased among elderly in rural areas in the South.
4. These racial differences persisted even when socioeconomic status was accounted for.
5. White elderly patients were favored at each stage in the course of diagnosis and treatment for coronary artery disease.

Values

The history of slavery for African Americans contributes to the suspiciousness and conflict that African Americans experience today toward the dominant culture. The capture of their ancestors and involuntary transportation to another continent is a part of their view of the world as hostile and dangerous. This world view has been important to their survival as subsequent experiences of racism and prejudice prove and reinforce the value of staying vigilant and guarded toward the dominant culture. Jones (1985) identifies several coping and defense mechanisms that African Americans have used to deal with racism. Health providers need to be aware of and be comfortable with exploring this area, if necessary, and be able to assist the patient in identifying and expanding options in coping with perceived racism in the health care system.

The nontraditional family arrangements that typify African American families can be viewed as a strength (Sue & Sue, 1990). Among lower socioeconomic African Americans, over 70 percent of families are headed by females (Jenkins, 1985). Partners, extended family members, and friends extend the social network and help raise children when resources are limited. When working with African American families, it is important to solicit information about who is living in the home, what children are living outside the home, and who helps out (Sue & Sue). In addition, it is important to strive to work toward restoring functional structure rather than changing the original family structure.

African Americans, like mainstream White Americans, value assertiveness (Thomas & Dansby, 1985). This is a strength that can be utilized in assisting African American clients in their communications with others. In addition, respectful assertive communication from the provider is valued as well. Other values similar to the dominant culture are a preferred mode of activity that involves "doing" and perceiving the nature of man as both good and bad (Ho, 1987; Sue & Sue, 1990).

Many African Americans are extremely church-oriented. Spirituality and church attendance are important aspects of their lives (Sue & Sue, 1990). The church serves as another support, providing for spiritual and social needs. Eliciting information about spiritual needs and how they are met, the importance of church attendance for the client, and the support received from the minister and the congregation can supply meaningful data. Exploring what aspects of church attendance are valued can also provide clues as to how to create meaningful interventions couched within the client's cultural context. For example, since meditation has been found to be helpful with lowering blood pressure, is there a similar response that may be obtained with meditative prayer? Church-oriented African Americans may be more willing to consider meditative prayer than transcendental meditation; further, prayer is a cost-free and culturally appropriate solution.

Healing System

Traditional healers in the African American culture tend to be women. Traditional healing tends to be a mixture of several overlapping healing systems, including classical medicine of an earlier time, selected contemporary medical beliefs, fundamental Christianity, and magical practices (Aponte et al., 1995). Magical practices are referred to as voodoo, hoodoo, crossing up, hexing, and witchcraft. Life is viewed as a process rather than a state, and the nature of a person is viewed as an energy force rather than matter; therefore, health, mind, body, and spirit are one. There is no distinction between psyche and soma. Consequently, one cure may benefit everything and anything.

Disease has several causative agents, including Divine punishment, unhealthy lifestyles or excesses, and unnatural causes, such as nonproductive worry, evil influences, or sorcery (Aponte et al., 1995). Appropriate treatment demands knowing the cause of illness so that the right healer might be consulted. Although clear estimates about the use of traditional healers in the African American population are not readily available, estimates from Detroit indicated that 41 percent of the African American women would use traditional folk healing treatments, compared with 14 percent of White American women; and 24 percent of the women and 10 percent of the men indicated having used folk treatments (Bailey, 1991).

Asian/Pacific Islander Americans

Asian/Pacific Islanders are a highly diversified group comprising the third largest of the racial/ethnic groups and 3 percent of the total United States population (United States Bureu of Census, 1991). Over 75 percent of Asian Americans are immigrants, mostly from Southeast Asia, and many are refugees. According to the United States Bureau of Census (1990), Chinese Americans comprise 22 percent of this population, followed by Filipino Americans (21 percent), Japanese Americans (19 percent), Korean Americans (10 percent), and Asian Indians (10 percent). This is a highly diverse group having over 30 different languages. Their median age is 29.9 years compared to 33 years in the total population and 34.4 years for Whites (United States Bureau of Census, 1992b). By the year 2000, it is projected that Asian/Pacific Islanders will be older than any racial/ethnic group except White Americans. At that time they are expected to have a median age of 31.2 years, compared with median ages of 29.8 for African Americans and 37.0 for White Americans (United States Bureau of Census, 1992a). Asian/Pacific Islanders have lower birth rates than the other racial/ethnic groups but higher than White Americans. Subgroup variations exist, however, with Vietnamese, Laotians, and Cambodians having higher birth rates than the other subgroups (O'Hare & Felt, 1991).

The highest concentrations of Asian/Pacific Islanders occur in the western states: California with 40 percent, Hawaii with 11 percent. There are 16 percent in the states of New York, Illinois, and New Jersey (United States Bureau of Census, 1991). Most Asian/Pacific Islanders live in urban areas, usually large metropolitan areas. About equal numbers live in inner cities and suburban areas, and only 6 percent live outside metropolitan areas (United States Bureau of Census, 1991).

Healthwise, the native-born Asian/Pacific Islanders are indistinguishable from the population as a whole; however, some distinctions exist with regard to socioeconomic level. The median income for Asian/Pacific Islanders is higher than the national median income, with Japanese Americans earning 38 percent more. Asian/Pacific Islanders have the highest mean household income (United States Bureau of Census, 1992c); however, O'Hare and Felt (1991) argue that when mean per capita income is considered, Asian/Pacific Islanders fall behind White Americans, due mainly to larger households among Asian/Pacific Islanders. Another factor frequently ignored is that Asian/Pacific Islander households contain more wage earners under one roof than in White American households. Again, as in other areas, great variation exists within the Asian/Pacific Islander subgroups. For example, Chinese Americans earn four times as much as Laotian Americans. Asian/Pacific Islanders are almost identical to White Americans in the United States with regard to high school and college education (O'Hare, 1992).

Health Status

- Breast cancer is higher in Hawaiian women than in White Americans with a rate of 111 and 86 per 100,000, respectively (Asian American Health Forum, 1989).
- Lung cancer is also 18 percent higher in Southeast Asian males than in the White American population, while liver cancer is 12 times higher (Asian American Health Forum, 1989; Schwartz & Thomas, 1987).
- Hypertension among Filipinos in California over the age of 50 occurs at a higher rate compared to other Californians, 61 percent and 47 percent, respectively (USDHHS, 1985).
- Tuberculosis and hepatitis B are serious health problems for Asians in large American cities, with a tuberculosis incidence 40 times higher than the total population and an estimated hepatitis B carrier rate of 4 percent compared to 0.3 percent (Asian American Health Forum, 1989). The high levels of these infectious diseases are generally thought to be a direct result of immigration with new immigrants being the primary carriers.
- Smoking is another major concern for Southeast Asians. Approximately 92 percent of Laotian men and 65 percent of Vietnamese men smoke, compared to 30 percent for the overall United States population (Asian American Health Forum, 1989).

Asian/Pacific Islanders have low utilization rates of outpatient and inpatient mental health services (Snowden & Cheung, 1990). The low utilization rates are thought to be due to the cultural sanctioning of handling problems within the family and thus avoiding shaming the family (Sue & Sue, 1990).

Values

Family relationships in traditional Asian/Pacific Islander families are influenced in varying degrees by Confucianism, which places a heavy emphasis on specified roles, hierarchical family structure, and propriety, and by Buddhism, which places an emphasis on harmonious living, respect for life, moderation in behavior, self-discipline, modesty, and selflessness (Ho, 1987). These values are behaviorally manifested in deference to authority and in emotional self-restraint. Tradition and family ancestry are highly valued, while obligation, respect, and obedience to parents are emphasized, reinforced, and expected, regardless of what a parent may say or do. Traditional families are patriarchal with power belonging to the father, husband, and oldest son in that order. Shame is frequently used to reinforce proper behavior. Shameful behavior causes a person and his or her family to lose face and may lead to withdrawal of confidence and/or support. To form strong therapeutic alliances with traditional Asian/Pacific Islanders, these values must be acknowledged and honored.

Healing System

Traditional healing systems among Asian/Pacific Islanders vary; however, all systems appear to adhere to the use of herbal remedies. Health is viewed as a state of spiritual and physical oneness with nature (Spector, 1996). Foundational to Chinese traditional healing practices, one of the oldest systems dating back to 300 BC, is the concept of the balance between yin (negative energy) and yang (positive energy). Everything in the universe contains these two aspects and herbal properties are classified as to their yin or yang nature. Health is dependent on harmony and blocked energy flow leads to disease. Good health is dependent internally on the equilibrium between basic emotions and organs and externally on harmony with the universe (Aponte et al., 1995). Techniques such as acupuncture, acupressure, moxibustion, and massage are used to restore balance and treat illness. Acupuncture and acupressure are used to rebalance energy flows. Acupuncture uses needles inserted into the skin, and acupressure uses finger pressure on the skin. Moxibustion uses heated, pulverized wormwood directly on the skin.

Vietnamese folk medicine tends to view illness as caused by natural causes, such as spoiled food or poisonous water, or supernatural causes in which dieties cause the illness as retribution for violations of religious ethics or acts of omission, or in a combination of ying-yang, hot-cold imbalances (Tran, 1980).

The Tibetan model of health postulates that distortions in one's world view, caused by failure to recognize one's interdependency and/or that everything changes (cold disorders), lead to emotional problems of overattachment (desire) or underattachment (aversion). These are labeled wind disorders and lead to physical disorders called heat disorders, caused by secondary emotions such as anger and pride (Brown, 1997).

Native Americans

Although highly diversified, American Indians and Alaska Natives are the smallest in numbers of the racial/ethnic groups. There are over 400 federally recognized Indian nations within the United States, each with its own traditions. Approximately one-third of Native Americans live on reservations and one-half live in urban areas. Twenty-eight percent of American Indians live in the midwest, mostly Oklahoma with 12.9 percent. Forty-seven percent reside in western states with the highest concentrations in California (12 percent), Arizona (10 percent), and New Mexico (6 percent) (O'Hare, 1992; U.S. Bureau of Census, 1991).

Native Americans are a young group with a median age of 23. As opposed to Latinos who are also a young group due to a high fertility rate, the youthfulness of Native Americans is due to excessive deaths before the age of 45. A high poverty rate of 31 percent (Indian Health Service, 1993), high unemployment rates ranging from 25 to 87 percent (Honingfeld & Kaplan, 1987), and harsh and substandard living environments contribute to health problems (Nichols, 1994; Rhoades, Hammond, Welty, Handler, & Amler, 1987). The educational level of Native Americans is also low, with less than 8 percent of the group having college degrees (Indian Health Service, 1988).

Health Status

The leading causes of death are heart disease and cancer; however, rates are lower than the overall population. The exception is the Oklahoma Indians, who have an incidence of lung cancer that is twice the national average (USDHHS, 1985). Native Americans of the southern United States have higher rates of gallbladder cancer and Alaska Natives have higher rates of liver cancer (USDHHS, 1985). The lower rates of heart disease and cancer may simply reflect that Native Americans do not live long enough to contract these diseases. Both heart disease and cancer are generally considered diseases of old age.

The six major causes of excess death are: unintentional injuries, cirrhosis, homicide, suicide, pneumonia, and diabetic complications (USDHHS, 1985). Alcohol-related injuries make up about 75 percent of the deaths from unintentional injuries, with 54 percent of these involving vehicular accidents. Alcohol is also implicated in the 60 percent higher homicide rate, and in suicide rates that are 28 percent higher than the national average, but in some tribes suicide occurs at rates ten times higher.

Infant deaths are twice as likely to occur during the first year of life and Native American infants are at higher risks for health problems than are non-Indian infants (Honingfeld & Kaplan, 1987; Rhoades et al., 1987). Fetal alcohol syndrome (FAS) occurs six times more frequently (Rhoades et al., 1987) and more than half of the mothers who produce a child with FAS will produce another child with FAS (Honingfeld & Kaplan, 1987). Sudden infant death syndrome occurs twice as much as in the non-Indian population (Indian Health Service, 1992) and the leading causes of death among American Indian infants are respiratory complications, intestinal infections, injuries, and poisoning (Honingfeld & Kaplan, 1987; Rhoades et al., 1987).

Cirrhosis and diabetes are two prevalent chronic diseases. Cirrhosis deaths occur three times more than in the total population. Diabetes is prevalent and in many tribes more than 20 percent of the members have contracted diabetes. In two Arizona tribes, over 40 percent of the tribal members have diabetes (Rhoades et al., 1987). Obesity is also a problem, which contributes to the high rates of diabetes experienced by Native Americans. Inpatient psychiatric admissions constitute only 1 percent of all psychiatric service admissions (Cheung, 1991). Although Indian Health Service (IHS) serves tribal members living on reservations or near urban IHS facilities, many living in rural areas still find it difficult to obtain adequate health care.

Values

Traditionally the extended family has been the norm, and the role and function of the extended family was to support and enable self-sufficiency. The American Indian family, however, is becoming increasingly disorganized due to outside influences and socioeconomic constraints (Nichols, 1994). The experience of Native Americans and Alaska/Aleutian Natives in the United States is likened to being "immigrants in their own land" (Atteneave, 1982). Although they are the original human inhabitants of this country and, therefore, owned the land, their land was taken away, and they were relegated to reservation living. This sociopolitical history contributes to what they are today. Their subjective culture and worldview continue to contain elements of suspiciousness, alienation, conflict, and perhaps fear of the dominant culture, along with elements of the traditional culture involving harmony and balance with self, others, and nature.

The worldview of Native Americans includes a present-time orientation in which time is cyclical and rhythmic and not organized by clocks or calendars (Atteneave, 1982). Native Americans value being in harmony, with oneself, with others, and especially with nature. One should respect oneself, others, and Mother Earth. Many of the traditional ceremonies are designed to regain harmony and balance with Mother Earth and collateral relationships. Native Americans have a high value for sharing, consequently, material possessions are not as important. It is more important that harmony be maintained with family, tribe members, nature, and oneself.

Healing System

To many traditional Native Americans, illness and disease have a spiritual causation. For example, to the Navajos, disease is traced back to something that should not have been done, such as breaking a taboo or contact with a ghost or witch. The Hopi believe evil spirits cause illness. Most traditional American Indians believe that everyone and everything has a spiritual nature (Spector, 1996); therefore, there is an alternative explanation for the causation of disease than what is practiced in mainstream United States culture. There are many different treatments that vary from tribe to tribe. Most treatments require the help of a medicine man or woman (shaman) who is the traditional healer of the tribe and is wise in the ways and relationships of men and nature. Special ceremonies may be dedicated to assessment and diagnosis, followed by ceremonies for treatment. Common treatments include purification by immersion in water and/or use of sweat lodges, chants, herbs. All treatments are administered reverently and with respect by the healer and the identified patient.

Whether or not traditional healers are used for health care, most Native Americans retain a belief in the wisdom and powers of the native healer. This is evident in Webster's (1996) study of alcoholism treatment programs. One of the most devastating problems for Native Americans is the abuse of alcohol and other drugs, such as glue and paint (Gloria & Peregoy, 1996). Many programs are now available for dealing with this issue with variable success as in the dominant society. Webster did a comparative qualitative analysis of two types of alcoholism treatment programs: standard Alcoholic Anonymous based programs and culturally sensitive programs designed around Native American traditions and ritual. Participants in the standard programs identified the Alcoholics Anonymous and Alanon portions of the programs as the most helpful treatment modalities as they allowed the participants to reconnect with the power source of God, faith, and spirituality. In the culturally sensitive treatment programs, the Native American ceremonies and rituals were viewed as necessary to reconnect to their native culture, identity, strength, faith, and philosophy. Participants in both programs, then, seemed to focus on the spiritual aspects of the programs.

Native American traditions spring from sharing rather than owning, accepting rather than dominating, and flowing with rather than intruding into the flow of life and growth (Hoffman, 1981). These processes are very evident in Nichols' (1994) qualitative research on similarities and differences between Cherokee mothers and non-Indian mothers. Nichols reported that all cultures include mothering functions to ensure physical survival of the infant, development of the infant's capacity for self-maintenance, and socialization into the culture. Cherokee mothers must also pass on clan membership, spread the care of the infant to other caretakers, and promote the harmony and natural rhythm of the infant's well-being by using techniques such as passive forbearance and not controlling or interfering with the natural rhythm of life.

Because of the widespread belief in the spiritual causation of disease, when working with Native Americans it is wise to elicit preferred modes of healing and how they might address the types of problems presented. It may be possible to refer to a traditional healer or to have the client incorporate some of the native traditions as part of the treatment regimen. Sometimes, assisting clients to explore what has kept them from pursuing traditional solutions that have worked in the past can be a powerful tool. This is especially true for Native Americans who were raised traditionally, perhaps on a reservation, and have now assumed an urban lifestyle where harmony with nature becomes extremely difficult. As with the other racial/ethnic groups, questions of identity may surface and must be sensitively dealt with.

Implications for Practice

Health providers must recognize the great diversity within all the racial/ethnic groups in the United States. Failure to adequately account for within-group variability with precise definition of the group being targeted has resulted in much criticism of the literature on cross-cultural differences (Betancourt & López, 1993; Triandis, 1994) and contributed to confusion in practice about how to work in a culturally competent manner with racial/ethnic groups. Although information is by necessity conveyed through the use of generalizations about racial/ethnic groups in the literature, it is important to guard against stereotyping and to maintain awareness of the great diversity within all racial/ethnic groups. It is also important to remember the similarities that bind all human beings.

In addition to the obstacles to health encountered by the mainstream population, racial/ethnic groups are subjected to distinct stressors which increase their vulnerability to disease and illness. Low education levels contribute to limited job market skills, which in turn contribute to underemployment, high unemployment, decreased income and economic opportunity, and decreased social capital (prestige) as well. Racial/ethnic individuals are more susceptible to violence against them and must learn to cope with it. The lack of social capital among the racial/ethnic poor youth makes gang participation and the concomitant gang violence especially attractive as a means of coping with prestige and turf issues.

Child-bearing, child-rearing, family structure, and marriage patterns among racial/ethnic individuals can be significantly different from those of the White American culture (Aponte et al., 1995). Within these structural patterns, racial/ethnic parents must teach their children how to deal with the discrimination, racism, and oppression they will encounter. Struggles around racial/ethnic identity are not uncommon at some point in a racial/ethnic individual's life, and frequently resurface throughout his or her life.

High rates of poverty contribute to numerous health issues, such as nutritional deficiencies, sanitation problems, limited medical accessibility, and high-risk behaviors, including alcoholism, drug abuse, violence, and AIDS. While the relationships between physical and mental health and socioeconomic level are well established (Adler et al., 1994; Aponte et al., 1995; Dohrenwend & Dohrenwend, 1969), attention to how economic development and political policies affect the quality of life and health issues for groups with high rates of poverty, such as racial/ethnic groups, has not been a priority issue for many health providers.

The association of psychological distress and changes in the neuroendocrine and immune systems is being rigorously investigated (McBride & Austin, 1996; O'Leary, 1990; Rossi, 1993). Factors that contribute to and enhance immunocompetence, such as personality traits, adaptation to disease strategies, and attribution responses, have been identified (McBride & Austin, 1996). Understanding and respecting each client's unique style of coping is stressed as being of paramount importance in successfully manipulating immunocompetence. Toward that end, the following considerations are offered to help health psychologists and other providers in increasing their competence in assessment and intervention with diverse racial/ethnic individuals.

Assessment Considerations

- Health providers need to be prepared to deal with psychosociocultural issues identified in a sensitive, competent manner that enhances the esteem and the functioning of the patient.
- Eliciting information about racial/ethnic identity, acculturation, language, nontraditional family arrangements, support networks, future aspirations, migration history, socioeconomic issues, and alternative healing systems will enhance problem identification and assessment and treatment planning and implementation.
- Healthy ways of coping with disease involve taking into account cultural strategies used by the client and the client's referent group.

Intervention Considerations

- Health providers need to be aware of how the client's unique psychosociocultural factors affect the utilization of health care and treatment adherence, as well as how to incorporate treatment options/procedures that are culturally congruent with the client's belief system.
- Providers must become experts in working with multisystems: the individual, family and support systems, service delivery systems, and the sociopolitical system.
- Understanding how lifelong social problems contribute to racial/ethnic clients' differential vulnerability to physical and mental health problems strengthens provider understanding and creativity in uniting with the client to tackle difficult problems, decrease learned helplessness, and collaborate toward health.
- Competent health providers will learn to elicit, accept, and use nontraditional family arrangements, which may include partners, extended family members, neighbors, and friends in the service of the client.
- Personal stories may offer clues as to what is important to a client. An astute provider will identify these elements and incorporate them into the intervention plan.
- Integration of cultural coping strategies into health treatment will enhance the immunocompetence of racial/ethnic individuals, decrease

the ethnocentrism of the United States' health culture, and begin to address a major limitation of health treatment today—the provision of culturally sound services.

Suggested Resources

A number of good books on counseling with ethnic minorities exist. Both *Psychological Interventions and Cultural Diversity* (Aponte, Rivers, & Wohl, 1995) and *Counseling the Culturally Different: Theory and Practice* (Sue & Sue, 1990) focus on counseling issues specific to the four major racial/ethnic groups: African, Latino, Asian, and Native Americans. The latter book is updated and reissued periodically.

Ethnicity and Family Therapy (McGoldrick, Giordano, & Pearce, 1996) provides a snapshot of family relationships and identifies dynamics and issues of 20 diverse racial/ethnic families. *Family Therapy with Ethnic Minorities* (Ho, 1987), another family therapy text, specifies interventions to increase effectiveness when counseling ethnic minority families.

For the "big picture" on Latino health, consult *Latino Health in the U.S.: A Growing Challenge* (Molina & Aguirre-Molina, 1994). This text provides a comprehensive coverage of the heterogeneity within the Latino culture and the interplay of health issues and the factors of migration and economic status.

Discussion Questions

1. What is the significance of the sickle cell trait and its impact on African Americans?
2. What is the relevance of acculturation level? What impact does acculturation level have on the health of racial/ethnic minorities?
3. Think of the last racial/ethnic individual you worked or interacted with. How did their ethnic identity surface? As you think back, can you identify what or how you might have enhanced the interaction if you had attended to ethnic identity (theirs and yours)?
4. Mortality by homicide is a major concern for at least three of the racial/ethnic groups discussed. How can you as a health provider make a positive impact on this complex issue?

5. American Indians and Alaskan Aleuts are the true United States natives. This country was subsequently populated by immigrants, mostly from western Europe. What are the factors that have contributed to the recent anti-immigrant position?

6. Since there is so much diversity within and between racial/ethnic groups in the United States, of what importance is it to attempt to learn about the culture and values of the different racial/ethnic groups?

7. The author talks about downstream and upstream approaches to poverty which significantly affect the health of racial/ethnic groups. What are some examples of upstream approaches?

8. What are the similarities and differences among the United States' health culture and the traditional healing systems of the four racial/ethnic groups?

References

Adler, N. E., Boyce, T., Chesney, M. A., Cohen, S., Folkman, S., Kahn, R. L., & Syme, S. L. (1994). Socioeconomic status and health: The challenge of the gradient. *American Psychologist, 49,* 15–24.

Alexander, C. N., Schnieder, R. H., Staggers, F., Sheppard, W., Clayborne, B. M., Rainforth, M., Salerno, J., Kondwani, K., Smith, S., Walton, K. G., & Egan, B. (1996). Trial of stress reduction for hypertension in older African Americans. *Hypertension, 28,* 228–237.

Amler, R. W., & Dull, H. B. (1987). *Closing the gap: The burden of unnecessary illness.* New York: Oxford University.

Aponte, J. F., Rivers, R. Y., & Wohl, J. (1995). *Psychological interventions and cultural diversity.* Boston: Allyn & Bacon.

Arnold, E., & Boggs, K. (1995). *Interpersonal relationships.* Philadelphia: Saunders.

Asian American Health Forum. (1989). *Year 2000 strategic health development program for Asian and Pacific Islander Americans.* Washington, DC: Author.

Atteneave, C. (1982). American Indians and Alaska Native families: Emigrants in their own homeland. In M. McGoldrick, J. K. Pearce, & J. Giordano (Eds.), *Ethnicity and family therapy* (pp. 55–83). New York: Guilford.

Bailey, E. J. (1991). Hypertension: An analysis of Detroit African-American health care treatment patterns. *Human Organization, 50,* 287–296.

Balcazar, H., Castro, F. G., & Krull, J. L. (1995). Cancer risk reduction in Mexican American women: The role of acculturation, education, and health risk factors. *Health Education Quarterly, 22,* 6–184.

Baptiste, D. A. (1987). Family therapy with Spanish-heritage immigrant families in cultural transition. *Contemporary Family Therapy, 9,* 229–250.

Berry, J. W. (1980). Acculturation as varieties of adaptation. In A. M. Padilla (Ed.), *Acculturation: Theory, model, and some new findings* (pp. 9–25). Boulder, CO: Westview.

Berry, J. W., & Kim, U. (1988). Acculturation and mental health. In P. R. Dasen, J. W Berry, & N. Sartorius (Eds.), *Health and cross-cultural psychology: Toward applications* (pp. 207–236). Newbury Park, CA: Sage.

Betancourt, H., & López, S. R. (1993). The study of culture, ethnicity, and race in American psychology. *American Psychologist, 48,* 629–637.

Black, S. A., & Markides, K. S. (1993). Acculturation and alcohol consumption in Puerto Rican, Cuban-American, and Mexican-American women in the United States. *American Journal of Public Health, 83,* 890–893.

Brown, C. (1997, February 18). *Traditional Oriental medicine.* Paper presented at Arizona State University, College of Nursing, Tempe, Arizona.

Butterfield, P. (1990). Thinking upstream: Nurturing a conceptual understanding of the societal context of human behavior. *Advances in Nursing Science, 12,* 1–8.

Carter, R. T. (1995). *The influence of race and racial identity in psychotherapy.* New York: Wiley.

Castro, F. G., & Gutierres, S. (1997). *Drug and alcohol use among rural Mexican Americans.* NIDA Research Monograph no. 168 (pp. 498–533). Rockville, MD: National Institute on Drug Abuse.

Chapa, J., & Valencia, R. R. (1993). Latino population growth, demographic characteristics, and educational stagnation: An examination of recent trends. *Hispanic Journal of Behavioral Sciences, 15,* 165–187.

Cheung, F. K. (1991). The use of mental health services by ethnic minorities. In H. F. Myers, P. Wolhford, L. P. Guzman, & R. J. Echemendia (Eds.), *Ethnic minority perspectives on clinical training and services in psychology* (pp. 23–31). Washington, DC: American Psychological Association.

Chilman, C. S. (1988). Never-married, single, adolescent parents. In C. S. Chilman, E. W. Nunnally, & F. M. Cox (Eds.), *Variant family forms* (pp. 17–37). Newbury Park, CA: Sage.

Cowie, M. R., Fahrenbruch, C. E., Cobb, L. A., & Hallstrom, A. P. (1993). Out-of-hospital cardiac arrest: Racial differences in outcome in Seattle. *American Journal of Public Health, 83,* 955–959.

Crawford, R. (1990). Individual responsibility and health policy. In P. Conrad, &. R. Klein (Eds.), *The sociology of health and illness: Critical perspectives* (pp. 387–397). New York: St. Martin's.

Decker, S. H., & Winkle, B. V. (1996). *Life in the gang.* New York: Cambridge University.

Devereaux, D. M., & Pickens, J. M. (1996). The health status of Arizona's Black children: Building a stronger foundation for the future. In K. Kyle, & A. L. Schneider (Eds.), *Profile and status of Black children in Arizona* (pp. 81–102). Tempe, AZ: Arizona State University.

Dohrenwend, B. P., & Dohrenwend, B. S. (1969). *Social status and psychological disorder: A casual inquiry.* New York: Wiley.

Escarce, J. J., Epstein, K. R., Coby, D. C., & Schwartz, J. S. (1993). Racial differences in the elderly's use of medical procedures and diagnostic tests. *American Journal of Public Health, 83,* 948–954.

Espin, O. M. (1987). Psychological impact of migration on Latinas: Implications for psychotherapeutic practice. *Psychology of Women Quarterly, 11,* 489–503.

Fernandez, D. M., & Sanchez, J. I. (1993). Acculturative stress among Hispanics: A bidimensional model of ethnic identification. *Journal of Applied Social Psychology, 23,* 654–668.

Figueira-McDonough, J. (1996). Teenage sexuality, pregnancy, and motherhood in Arizona's Black community. In K. Kyle & A. L. Schneider (Eds.), *Profile and status of Black children in Arizona* (pp.102–124). Tempe, AZ: Arizona State University.

Freeman, H. (1994, September). *The impact of values and beliefs on health.* Paper presented at the Implications of Cultural Values, Beliefs, and Norms for Health Research Conference, Milwaukee, WI.

Gloria, A. M., & Peregoy, J. J. (1996). Counseling Latino alcohol and other drug abusers: Cultural issues for consideration. *Journal of Substance Abuse Treatment, 8,* 1–8.

Goldberg, K. C., Hartz, A. J., Jacobsen, S. J., Krakauer, H., & Rimm, A. A. (1992). Racial and community factors influencing coronary artery bypass graft surgery rates for all 1989 Medicare patients. *JAMA, 267,* 1473–1477.

Golding, J. M., Karno, M., & Rutter, C. M. (1990). Symptoms of major depression among Mexican-Americans and non-Hispanic Whites. *American Journal of Psychiatry, 147,* 861–866.

Griffith, J., & Villavicencio, S. (1985). Relationships among acculturation, sociodemographic characteristics and social supports in Mexican American adults. *Hispanic Journal of Behavioral Sciences, 7,* 75–92.

Hayes-Bautista, D. E. (1994, July). *Latino health care in the US.* Paper presented at the annual meeting of the National Asssociation of Hispanic Nurses, Costa Mesa, CA.

Hibbeln, J. A. (1996). Special populations: Hispanic migrant workers. In S. Torres (Ed.), *Hispanic voices: Hispanic health educators speak out* (pp. 162–192). New York: NLN.

Ho, M. K. (1987). *Family therapy with ethnic minorities.* Newbury Park, CA: Sage.

Hoffman, F. (Ed.). (1981, April). *The American Indian family: Strengths and stresses.* Paper presented at the American Indian Social Research and Development Associates Conference, Phoenix, AZ.

Honingfeld, L. S., & Kaplan, D. W. (1987). Native American postneonatal mortality. *Pediatrics, 80,* 575–578.

Hovey, J. D., & King, C. A. (1996). Acculturative stress, depression, and suicidal ideation among immigrant and second-generation Latino adolescents. *Journal of the American Academy of Child Adolescent Psychiatry, 35,* 35–39.

Ibrahim, F. A. (1991). Contribution of cultural worldview to generic counseling and development. *Journal of Counseling & Development, 70,* 13–19.

Indian Health Service. (1988). *Indian Health Service chart series book.* Washington, DC: U.S. Department of Health and Human Services.

Indian Health Service. (1992). *Regional differences in Indian health—1992.* Washington, DC: U.S. Department of Health and Human Services.

Indian Health Service. (1993). *Regional differences in Indian health—1993.* Washington, DC: U.S. Department of Health and Human Services.

Jenkins, Y. M. (1985). The integration of psychotherapy-vocational interventions: Relevance for Black women. *Psychotherapy, 22,* 394–397.

Jones, E. E. (1985). Psychotherapy and counseling with Black clients. In P. B. Pedersen (Ed.), *Handbook of cross-cultural counseling and therapy* (pp. 173–179). Westport, CT: Greenwood.

Julian, T. W., McKenry, P. C., & McKelvey, M. W. (1994). Cultural variations in parenting: Perceptions of Caucasian, African-American, Hisapnic, and Asian-American parents. *Family Relations, 43,* 30–37.

Keefe, S. E. (1980). Acculturation and the extended family among urban Mexican Americans. In A. Padilla (Ed.), *Acculturation: theory, models, and some new findings* (pp. 85–110). Boulder, CO: Westview.

Klag, M. J., Whelton, P. K., Coresh, J., Grim, C. E., & Kuller, L. H. (1991). The association of skin color with blood pressure in United States Blacks with low socioeconomic status. *JAMA, 265,* 599–602.

Kleinman, A. (1980). *Patients and healers in the context of culture.* Berkeley: University of California Press.

Kleinman, A. (1987). Anthropology and psychiatry: The role of culture in cross-cultural research on illness. *British Journal of Psychiatry, 151,* 447–454.

Kutscher, R. E. (1990). Outlook 2000: The major trends. *Occupational Outlook Quarterly, 34,* 2–7.

Lieu, T. A., Newacheck, P. W., & McManus, M. A. (1993). Race, ethnicity, and access to ambulatory care among US adolescents. *American Journal of Public Health, 83,* 960–965.

Louis Harris Associates. (1985). *A study of the sources, correlates and manifestations of perceived and experienced stress in the United States.* Rockville, MD: U.S. Department of Health and Human Services.

Marín, B. V., Marín, G., Perez-Stable, R., & Sabogal, F. (1990). Cultural differences in attitudes toward smoking: Developing messages using the theory of reasoned action. *Journal of Applied Social Psychology, 20,* 478–493.

Marín, G., & Marín, B. V. (1991). *Research with Hispanic populations.* Newbury Park, CA: Sage.

McBride, A. B., & Austin, J. K. (1996). *Psychiatric-mental health nursing: Integrating the behavioral and biological sciences.* Philadelphia: Saunders.

McGoldrick, M., Pearce, J. K., & Giordano, J. (Eds.). (1996). *Ethnicity and family therapy* (2nd ed.). New York: Guilford.

McGovern, T. V., Furumoto, L., Halpern, D. F., Kimble, G. A., & McKeachie, W. J. (1991). Liberal education, study in depth, and the arts and sciences major—Psychology. *American Psychologist, 46,* 598–605.

Mendoza, R. H. & Martinez, J. L. (1981). The measurement of acculturation. In A. Baron, Jr. (Ed.), *Explorations in Chicano psychology* (pp. 71–82). New York: Praeger.

Moccia, P., & Mason, D. J. (1986). Poverty trends: Implications for nursing. *Nursing Outlook, 34,* 20–24.

Molina, C. W., & Aguirre-Molina, M. (1994). *Latino health in the US: A growing challenge.* Washington, DC: American Public Health Association.

Moyerman, D. R., & Forman, B. D. (1992). Acculturation and adjustment: A meta-analytic study. Hispanic *Journal of Behavioral Sciences, 14,* 163–200.

National Center for Children in Poverty. (1990). *A statistical profile of our poorest young citizens.* New York: Author.

National Center for Health Statistics, Centers for Disease Control, Public Health Service. (1990). *National health interview survey.* Hyattsville, MD: U.S. Department of Health and Human Services.

National Coalition of Hispanic Health and Human Services Organizations (NCHHSO). (1988). *Delivering preventive health care to Hispanics: A manual for providers.* Washington, DC: Author.

National Heart, Lung, and Blood Institute. (1990). *National cholesterol education program: Report of the expert panel on population strategies for blood cholesterol reduction.* Washington, DC: U.S. Department of Health and Human Services.

National Migrant Resource Program. (1990). *Seasonal farmworker objectives for the year 2000.* Austin, TX: Author.

Neff , J. A., Hoppe, S. K., & Perea, P. (1987). Acculturation and alcohol use: Drinking patterns and problems among Anglo and Mexican American male drinkers. *Hispanic Journal of Behavioral Sciences, 9,* 151–181.

Negy, C., & Woods, D. J. (1992). A note on the relationship between acculturation and socioeconomic status. *Hispanic Journal of Behavioral Sciences, 14,* 248–251.

Nichols, L. A. (1994). *The infant caring process among Cherokee mothers.* Unpublished dissertation, University of Arizona, Tucson.

Norton, D. G. (1983). Black family life patterns, the development of self and cognitive development of Black children. In G. J. Powell, J. Yamamoto, A. Romero, & A. Morales (Eds.), *The psychosocial development of minority group children* (pp. 183–191). New York, Brunner/Mazel.

O'Hare, W. P. (1992). America's minorities: The demographics of diversity. *Population Bulletin, 47,* 1–47.

O'Hare, W. P., & Felt, J. C. (1991). *Asian Americans: America's fastest growing minority group.* Washington, DC: Population Reference Bureau.

O'Leary, A. (1990). Stress, emotion, and human immune function. *Psychological Bulletin, 108,* 363–382.

Padilla, A. M., Wagatsuma, Y., & Linholm, K. J. (1985). Generational and personality differences in acculturative stress among Mexican-Americans and Japanese Americans. *Spanish Speaking Mental Health Research Center Occasional Papers, 20,* 15–38.

Public Health Service. (1988). *The surgeon general's report on nutrition and health.* Washington, DC: U.S. Department of Health and Human Services.

Rhoades, E. R., Hammond, J., Welty, T. K., Handler, A. O., Amler, R. W. (1987). The Indian burden of illness and future health interventions. *Public Health Reports, 102,* 361–368.

Rodriguez, E. R. (1994). *The role of psychological separation, ethnic identity, and worldview in college adjustment.* Unpublished doctoral dissertation, Arizona State University.

Rodriguez, E. R. (1996). The sociocultural context of stress and depression in Hispanics. In S. Torres (Ed.), *Hispanic voices: Hispanic health educators speak out* (pp. 143–158). New York: NLN.

Rogler, L. (1994). International migrations. *American Psychologist, 19,* 701–708.

Rosenthal, D. A., & Feldman, S. S. (1992). The nature and stability of ethnic identity in Chinese youth. *Journal of Cross-Cultural Psychology, 23,* 214–227.

Rossi, E. L. (1993). *The psychobiology of mind-body healing* (2nd ed.). New York: Norton.

Russell, D. M. (1988). Language and psychotherapy: The influence of nonstandard English in clinical practice. In L. Comas-Díaz, & E. H. Griffith (Eds.), *Clinical guidelines in cross-cultural mental health* (pp. 33–68). New York: Wiley.

Sabogal, F., Marín, G., Otero-Sabogal, R., VanOss Marín, B., Perez-Stable, E. J. (1987). Hispanic familism and acculturation: What changes and what doesn't. Hispanic Journal of *Behavioral Sciences, 9,* 397–412.

Salgado de Synder, V. N. (1987). Factors associated with acculturative stress and depressive symptomatology among married Mexican immigrant women. *Psychology of Women Quarterly, 11,* 475–488.

Sanchez, A. M., Demmler, J., & Davis, M. (1990). *Toward pluralism in the mental health disciplines.* Boulder, CO: Western Interstate Commission for Higher Education.

Schwartz, G. E. (1984). Psychobiology of health: A new synthesis. In B. L. Hammonds, & C. J. Scheirer (Eds.), *Psychology and health* (pp. 145–193). Washington, DC: American Psychological Association.

Schwartz, S. M., & Thomas, D. B. (1987, October). *Estimates of cancer incidence among Southeast Asian refugees in the United States.* Paper presented at the Annual Meeting of the American Public Health Association, New Orleans, LA.

Selik, R. M., Castro, K. G., & Papaionnou, M. (1988). Racial/ethnic differences in the risk of AIDS among Hispanics in the United States. *American Journal of Public Health, 78,* 1539–1544.

Selik, R. M., Castro, K. G., Papaionnou, M., & Ruehler, J. W. (1989). Birthplace and the risk of AIDS among Hispanics in the Unites States. *American Journal of Public Health, 79,* 836–839.

Sickle Cell Disease Guideline Panel. (1993). *Sickle cell disease: Screening, diagnosis, management, and counseling in newborns and infants.* Rockville, MD: U.S. Department of Health and Human Services.

Smart, J. F., & Smart, D. W. (1994). The rehabilitation of Hispanics experiencing acculturative stress: Implications for practice. *Journal of Rehabilitation, 60,* 8–12.

Smith, J.C., Mercy, J. A., & Rosenberg, M. L. (1986). Suicide and homicide among Hispanics in the Southwest. *Public Health Reports, 101,* 265–270.

Snowden, L. R., & Cheung, F. K. (1990). Use of inpatient mental health services by members of ethnic minority groups. *American Psychologist, 45,* 347–355.

Sodowsky, G. R., Lai, E. W. M., & Plake, B. S. (1991). Moderating effects of sociocultural variables on acculturation attitudes of Hispanics and Asian Americans. *Journal of Counseling & Development, 70,* 194–204.

Spector, R. E. (1996). *Cultural diversity in health & illness.* Stamford, CT: Appleton & Lange.

Spencer, G. (1989). *Projections of the population of the United States, by age, sex, and race: 1988 to 2080.* Current population reports, population estimates and projections. Series P-25, No. 1018. Washington, DC: U.S. Department of Commerce, Bureau of the Census.

Subcommittee on Definition and Prevalence, Joint National Committee on Detection, Evaluation, and Treatment of High Blood Pressure. (1985). Hypertension prevalence and the status of awareness, treatment and control. *Hypertension, 7,* 460.

Sue, D. W., & Sue, D. (1990). *Counseling the culturally different: Theory and practice.* New York: Wiley.

Szapocznik, J., & Kurtines, W. (1980). Acculturation, biculturalism, and adjustment among Cuban Americans. In A. M. Padilla (Ed.), *Acculturation theory, models, and some new findings* (pp.139–159). Boulder, CO: Westview.

Thomas, M. B., & Dansby, P. G. (1985). Black clients: Family structures, therapeutic issues, and strengths. *Psychotherapy, 22,* 398–407.

Tjafel, H. (1981). *Human groups and social categories.* Cambridge, England: Cambridge University.

Tran, T. M. (1980). *Indochinese patients.* Fall Church, VA: Action for Southeast Asians.

Triandis, H. C. (1994). *Culture and social behavior.* New York: McGraw Hill.

Triandis, H. C., Lambert, W., Berry, J., Lonner, W., Heron, A., Brislin, R., & Draguns, J. (1980). *Handbook of cross-cultural psychology* (Vol. 1–6). Boston: Allyn & Bacon.

U.S. Bureau of Census. (1990). *Census of population and housing—Summary tape file 1: Summary population and housing characteristics.* Washington, DC: U.S. Government Printing Office.

U.S. Bureau of Census. (1991). *Race and Hispanic origin. 1990 Census Profile, 2,* 1–8.

U.S. Bureau of Census. (1992a). *Current population reports, P25-1092, Population projections of the United States by age, sex, race and Hispanic origin: 1992–2050.* Washington, DC: U.S. Government Printing Office.

U.S. Bureau of Census. (1992b). 1990 *Census of population, 1990, CP-1-4, General population characteristics.* Washington, DC: U.S. Government Printing Office.

U.S. Bureau of Census. (1992c). 1990 *Census of population and housing, 1990 CPH-1-1, Summary population and housing characteristics.* Washington, DC: U.S. Government Printing Office.

U.S. Department of Health and Human Services. (1985). *Report of the secretary's task force on Black and minority health.* Washington, DC: Author.

U.S. Department of Health and Human Services. (1990). *Report of the Secretary's Task Force on Black and minority health.* Washington, DC: U.S. Government Printing Office.

Webster, S. C. (1996). *Analysis of culturally sensitive and traditional alcohol treatment as perceived by Native American clients.* Unpublished thesis, Arizona State University, Tempe.

Wenneker, M. B., & Epstein, A. M. (1989). Racial inequalities in the use of procedures for patients with ischemic heart disease in Massachusetts. *JAMA, 261,* 253–257.

Williams, C. L., & Berry, J. W. (1991). Primary prevention of acculturative stress among refugees. *American Psychologist, 46,* 632–641.

Wilson, W. J. (1987). *The truly disadvantaged.* Chicago: University of Chicago.

Worley, N. K. (1997). *Mental health nursing in the community.* St Louis, MO: Mosby.

Zamanian, K., Thackrey, M., Starrett, R. A., Brown, L. G., Lassman, D. K., & Blanchard, A. (1992). Acculturation and depression in Mexican-American elderly. In T. L. Brink (Ed.), *Hispanic aged mental health* (pp. 109–112). New York: Haworth.

IV
SPECIAL ISSUES

16
Perspectives from Psychiatry

Jesse R. Fann

Psychiatrists and psychologists have traditionally worked quite separately from one another. In fact, differences in professional beliefs and practices, stemming from longstanding guild issues and competition resulting from ideological and economic sources, created a chasm that prevented the two disciplines from working together comfortably (Berg, 1986). Today, the field of mental health care has shifted to an environment of integration and cooperation. While more work is needed to better define the roles of psychiatrists, psychologists, psychiatric nurse practitioners, social workers, and other mental health counselors in our health care system, there is little doubt that all disciplines will be working more closely with other health care providers in multidisciplinary teams. This chapter specifically looks at how psychiatrists and psychologists can work together in clinical and research settings to achieve optimal care for patients and a productive and rich working collaboration.

What Is a Psychiatrist?

Psychiatrists are medical doctors who have completed four years of medical school, one year of internship training, and three years of psychiatric residency training. Internship includes training in internal medicine, family practice, and/or pediatrics, neurology, and often some psychiatric training. Psychiatric residency training usually includes one year of inpatient adult psychiatry, at least two months of consultation-liaison psychiatry in a general hospital, at least two months of child and adolescent psychiatry, at least one month of emergency psychiatry, and at least one year of outpatient psychotherapy training, which includes cognitive-behavioral and psychodynamic techniques. The remainder of the residency involves electives, which may include more advanced psychotherapy training, consultation work, administration, research, or other specialty clinical rotations, such as drug and alcohol treatment, community psychiatry, forensic psychiatry, and psychopharmacology (Accreditation Council for Graduate Medical Education, 1997).

Like training in other medical specialties, psychiatric training emphasizes use of the medical model. This model involves first taking a detailed medical/psychiatric history. Such a history includes a "chief complaint," history of present illness, past medical/psychiatric history, medication history, family history, and social history. Next, a complete physical and mental status exam is obtained. Based on this information, a diagnosis is made using the multiaxial system outlined in the American Psychiatric Association's *Diagnostic and Statistical Manual, 4th edition (DSM-IV)* (American Psychiatric Association, 1994). Of course, the diagnosis should not merely pigeonhole a patient into a diagnostic category from which a prescribed treatment should follow; instead, a complex formulation must be constructed using a *biopsychosocial model* (Engel, 1980). The biopsychosocial model dictates that for every illness and every patient, biomedical, psychiatric, psychological, and social considerations for assessment, treatment, and follow-up are required. When arriving at a diagnosis and formulating a treatment plan, modern psychiatric training emphasizes the need to consider the biomedical, psychological, and sociocultural contributions to the patient's problems, coping styles, and behaviors.

Most of psychiatric training focuses on the choice and implementation of appropriate treatment modalities. Again, the biopsychosocial model is employed. Biological modalities include medications and electroconvulsive therapy. Psychological modalities include the various forms of individual, couple, family, and group psychotherapy. Social interventions include the manipulation of social support, vocational, and avocational systems.

The American Psychiatric Association has formulated guidelines for psychiatrists when working with nonmedical mental health practitioners (Official Actions, 1980). As mental health care delivery is increasingly provided by nonmedical practitioners, psychiatrists practice less in isolation and more within the framework of an organized health care delivery framework.

While this increase in collaboration can lead to an improved environment of collegiality between psychiatrists and nonmedical practitioners, such collaboration must be carried out within certain limits. For example, psychiatrists should not undertake the supervision of nonmedical practitioners unless they are fully prepared to assume medical responsibility for the patient. Psychiatrists may not be supervisors in name only, nor should they allow themselves to be used solely as a means for obtaining insurance payment for nonmedical providers.

What Is a Consultation-Liaison Psychiatrist?

Consultation-liaison psychiatrists often work closely with counseling psychologists. Many consultation-liaison psychiatrists have had one to two years of postresidency specialty training. They are responsible for evaluating and treating patients outside of the inpatient and outpatient psychiatry setting. Examples of such settings include medical, surgical, and obstetrical-gynecological units in a general hospital, outpatient primary care clinics, and interdisciplinary pain and rehabilitation units.

Consultation-liaison psychiatrists are especially attuned to the mind-body continuum. When they are asked to evaluate a patient for depression, for example, a myriad of possibilities must immediately be considered. Does the patient really have depression, or are his or her symptoms actually a symptom of a medical illness or medication, such as bradykinesia and mask-like facies from Parkinson's disease? Thus, the consultation-liaison psychiatrist must be familiar with all the potential psychiatric effects of medical illness and nonpsychiatric medications.

Furthermore, the psychodynamic meaning of the medical illness must be explored in the context of the patient's psychiatric symptoms and signs. Because a patient's developmental history will clearly color the way one copes with and experiences a physical illness, careful exploration of such past experiences as significant relationships, traumas, and losses is critical. This needs to be done in a manner that does not alienate a patient who may not be accustomed to speaking with mental health professionals or who may not have been told why such a person was consulted. Often, patients will assume that the medical team has given up on them and think that their complaints are "all in their mind."

The process of somatization, the physical manifestation of psychic stress and conflict, is a central concern of the consultation-liaison psychiatrist. Often, a medical team will ask a psychiatrist to evaluate a patient who complains of physical symptoms that the team cannot explain. Unfortunately, mental health professionals are often not consulted until an exhaustive and futile, and often extremely expensive and uncomfortable, medical workup has been performed. It is only at this time that the concept of somatization is entertained. In reality, however, this concept is not an all-or-none phenomenon, and it is up to the consultation-liaison psychiatrist to explain to the patient as well as the medical team that physical symptoms arise simultaneously with physiologic dysfunction and injury as well as with psychological distress and illness.

The consultation-liaison psychiatrist must bear in mind the medical consequences of the psychiatric treatment. For example, prescribing a tricyclic antidepressant to a patient with a cardiac conduction defect or recommending cognitive-behavioral therapy for a patient with cognitive deficits from a recent stroke would likely be both dangerous and distressing to the patient. Behavioral plans and assistance with family and social systems are key elements of the consultation-liaison psychiatrist's job.

The Role of Psychiatrists and Psychologists in the Clinical Setting

The managed care environment has contributed to a major shift in the role of the psychiatrist in the clinical setting. Psychiatrists now work more closely with other medical and mental health practitioners than they have in the past. They function more as consultants than as solo practitioners in specialized inpatient psychiatric units and outpatient psychiatric practices. Within the primary care setting, for example, several effective models can be utilized in the teaching and delivery of mental health care (Rand & Thompson, 1997).

In such an environment, the tasks that psychiatrists perform have become more restricted. While they are trained in psychotherapy, many do not have the time or freedom to practice it. Instead, psychiatrists are asked to focus their efforts on rapid diagnosis and psychopharmacological treatment. Effective collaborations with psychologists and other mental health professionals have become essential in these settings. Such collaboration is perhaps an example of "a good thing happening for the wrong reason."

The Consultation-Liaison Setting

The consultation-liaison setting affords a unique opportunity for psychiatrists and psychologists to work together (Goldberg, Tull, Sullivan, Wallace, & Wool, 1984). The traditional consultation service, where patients are seen by the mental health professional only upon a request for consultation made by the medical team, is being replaced in many settings by a liaison service, where the presence of the mental health professional in the medical team leads to early detection and treatment of mental illness and to shared knowledge and skills regarding mental health with other health care professionals. While liaison services are not yet universally utilized, they will have growing importance in this era of national health care reform, where prevention is a top priority. Psychiatrists and psychologists must work together to forge their place in the inpatient and outpatient health care setting; otherwise, the majority of patients with comorbid psychiatric problems will remain undetected, unreferred, and untreated (Schulberg, Magruder, & deGruy, 1996). Combining forces also gives the medical patient who, for whatever personal reason, may prefer a psychologist over a psychiatrist or vice versa, a higher likelihood of getting the all-important first contact with a mental health practitioner.

On a consultation-liaison service, both psychiatrists and psychologists can perform the initial consultation. However, each discipline has its unique expertise that complements the other to provide a comprehensive assessment and care plan. Both disciplines must become part of the multidisciplinary medical team, helping with emotional and behavioral aspects of all facets of medical care (e.g., medical, nursing, dietary, social, vocational, disposition issues). To achieve this, weekly meetings to discuss clinical, administrative, and educational matters are recommended. While referring physicians expect the consultant to help clarify the diagnosis to treat the symptoms and to help the medical and surgical staff in managing the patient, the priorities of the consulting service vary from service to service. Detailed psychodynamic formulations with psychological jargon are seldom useful and of little interest to the referring physician. The psychiatrist, who has gone through medical training and has been on the "other side" of the consultation, can help to clarify the goals of primary physicians who ask for consults.

While psychiatrists and psychologists are trained in arriving at diagnostic and treatment formulations from somewhat different orientations (e.g., psychiatrists' training may emphasize categorical and medical diagnoses while psychologists' training may emphasize more dimensional and behavioral diagnoses), the roles of the psychiatrist and psychologist in the diagnostic treatment formulation can focus on their respective strengths. While there is much overlap in skills, it is important that each discipline recognize its particular expertise and defer to the other when appropriate. Through mutual education, for example, the psychologist must recognize situations when a pharmacologic intervention may be indicated. Conversely, psychiatrists must consider situations such as when neuropsychological testing is needed when cognitive deficits are suspected. Such a model of integration is illustrated in the following case.

The psychiatry/psychology consult team is asked to see a 32-year-old male inpatient who is recovering from a bone marrow transplant for leukemia. The medical team is concerned about his poor memory and periods of disorientation and requests neuropsychological testing. The patient's behavior consists of periods of severe agitation, impulsivity, grandiose thinking, and rapid speech. When he is less agitated, he appears depressed, anxious, and withdrawn from staff and family members.

The psychologist performs the initial evaluation and, from the medical chart and interviews with the patient, family, and staff, makes a diagnosis of major depressive disorder and delirium. The psychiatrist on the service is then asked to assist with the treatment of the delirium. The psychiatrist determines that the delirium is due to corticosteroids and excessive benzodiazepine anxiolytic medications. He also discovers that the patient is suffering from severe nausea and vomiting, resulting from various medications and anxiety, as well as from longstanding familial conflicts and maladaptive coping mechanisms that contribute to the patient's mood and anxiety problems. After recommending to the medical team an expedited taper of his steroids and benzodiazepines, the psychiatrist and psychologist coordinate an integrated longitudinal treatment plan.

It is determined that when the delirium begins to clear, an antidepressant will be started and the psychologist will meet with the patient for cognitive-behavioral therapy to help combat the nausea. In addition, the psychologist will meet with the patient, his mother, and his primary caregiver on a regular basis to address interpersonal conflicts and to develop a behavioral plan. Because the patient is not sophisticated in psychological issues, possibly due to cognitive side effects of the transplant and of chemotherapy, he tends to focus on pharmacologic issues and is resistant to discussing psychosocial issues. By delegating the pharmacologic treatment to the psychiatrist and the psychotherapy and family treatment to the psychologist, a therapeutically effective and efficient plan is achieved. To guarantee a team approach, the psychiatrist and psychologist occasionally meet jointly with the patient and mother to discuss the overall treatment plan. Neuropsychological testing is also performed by the psychologist and reveals cognitive deficits that are addressed in both behavioral and pharmacologic treatment.

The Psychiatric Inpatient Unit

As in the outpatient case just described, psychiatrists and psychologists can also work together to provide a complementary set of services in the psychiatric inpatient and partial day hospital setting. With the ever-shortening length of stay for psychiatric hospitalizations, intensive, efficient, and comprehensive care has become both increasingly essential as well as increasingly challenging.

Psychiatrists and psychologists, whether full-time staff or residents and interns, can work in tandem, each following their own patients. The psychiatrist must ultimately be responsible for medication decisions. The optimal arrangement in a teaching hospital setting is an attending psychiatrist supervising both psychiatry residents and psychology interns. If medical students are present, both psychiatry residents and psychology interns can contribute to their education. Patients who are particularly suited for psychotherapeutic intervention can be preferentially selected for a psychology intern, while those who are not, such as severely psychotic or manic patients, can be preferentially selected for a psychiatry resident.

Psychologists can also be valuable group leaders in the inpatient and partial day hospital setting. Such group interventions as cognitive-behavioral therapy and psychoeducational groups are particularly suited for the psychologist. Joint psychologist/psychiatrist-led groups are an efficient and team-building way to combine the expertise of both disciplines on the inpatient unit.

The Outpatient Setting

Historically the mainstay model of practice for both psychiatrists and psychologists, the solo practice model, has given way to more group practices, where psychologists, psychiatrists and other mental health professionals share a common suite or "virtual" group practice, and refer patients to each other and cover for each other. Many such practices are located in buildings that house a myriad of medical specialties, facilitating rapid referrals and communication. Commonly, psychiatrists and psychologists will share the same patient, where the psychiatrist manages the medications and the psychologist manages the psychotherapy. While this split is convenient, it is artificial and suboptimal in some respects. Medication management has its own psychodynamic implications, conversely, psychotherapy cannot be conducted without consideration of the patient's somatic and medical symptoms and condition.

The Role of Psychiatrists and Psychologists in the Research Setting

A particularly exciting setting in which psychiatrists and psychologists can collaborate is in the research arena. The same skills that complement each other in the clinical setting do so in the research setting. Of particular value to mental health research is the psychologist's expertise in psychotherapeutic intervention, testing, and research methodology. These skills, coupled with the psychiatrist's expertise in biomedical diagnosis, evaluation, and treatment, and experience in working within the medical system, provide a rich and boundless array of potential research endeavors. Following is an example of such a collaboration.

During a routine weekly clinical meeting among the psychiatrists and psychologists of a psychiatry/psychology consult team in a general hospital, one psychologist made the observation that many consultations for depression and anxiety had been turning out to actually be cases of delirium. A research project was thus proposed to study the incidence, risk factors, and consequences of delirium in a hospital setting.

In designing the study, both psychiatrists and psychologists contributed to each aspect of the design, with a psychiatrist and a psychologist as coprincipal investigators. While the psychiatrists were particularly attuned to the potential medical risk factors for and medical sequelae of delirium, the psychologists were more familiar with the affective and neuropsychological tests that would best capture the neuropsychiatric sequelae of the delirium. Each discipline lent their expertise to the collaborative development and implementation of the study.

Lessons Learned in Working with Psychologists

Unique Contributions

Psychiatrists and psychologists have unique clinical and research training and experiences that must be creatively utilized to maximize the care of patients, the search for new knowledge, and the development of a more efficient, effective, and equitable mental health care system. Old and divisive guild issues must be abandoned for mutual respect and communication. Although psychologists cannot prescribe medications, they can learn more about psychopharmacology so that they can more knowledgeably inform patients of their treatment options and make appropriate and timely referrals to psychiatrists. Conversely, although psychiatrists are not trained in neuropsychological and psychological testing and in other treatment modalities, such as relaxation and imagery, they should become familiar with their indications and uses.

Communication

Communication between psychiatrists and psychologists presents unique challenges and rewards. When working with psychiatrists, it is helpful to remember that they are trained to gather whatever information is necessary to arrive at an initial diagnosis, or at least a differential diagnosis, according to the *DSM-IV.* As taught in medical school, such information is usually gathered and presented in a structured manner, that is, chief complaint, history of present illness, past psychiatric and medical history, medications, family history, social history, and mental status and physical examination. While experienced psychiatrists are able to gather data and to formulate diagnoses and treatment plans without loyally confining themselves to such a structured, linear schema, knowledge of such a framework is helpful in communicating with psychiatrists. As with any form of communication, "speaking the same language" facilitates communication between psychologists and psychiatrists. *DSM-IV* nosology, while only scratching the surface of describing mental illness, is a good place to start. Presenting a differential diagnosis when presenting a case to a psychiatrist will get the ball rolling in the right direction.

It is important to remember the limitations on practice that managed care is imposing on both psychologists and psychiatrists. While psychiatrists are aware of the importance of psychotherapy and other psychosocial treatments, they are often confined to 15- to 30-minute sessions with patients that often allow them only to address medication issues. Nonetheless, psychiatrists welcome information on other psychosocial aspects of the patient's problems and treatment that help to complete the clinical picture and to facilitate the overall care of the patient. Obviously, patient confidentiality must be respected and proper releases of information must be obtained.

Summary

How health care professionals approach patients and their problems is influenced by the conceptual models in which they learn and experience their professional tasks. These conceptual models, while often not made explicit, can exert considerable power over one's professional practice and interactions. It is paradoxical that psychiatrists and psychologists go through their training in relative isolation from each other and yet are thrown together afterward to treat similar patients and problems. The scientific method and its application to the human endeavor of finding a patient's problem, finding its cause, and finding a treatment appear to be the common ground upon which physicians and psychologists build their knowledge and practice. Given such a foundation, the psychiatrist and psychologist should be able to work together as a team toward stronger collaboration. With the political and economic forces acting upon the health care system, the survival of a strong mental health system depends on all mental health professionals working together to show their value to the medical community.

Suggested Resources

The *DSM-IV* (American Psychiatric Association, 1994) provides diagnostic criteria, epidemiologic data, and differential diagnoses for the mental disorders. It is an invaluable reference that is used by nearly all mental health professionals.

"Toward a Diagnostic Alliance Between Psychiatrist and Psychologist" (Berg, 1986) describes some of the pitfalls that can lead to conflict between psychiatrists and psychologists in the clinical setting. Recommendations are cited to improve collaboration between the two specialties.

"The Clinical Application of the Biopsychosocial Model" (Engel, 1980) presents historical and theoretical background and practical applications of the biopsychosocial model for use in modern medicine.

The roles of the psychiatrist, psychologist, nurse-clinical specialist, and social worker in the team approach in the oncology setting are described in detail in "Defining Discipline Roles in Consultation Psychiatry: The Multidisciplinary Team Approach to Psychosocial Oncology" (Goldberg et al., 1984). The biopsychosocial model is applied.

The "Official Actions" (1980) summarizes the general role, responsibilities, and limitations of psychiatrists when working with nonmedical mental health professionals.

"Using Successful Models of Care to Guide the Teaching of Psychiatry in Primary Care" (Rand & Thompson, 1997) presents several models within which to teach psychiatry to primary care physicians. These models can be used by psychiatrists and psychologists to improve collaboration and communication with primary care practitioners.

"Major Depression in Primary Medical Care Practice: Research Trends and Future Priorities" (Schulberg et al., 1996) reviews factors that lead to suboptimal recognition and treatment of depression in primary care settings.

Discussion Questions

1. What are some similarities and differences between the training of psychiatrists and psychologists? How can they be used to facilitate collaboration?
2. What are the advantages of psychiatrists and psychologists working together in the clinical and research settings?
3. What steps can be taken to improve collaboration between psychiatrists and psychologists in the managed care setting?
4. How can psychologists contribute to the training of psychiatry residents?
5. How can psychiatrists contribute to the training of psychology students and interns?

References

Accreditation Council for Graduate Medical Education. (1997). Program requirements for residency education in psychiatry. *In Graduate Medical Education Directory 1997-98* (pp. 261–268). Chicago: American Medical Association.

American Psychiatric Association. (1994). *Diagnostic and statistical manual of mental disorders* (4th ed.). Washington, DC: Author.

Berg, M. (1986). Toward a diagnostic alliance between psychiatrist and psychologist. *American Psychologist, 41,* 52–59.

Engel, G. L. (1980). The clinical application of the biopsychosocial model. *American Journal of Psychiatry, 137,* 535–544.

Goldberg, R. J., Tull, R., Sullivan, N., Wallace, S., & Wool, M. (1984). Defining discipline roles in consultation psychiatry: The multidisciplinary team approach to psychosocial oncology. *General Hospital Psychiatry, 6,* 17–23.

Official actions: Guidelines for psychiatrists in consultative, supervisory, or collaborative relationships with nonmedical therapists (1980). *American Journal of Psychiatry, 137,* 1489–1491.

Rand, E. H., & Thompson, T. L. (1997). Using successful models of care to guide the teaching of psychiatry in primary care. *Psychosomatics, 38,* 140–147.

Schulberg, H. C., Magruder, K. M., & deGruy F. (1996). Major depression in primary medical care practice: Research trends and future priorities. *General Hospital Psychiatry, 18,* 395–406.

17

Spirituality, Health, and Science: The Coming Revival?

Carl E. Thoresen

Everyone who is seriously involved in the pursuit of science becomes convinced that a Spirit is manifest in laws of the universe.

—Albert Einstein

The notion that our physiology and even our anatomy serve at the pleasure, if not the beck and call, of our cognition has surely arrived on the health care scene with increasing momentum (e.g., Goleman & Gurin, 1993). In today's terms, much of the practice of alternative or complementary medicine can be thought of as mind-body or bodymind conceptions of health and disease. While many have long suspected that the Cartesian split of mind from body left too much out, the biomedical model that emerged in the past century left little space for the mind, that is, for social and cognitive factors. Engel's (1977) seminal article in *Science,* which advocated a biopsychosocial model, offered an antidote for the biomedical perspective and provided the kind of high-status intellectual boost needed for some researchers to justify their mind-body beliefs and go forward with their research.

Preparation of this chapter was aided by the National Institute for Healthcare Research and the John M. Templeton Foundation in supporting the Scientific Research in Spirituality Forum. The contributions to my thinking from my group work with hundreds of women and men as well as the work of many are gratefully acknowledged, especially Robert Bellah, Eknath Easwarsan, Meyer Friedman, James Gill, Harold Koenig, David Larson, Joel Levin, Frederic Luskin, Dan McAdams, Michael McCullough, John Martin, Dale Matthews, William Miller, Kenneth Pargament, Houston Smith, Kay Thoresen, and David Wolf. I remain, however, solely responsible for what is presented here.The assistance of Jennifer Hoffman Goldberg and Annie Craft Kincheon in preparing this manuscript is also gratefully acknowledged.

The earlier work of Neil Miller and Herbert Benson in the 1960s on the physiological effects of conditioning and transcendental meditation, respectively, suggested that focusing attention and using specific cognitions (or mental states) could alter specific physiological processes. Meyer Friedman and Ray Rosenman, two cardiologists, also showed at this time that serum cholesterol levels of accountants sharply increased as the April 15 tax deadline approached, then sharply declined in May, without any change in their diet, exercise, smoking, or other known risk factors for higher cholesterol levels (Friedman, Rosenman, & Carroll, 1958).

These findings seemed extraordinary at the time, in part because they exceeded the boundaries of the existing biomedical model. Currently such data seem ordinary, in terms of the brain constantly influencing and being influenced by the body, although we are a long way from understanding just how this works (Goleman & Gurin, 1993; Roush, 1997).

Talk of mind-body relationships has understandably rekindled notions of consciousness, including matters of spirituality and religion, and how expanding consciousness can reduce disease and promote health (e.g., Marwick, 1995). In some ways, once the transactional nature of the mind-body relationship became recognized, the possible role of spiritual and religious factors in health seemed more plausible (Walsh & Vaughn, 1993).

In this chapter I first explore the concept of spirituality followed by the findings of several reviews of the scientific literature on spirituality/religion and health, especially intervention studies. I end with a discussion of current controversies and some conclusions.

Why the Current Interest?

The growing interest in spiritual and religious (SR) factors may lie in the convergence of several themes in American culture:

- Ninety-six percent of Americans currently believe in a God or a universal Spirit, 75 percent pray regularly, 42 percent attend religious worship service almost weekly, 67 percent are members of a local religious body, and 67 percent feel that religion is "very important in their lives" (Gallup, 1995; Matthews, Larson, & Barry, 1993).
- People are working longer hours under greater pressure to perform with less time to focus on living more consciously in the present (e.g., Covey, Merrill & Merrill, 1995; Schor, 1991).

- People are being denied or feel threatened about career security, with downsizing and redundancies commonplace, and are working under increasingly competitive conditions (e.g., Frank & Cook, 1995).
- People are living longer, often with major chronic diseases, and in their later years are becoming more concerned about spiritual issues (e.g., Erikson, Erikson, & Kivnick, 1986; Remen, 1996).
- People of all ages are suffering more from emotional disorders, such as depression, as well as hostility and a range of fears and anxieties (e.g., Booth-Kewley & Friedman, 1987; Seligmann, 1991).
- People born after 1950 may be less likely to have had moral, emotional, religious, or spiritual preparation or "intelligence" (acquired under-standings and learned capabilities) to cope with life in today's fast-paced, postmodern information culture (e.g., Coles, 1996; Damon, 1995; Goleman, 1995).

The popularity of spiritually oriented books, besides the Bible, on best-selling lists has been impressive, including Peck's (1978) *The Road Less Traveled,* Moore's (1992) *Care of the Soul,* and Armstrong's (1993) *A History of God.* This popularity may attest to what may be called the "spiritual hunger" felt by many (see Borysenko, 1993; Keen, 1994).

Evidence of this spiritual void can be found in studies of the American character. Bellah, Madsen, Sullivan, Swidler, and Tipton (1985) noted in their four-year in-depth interview study that the growing sense of feeling isolated and lacking community stemmed in part from a lack of spiritual and religious experiences. Those studied suffered from what might be called an extreme, self-absorbed individualism or "individualism gone berserk" (Bracke & Thoresen, 1996).

A closely related perspective concerns the health effects of perceived social and emotional isolation in American life. Several long-term epidemiological studies have shown that people who report feeling unsupported emotionally are at substantially higher risk for death from all causes (House, Landes, & Umbertson, 1988). This risk of death, roughly two to three times greater, holds for men and women from different social and ethnic groups and for people in other western cultures. A strong overlap seems probable between SR factors and perceiving that others, including a higher power, are there to help you cope with life's many pressures and demands. Although not yet documented, it seems highly likely that the observed benefits of higher levels of perceived social support, particularly emotional support, may be explained in part by the role of SR factors.

Several other growing social and cultural problems highlighting interest in spirituality and health could be cited, such as depression, inner-city violence, poverty, alcohol and substance abuse, job strain, work addiction, anger/hostility, chronic stress, hopelessness, and anxiety-related disorders.

What *Is* Spirituality?

One of the many origins of the word *spirit* (from *spiritus* in Latin) referred literally to the breath or breathing, that is, to something unquestionably vital or animating in people, not something physical or material, thus something not readily observed by the senses. The closely related term *soul* was initially thought to be a spiritual entity, distinct from the body, that gave the person the capacity to transcend what might be called animal or survival instincts. As Keen (1994) speculates, our earliest ancestors were trying to discover and understand just how people differed between being alive and being dead. Immediately after people died, they probably looked much the same to our ancestors, but something was missing. When persons died, they no longer breathed nor did they show any energy or vitality. In effect, they lacked spirit (breath) and soul (animating entity). In this chapter, the focus will be on spirituality, assuming as some do, that the soul may be viewed either as the locale of the spirit or as synonymous with the spiritual (Keen, 1994).

Clearly the term *spirit* has evolved over the centuries, yet the underlying essence of spirituality still alludes to a search or quest for the sacred in life and beyond, a seeking of answers to life's most meaningful and vital questions. As such, any crisp, tightly bounded definition that readily captures the breadth and depth of spirituality creates problems. As we shall see, spirituality as a concept involves several complexities.

Aldridge (1993), for example, presented 13 definitions focused primarily on spirituality and healing. Most definitions cited mentioned or alluded to the following:

- the need to transcend or rise above everyday material or sensory experience
- one's relationship to God or some other higher universal power, force, or energy
- the search for greater meaning, purpose, and direction in living

- healing by means of non-physical kinds of intervention (e.g., prayer, meditation, religious beliefs)

Others have defined spirituality in terms of organized religions, that is, as part of the Judeo-Christian tradition that includes both institutional as well as personal factors (e.g., Koenig, 1993). In a recent comprehensive review of religion and counseling, Worthington, Kurusu, McCullough, and Sandage (1996) made the following distinction:

- *Religious* applies to any organized religion and concerns religious beliefs (propositional statements in agreement with some organized religion) and religious values (broad organizing statements about what is important in life).
- *Spiritual,* by contrast, is believing in, valuing, or being devoted to some power higher than what exists in the physical world.

Thus, a person may be spiritual, believing in a higher source (e.g., universal divine energy) without believing, for example, in the Christian God or Jesus and without holding any specific religious beliefs or values. Or the person could be both spiritual and religious, believing in and valuing a higher power, such as God, consistent with some organized religion. Furthermore, a person may also be religious but not very spiritual, accepting the doctrines of a religious organization but not experiencing or expressing much devotion to a higher power, other than intellectually agreeing that such a power exists.

Others, however, view spirituality more broadly. Bellingham, Cohen, Jones, and Spaniol (1989) suggest that feelings of connectedness with oneself, with others, and with a larger meaning or purpose in life captures the key feature of spirituality, a feeling not necessarily characteristic of someone who is religious or believes, for example, in God. Still others highlight the role of faith, hope, love, and commitment along with connectedness in defining spirituality (e.g., Hawks, Hull, Thalman, & Richins, 1995; Young, 1984). I suspect that the defining core of spirituality, seen as a latent, multidimensional construct with several facets (much like personality or health), lies in experiences and beliefs of a transcendent relationship with a power, spirit, or force greater than the individual, something beyond the confines of ego or self (Walsh & Vaughn, 1993).

Spirituality can also be thought of in terms of certain beliefs, motivation, and practices (Miller & Bennett, 1997). Examples might be beliefs about existence, nature, and higher power; motivation in terms of values, faith, positive expectations, and levels of confidence; and practices, such as prayer, serving others, and spending time alone in wilderness areas.

If we accept the multidimensionality of spirituality, that it has many facets and that some persons may agree on some of these facets but not others, then we can seek different ways to understand it. We can also accept the fact that an assessment of spirituality probably requires multifaceted approaches, making it difficult to capture spirituality, for example, in a simple, brief questionnaire. To increase spirituality also probably requires more than one kind of intervention. This does not preclude, however, attempts to create a relatively brief set of measures that could provide the major outlines of a multidimensional portrait of spirituality or of short-term interventions to alter some facets of spirituality.

Some Working Definitions

For our purposes, we can use some working definitions, mindful of the limitations in doing so. But let us be sensitive about two major points: First, as in small particle physics research and quantum theory, our efforts to assess spirituality could alter what we are seeking to measure more objectively. In physics this is called the Heisenberg Principle, which notes that trying to assess the speed and location of an electron alters its speed and location. We may not be able to capture in our measures all of what spirituality entails because trying to do so may alter the spiritual experience we are trying to measure (Glass & Mackey, 1988).

Second, we may not be able to capture features of spirituality simply because we cannot adequately describe or articulate just what they are. In the philosophy of science this is sometimes described as the "tacit" knowledge problem: We may "know" something but not be able to describe it to others (Polanyi, 1958). One thing is clear: We can at present assess some features of SR factors with existing measures and, in doing so, we can expand our understanding of their role in health and well-being.

Albert Einstein (1954) pondered, among many things, the issues of spirituality and religiousness. His wise dictum, "Science without religion is lame, religion without science is blind," bears noting. While Einstein remained skeptical about the science of his day being able to penetrate the complexities of spiritual and religious phenomena, he believed that we must recognize the place and existence of a higher power in understanding the universe.

Here then are some working definitions of religion and spirituality, derived in part from the National Institute for Healthcare Research conference papers on science and spirituality (Larson, Swyers, & McCullough, 1997), that may help clarify but not fully capture these concepts:

- *Religion.* An organized system of beliefs, practices, rituals, and symbols designed to facilitate a relationship to and understanding of a deity (or deities) as well as to promote understanding and harmony of a person's relationship to oneself and others in living together in community. Religion as a social institution involves many practices and procedures that can have both positive and negative effects.
- *Spirituality.* A person's unique search, which may or may not be as a member of a religion, over the lifespan for what is sacred in life, answers to life's ultimate questions (such as the meaning, purpose, and direction in life), as well as a feeling of connectedness to others and the environment. The defining characteristic, however, is the quality of one's transcendent relationship to some form of a higher power, spirit, or force. This search can at times involve suffering and pain as one explores and confronts beliefs, feelings, and actions. As such, spirituality involves expanding human consciousness and, as with religion, can have both positive and negative effects.

Note that the major distinction between these two terms may be the social and institutional nature of religion compared to the more individual thrust and experience of spirituality. Both involve the seeking of the sacred in living and both focus on a transcendent "beyond the ego" relationship with God or a higher universal power or spirit.

The issue of multiculturalism, now generally accepted as a major force in psychology (Worthington et al., 1996), reminds us that SR factors always exist within influential social contexts or settings. For example, not all Roman Catholics living in the United States (e.g., rural Florida versus Oregon coast) necessarily share identical beliefs, experiences, and behaviors. Local religious or spiritual "cultures" provide different settings that influence how people think and act religiously or spiritually. Despite these real differences, since the beginning of civilization, almost all spiritual and religious perspectives share the following core principles: humility, selflessness (serving others but not self-abasement), love in its many meanings, compassion, forgiveness, joy, feeling "alive" to life, and integrity (beyond only "telling the truth") (Thoresen, 1997, based on the work of Smith, 1989).

These themes may not, of course, correspond with the experience of a particular person or the practices of a religious institution at a particular point in history. They suggest, however, that a universality of needs and concerns exists, shared widely across many cultures for thousands of years. Let us now turn to empirical evidence from published research about SR and health.

What's the Evidence?

Over 200 empirical studies relating SR factors to health have been published since the 1960s (Jarvis & Northcott, 1987; Levin, 1994; Matthews et al., 1993; Worthington et al., 1996). In general, published reviews have found a positive, although at times modest, relationship between religious beliefs and practices and physical and mental health outcomes. This relationship is statistically significant in most studies, showing that religious commitment and practice relate to lower morbidity and mortality rates. However, finding statistically significant relationships between SR and reduced death and disability do not, by themselves, demonstrate that SR causes or best explains less death or disease. Furthermore, a statistically significant relationship between a spiritual factor (e.g., meditating daily) and a health outcome (e.g., reduced diastolic blood pressure) may not demonstrate a meaningful or clinically useful result. As discussed in chapter 5 with Goldberg, more practical or clinically significant tests should be used to determine whether an outcome or result has practical or clinical value (see Thoresen, Luskin, & Harris, in press).

Here is a simplified list of overall significant findings on SR factors reported by Levin (1994), who examined 250 studies conducted between the 1930s and late 1980s.

- Findings consistently found positive effects in terms of reduced coronary heart disease, high blood pressure, stroke, most cancers, and several health status indicators.
- Findings consistently showed reduced morbidity and mortality.
- Findings held, no matter how spirituality was defined or measured (i.e., beliefs, experiences, behavior, or attitudes).
- Findings were positive for Whites, Hispanics, and African Americans and for people in America, European, African, and Asian cultures.

The studies included the following parameters:

- Research designs varied from prospective, retrospective, case-control, and cohort types.
- Participants included Protestants, Catholics, Jews, Parsis, Buddhists, and Zulus.
- Studies included people with self-limiting, acute conditions, fatal chronic diseases, a variety of illnesses (from brief to lengthy), persons in remission for various diseases, and participants who had died during the research process.

In these studies SR factors were measured in a number of ways (e.g., belief in God, Bible reading, frequency of prayer). Overall, Levin (1994) concluded that while the evidence of a relationship is impressive, there was "only mixed evidence" that such relationships between SR factors and health were causal (e.g., spiritual meditation or prayer reduced cancer risk).

Recently, a group of more than 50 scholars from several areas (e.g., psychology, family medicine, theology) completed a series of research reviews on spiritual and religious factors in four major areas: physical health, mental health, alcohol and substance abuse, and biology and neurophysiology (Larson et al., 1997). Some of their review findings echo those already mentioned. Some, however, have not been covered in other reviews. Findings about the relationship of SR and mental health include higher rates of subjective well-being, higher life satisfaction, and higher marital satisfaction, along with lower rates of depressive symptoms, suicide, juvenile delinquency, alcohol and drug abuse, and divorce. More specifically, SR has been related to reduced cigarette smoking and so-called recreational drug use (e.g., Hardesty & Kirby, 1995). Meditation-type interventions have been associated with reduced alcohol/drug use and related problems and with longer life in the elderly (e.g., Alexander, Langer, Newman, & Chandler, 1989). Furthermore, participation in Alcoholics Anonymous (AA) relates to better health outcomes, but only after outpatient treatment and, to a lesser extent, only after in-patient treatment (Emerick, Tonigan, Montgomery, & Little, 1993).

Koenig and Futterman (1995) carefully examined SR with older persons in 89 empirical studies and, in general, found SR to be negatively related to indicators of poor mental or physical health. For example, in terms of overall mortality, one study (Zuckerman, Kasl, & Ostfeld, 1984) of 400 elderly poor people found that the odds of dying were 2.3 times higher for nonreligious versus religious persons (i.e., attended religious services, self-rated religiousness, and religiousness seen as source of strength), even when health status and gender were statistically controlled.

A well-designed study (Seeman, Kaplan, Knudsen, Cohen, & Guralnik, 1987) of 7,000 adults found that active involvement in church activities predicted longer survival for those 38–49 years old and those over 60. However, when smoking, physical activity, body weight, depression, and eating breakfast were controlled for, religious activity no longer predicted mortality. Since religious activity is related to all of the above factors (e.g., more church is related to less depression), the statistical analysis used in this study (and others) may lead to "squeezing out" the contribution of SR activities, even when such factors still play an indirect or moderator role in better health.

In contrast, Strawbridge, Cohen, Shema, and Kaplan (1997) found that among 5,286 adults studied over 28 years, those who attended religious services more frequently had significantly lower death rates (36 percent less) than infrequent attenders, even when several physical and mental health factors were statistically controlled. Women benefited more than men. Intriguing was the finding that during the 28 years, higher church attenders were more likely to reduce other harmful health behaviors (e.g., smoking, alcohol abuse) and to increase health-enhancing behaviors (e.g., increase physical exercise, number of close friends), compared to less frequent church attenders. Furthermore, those who did change these health-related practices reduced the relationship of religious attendance and mortality. That is, the improvement in health practices accounted for some of the reduced death rates in church attenders, strongly suggesting that the benefits of SR factors observed in this study may be accounted for by encouraging people to take better care of themselves. Note, however, that frequent religious attendance preceded the changes in health practices over time, implying that religious involvement may play a causal role in reduced mortality.

In a major 23-year study of 10,000 male Israeli civil servants, Goldbourt, Yaari, and Medalie (1993) found that orthodox religious practice (e.g., religious education, self-rated religious belief, frequency of attending services) was associated with 50 percent fewer deaths from all causes among religious males compared to nonreligious males. This difference held up even when all major coronary heart disease risk factors (e.g., smoking, blood pressure, cholesterol) were controlled for in the analysis. Another Israeli study (Friedlander, Kark, & Stein, 1986) found 4.2 to 7.3 times higher coronary heart disease death rates for nonreligious compared to religiously orthodox males, again with other coronary heart disease risk factors controlled.

In the first meta-analytic review of SR factors and all-cause mortality, McCullough, Larson, Hoyt, Koenig, and Thoresen (1998) found that in over 20 published studies (N=78,832) the weighted effect size (0.15, p<.001) of religious involvement (e.g., regularly attending religious service; prayer or meditation) on death was of the same magnitude as studies of social support or hostility in predicting mortality (accounting for 2–5 percent of deaths).

One of the most innovative studies to date examined the role of SR in caregivers of partners dying of AIDS (Folkman, in press; Richards & Folkman, in press). Using in-depth interviews of caregivers shortly after the partner's death, and again six months later, they analyzed transcripts of over 80 interviews and identified those who had spontaneously mentioned spiritual or religious themes. When this spiritual group was compared to the non-spiritual group (roughly equal in number), those who were more spiritually oriented reported more negative emotionality (e.g., depression, anxiety, physical stress symptoms) shortly after the partner's death. However, six months later they were functioning much better than the nonspiritual group in terms of reduced negative emotions and types of coping used (e.g., more problem-focused coping and less denial). Spiritually-minded caregivers also experienced more positive emotions, such as humor and seeing the comedy of everyday life, in trying to deal with the loss. Using a research design that combined both quantitative and qualitative assessments, repeated over time, especially in encouraging participants to describe their experiences ("tell their stories"), proved invaluable in discovering these unanticipated changes in caregivers' experience.

Intervention Studies: What Works Best?

Although the research literature offers generally positive results about the relationship of SR and health outcomes, these findings remain correlational (Thoresen et al., 1997). Lacking are controlled interventions in which a religious or spiritual factor(s) serves as the focus of the treatment or as part of the treatment. Demonstrating that *changes* in SR lead to .changes in health outcomes could provide much more convincing evidence that SR is responsible in part for improved health status.

While very few controlled intervention studies have been conducted (the exception to this has been a range of meditation studies [e.g., Alexander, 1994]), some clinical intervention studies have involved a spiritually-related component, even if it was not labeled as spiritual. Three studies come to mind: Ornish and colleagues (1990), Spiegel, Bloom, Kraemer, and Gottheil (1989), and Friedman and colleagues (1986). In all three, the overall intervention had several components, some with spiritual content. To varying degrees, the following issues were considered: direction, meaning, and purpose in life; feelings of connectedness to oneself, others, and with a higher power; clarifying what is trivial and what is truly vital in life; reducing self-critical and hostile cognitions; and fostering love, compassion, and forgiveness. Although such concerns were not typically called spiritual, often referred to as philosophy of life issues, the spiritual relevance seems clear.

To illustrate, in the Friedman and others (1986) study using group counseling with over 1,000 post-coronary patients, spiritually-related quotations and behaviors were used in a Participant Workbook to stimulate action, reflection, and discussion. Examples include asking participants to practice listening actively to others, telling your spouse (child) how much you loved him or her, and spending time alone in nature. They were also asked to reflect on various thoughts, such as this thought by a former coronary patient, "When all the clocks and calendars have stopped their counting for you, what then has your life counted up to?" or "It is only with the heart that one can see rightly. What is essential is invisible to the eye" (St. Exupery).

Well-controlled intervention studies are rare. In 146 empirical studies reviewed by Worthington and others (1996), only 6 percent were intervention studies. Of these, most involved small samples of less than 50, typically 15 or 20, and several did not use any kind of comparison or control group.

Two larger studies that used rigorous research designs deserve comment. Byrd (1988) studied 393 post-coronary patients who were randomly assigned to an intercessory prayer condition or to usual care (intercessory prayer is when someone prays for another person). In the prayer intervention, hospitalized patients were prayed for by three to seven Christians living in the area. Patients did not know they were being prayed for, nor did their physicians. Those who prayed only knew the patient's first name and his or her diagnosis and general condition. They also received periodic updates on the patient's condition. Those prayed for spent significantly fewer days in critical care units, in the hospital, required fewer medications in hospital and at discharge, developed fewer new symptoms, and were rated higher in their responsiveness to the course of treatment. Although this study employed an experimental design with adequate statistical power and produced interesting results, any single study clearly requires replication before findings can be viewed with any acceptance. Several efforts to do so are currently underway (see Benson, 1996).

In a second intervention, Propst, Ostrum, Watkins, Dean, and Mashburn (1992) used three forms of counseling (religious- or nonreligious-oriented cognitive-behavior therapy or pastoral counseling) and a waiting-list control group with 59 depressed clients all of whom were religious. Counseling was done by 10 counselors (5 religious and 5 nonreligious) over 18 one-hour weekly sessions. Assessments were made before treatment, at posttreatment, after 3 months, and after 24 months. Nonreligious counselors using religiously-focused cognitive-behavior therapy had the best results on a variety of psychosocial measures compared to religious counselors. The least effective treatment was nonreligious counselors using cognitive-behavior therapy. Recall that all clients were religious. Noteworthy is the finding that religious clients did better when the cognitive-behavior therapy interventions were more religiously focused. Worthington and colleagues (1996) commented that, in general, religiously-adapted cognitive and behavior therapies used with religious clients have been more effective.

The SR Coping Concept

The use of prayer and cognitive behavior therapy in the above studies highlights the concept of coping. In many ways a major function of religion and spirituality is helping people cope better with life, that is, assisting them in solving problems, making decisions, dealing with crisis, and creating more meaning and purpose in living. Pargament (1996) has conducted extensive research on religious coping, developing several scales that assess different forms of religious coping, including spiritually-based coping (e.g., "Experienced God's love and care," "My faith showed me different ways to handle the problem"), good deeds coping (e.g., "Confessed my sins"), and religious support coping (e.g., "Sought support from other church members"). Pargament provides solid psychometric evidence for measures used and offers a perspective that recognizes the need to consider and respect individual differences in conducting research and providing help to others.

While the many types of self-report questionnaires used in SR research cannot be discussed here, common examples of items used include: "How often do you go to religious services? (six choices from "more than once a week" to "never") and "Within your religious or spiritual tradition, how often do you meditate? (eight choices from "more than once a day" to "never"). Often only one or a few such items have been used in studies, thus severely limiting what we know about SR and health. Still, even with such limitations, studies have often yielded noteworthy results.

Some innovative assessment approaches, however, deserve mention. One innovation is to use a more qualitative, narrative approach, coupled with more common approaches, such as survey measures. The narrative approach (Folkman, in press; Richards & Folkman, in press) engages people to "tell their stories," providing a rich source of ideas and hypotheses about SR factors and health. McAdams (1993) speaks of "nuclear episodes," identified in narrative analyses as incidents in a person's life that serve as life history benchmarks around which persons often create the scripts and self-schema that powerfully influence their behavior. McAdams has successfully used narrative assessment to clarify various basic need themes in people's lives, such as power or intimacy. Table 17.1 presents a series of open-ended questions that

---

Table 17.1
Religious and Spiritual Assessment Interview

Religious Background and Beliefs
1. What religion did your family practice when you were growing up?
2. How religious were your parents?
3. Do you practice a religion currently?
4. Do you believe in God or a Higher Power?
5. What have been important experiences and thoughts about God/Higher Power?
6. How would you describe God/Higher Power? Personal or impersonal? Loving or stern?

Spiritual Meaning and Values
1. Do you follow any spiritual path or practice (e.g., meditation, yoga, prayer, solitude)?
2. What significant spiritual experiences have you had (e.g., mystical experience, near-death experience, 12-step spirituality, drug-induced dreams)?

Prayers/Meditation Experiences
1. Do you pray or meditate? When? In what way(s)?
2. How has prayer or meditation worked in your life?
3. Have your prayers been answered?
4. Has your meditation changed you?

---

can be used, for example, in a large group by breaking down into dyads or groups of three or four to stimulate reflection and discussion of SR factors.

Use of qualitative approaches that feature in-depth assessments can complement information currently available from questionnaires and demographic data (e.g., age, religious affiliation). Expanding the repertoire of assessment methods can expand our understanding of SR and health. For a comprehensive picture of existing spiritual and religious assessment measurements, see Hill and Hood (in press).

Controversies and Conclusions

Matters of the spirit, including religious beliefs, experiences, and practices, continue to provide ample opportunity for debate, disagreement, and controversy. While the twentieth century has seen a sharp decline in the role and influence of religion and spirituality in many Western industrialized cultures, survey evidence suggests that many people are concerned about spiritual issues. For example, most Americans believe in God and often pray or meditate in some way and many use spiritually- or religiously-oriented ways of coping with life problems and stresses. Importantly, in recognition of the normality of SR concerns, religious or spiritual experiences are no longer classified by the professional psychiatric community (*Diagnostic and Statistical Manual of Mental Disorders* or *DSM-IV*) as a sign of a mental dysfunction or a pathological disorder (Lukoff, Lu, & Turner, 1992). Rather, people are now seen as suffering at times from a range of various spiritual and religiously-based problems, sometimes termed "spiritual emergencies," such as acute distress associated with major life events, certain beliefs, or practices of a particular church, or a perceived crisis about one's life or one's relationship to a higher power. Sometimes religious or spiritual institutions, practices, or beliefs can create serious problems, something long recognized (e.g., James, 1902). Often such problems stem from authoritarian leadership and devious practices by those who prey on people who blindly accept the dogmatic dictates of some religious institutions and those in authority.

One of the controversies has been called the "religiosity gap." This refers to the small proportion of mental health care professionals who are actively religious or spiritual (in the 20–35 percent range) compared to the larger proportion of the general public (ranging from 40–75 percent) who attend services or view themselves as religious or spiritually focused (see Lukoff et al., 1992).

While only 1–5 percent of the general public describe themselves as atheists or agnostic, over 50 percent of psychologists and psychiatrists describe themselves as such (Gallup, 1985). This gap creates several problems, one being the failure of many health professionals to consider religious or spiritual factors in terms of assessment and treatment approaches. The "spirituality gap," as defined in this chapter, may be less but is still significant, especially since few professional training programs explicitly provide information and skills about spiritual beliefs and practices (Richards & Bergin, 1997).

Another controversy surrounds the many problems associated with the assessment of SR factors. If we continue to use very simplistic measures, such as only using one's religious affiliation as the sole measure of religion or relying solely on a brief self-report questionnaire to capture spirituality, then progress will be limited. At issue is how to capture the subtleties and nuances of spiritual experience, given its multidimensional nature. Various types of interviews, behavioral observations, self-ratings, logs, and diaries and journals, along with ambulatory monitoring of cognitions and emotional states and use of focus group methodology, seem fruitful approaches to explore in concert with some existing measures such as coping scales and standardized measures of emotional status.

Perhaps the most basic controversy concerns the perceived incompatibility of science and spirituality. Can we be scientific about spirituality or does trying to do so represent a fundamental contradiction? Studies cited in this chapter suggest that we have already been successful to some extent in bringing the essence of science to understanding the relationships of SR and health. These efforts have produced modest yet encouraging results; however, almost all data gathered in these studies are based on methods of assessment that can be challenged and do not demonstrate cause and effect. As a recent *Science* article (Roush, 1997) suggests, some scientists (but not all) strongly and vigorously dissent from accepting these SR relationships with health as scientifically valid. Some may also believe that science and spirituality are by definition not only inherently incompatible, but also that science may seriously misrepresent and distort the essence of religion and spirituality (e.g., Thomson, 1996).

Another controversy concerns how the influence of SR factors produces changes in health outcomes. In science, this issue is called the "mechanisms" issue. That is, what specific processes could possibly account for SR producing less disease and better health? Several possible if not plausible explanations exist:

- People who are spiritually or religiously focused may engage in fewer known risk factors for disease (e.g., high-fat diet, smoking), thus have better health.
- Such people may use cognitive coping strategies (e.g., meditation or self-affirmations) in ways that promote positive changes in emotional states (e.g., reduced anger or resentment) which in turn enhance immune functioning (e.g., elevated lymphocyte levels), thus reducing disease risk.
- Spiritual or religious beliefs or practices may directly mediate change or may serve as moderating factors that influence health status (e.g., feeling strength or comfort from belief in a higher power reduces or moderates the influence of higher fat diet on serum cholesterol levels).

Oxman, Freeman, and Manheimer (1995), for example, demonstrated a direct mediating effect in 232 patients of perceived strength and comfort from their religious beliefs and a fivefold reduction in death over six months after major coronary surgery. When social support (participating in groups regularly) was also considered, the combined benefit was a tenfold reduction in death (2 percent versus 23 percent). How do we explain the way that strength and comfort from religious beliefs and social support dramatically reduce death? Answers are not readily available, at least those acceptable to most in the scientific community.

At a more challenging level, spirituality concerns higher states of consciousness (e.g., experiencing God or profound inner peace). How do we study the possible processes involved in consciousness? Keeping in mind the notion of emergent concepts, that is, the idea that one level of complexity cannot fully explain a higher level of complexity (e.g., physiology per se cannot explain closeness to God), the answer may not be simply reducible to physical changes in neurochemistry, such as those observed in the brain from functional magnetic resonance imaging techniques (e.g., Mandell, 1980). Lacking plausible explanations for SR and health relationships creates powerful barriers for some in taking results of SR studies seriously, even if such studies are conducted with state-of-the art research methods. Still, the history of science is filled with unexplained findings of useful procedures that were eventually explained (the exact mechanisms of why aspirin works is but one example). Note also that many prescribed medicines, such as various antidepressants that have been demonstrated to reduce depression, are still somewhat of a mystery in terms of just why they work.

At this point we need to focus more on demonstrating that SR can lead to beneficial outcomes. In time, we may develop and adopt more integrative theories that can reveal causal mechanisms (see Schwartz & Russek, 1997, for a stimulating discussion of new theories).

For years, data have been consistently clear on one major point: Most Americans report being religious and/or spiritual. Couched in a medical metaphor, the negative side effects of SR on health appear limited while the potential benefits seem very worthwhile. The evidence available supports cautious optimism about the role of SR in health and disease. Even if a health professional personally is not spiritually or religiously active, the needs and experiences of those seeking help deserve to be respected. After all, it is the person with the disease or the disorder that we are trying to help, not just the disease or disorder itself.

Suggested Resources

The Power of Myth (Campbell, 1988) is an excellent record of several discussions between Joseph Campbell and Bill Moyers about the role of beliefs and spirituality in different cultures. This book is very readable and includes many insights.

An outstanding, beautifully written brief introduction to the practice of meditation is *Meditation* (Easwaran, 1991). Easwaran uses selections from the world's enduring spiritual and religious literature (e.g., Christian Saints, Hindu scriptures) to present a comprehensive eight-point program of spiritual growth and development (e.g., learning to slow down, practicing "one-pointed" attention, and putting others first).

One of the best reviews of studies available by a physician experienced with the topic is "Religion and Health: Is There an Association, Is It Valid, and Is It Caused?" (Levin, 1994). Focusing on physical health outcomes, it offers a conservative and well-reasoned appraisal of the relationship of spiritual and religious factors to health outcomes based on published research.

The World's Religions (Smith, 1989) is an impressive and invaluable text that provides a rare look at all of the major religions written in a very comfortable and readable style. Smith, a Methodist, actually lived in many countries and lived several religions, using Buddhist, Hindu, and Muslim religious practices. He demonstrates how all major religions, in their founding assumptions and philosophy, seek the same outcomes.

"Empirical Research on Religion and Psychotherapeutic Processes and Outcomes: A 10-Year Review and Research Prospectus" (Worthington et al., 1996) is the most comprehensive research review available that focuses primarily on religious factors and a broad array of topics (e.g., effects of religious counselors; effects of religious techniques and integrating religious techniques into general theoretical approaches). It also includes a list of all journals that publish religious or spiritual research.

Discussion Questions

1. How do you personally think about spirituality in your own life? For you, what are its major features?
2. If you were to defend the position that spiritual and religious factors help promote health and prevent disease, what would you cite as evidence to support your position?
3. Assume that you as a health professional (e.g., physician, counseling psychologist, clinical social worker, coronary care nurse) have been given the responsibility to help develop a new program for people with a chronic and incurable disease. What would you do to explore the possibility of including some type of spiritual or religious component to this program?
4. What spiritual or religious issues do you believe are most important to consider in helping people with their health problems and concerns? How would you try to justify including these issues?
5. What do you see as the biggest barrier to conducting scientific research that examines spiritual/religious factors and health issues? What might help reduce this barrier?
6. If someone, with your approval, planned to assess your spiritual/religious health and well-being, what do you think would be the most effective way of doing so? If the assessment had to be done under strict limits of time and resources, what would work best for you?

References

Aldridge, D. (1993). Is there evidence for spiritual healing? *Advances, 9,* 4–21.

Alexander, C. N. (1994). Treating and preventing alcohol, nicotine and drug abuse through transcendental meditation: A review and meta-analysis. *Alcoholism Treatment Quarterly,* 11, 13–87.

Alexander, C. N., Langer, E. J., Newman, R. I., & Chandler, H. M. (1989). Transcendental meditation, mindfulness and longevity: An experimental study with the elderly. *Journal of Personality and Social Psychology, 57,* 950–964.

Armstrong, K. (1993). *A history of God.* New York: Knopf.

Bellah, R. N., Madsen, R., Sullivan, W., Swidler, A., & Tipton, S. (1985). *Habits of the heart: Individualism and commitment in American life.* Berkeley, CA: University of California. Bellingham, R., Cohen, B., Jones, T., & Spaniol, L. (1989). Connectedness: Some skills for spiritual health. *American Journal of Health Promotion, 4,* 18–31.

Benson, H. (1996). *Timeless healing: The power and biology of belief.* New York: Scribner.

Booth-Kewley, S., & Friedman, H. S. (1987). Psychological predictors of heart disease: A quantitative review. *Pyscological Bulletin, 101,* 343–362.

Borysenko, J. (1993). *Fire in the soul.* New York: Warner.

Bracke, P., & Thoresen, C. E. (1996). Reducing Type A behavior patterns: A structured group approach. In R. Allan, & S. Scheidt (Eds.), *Heart and mind* (pp. 255–290). Washington, DC: American Psychological Association.

Byrd, R. B. (1988). Positive therapeutic effects of intercessory prayer in a coronary care unit population. *Southern Medical Journal, 81,* 826–829.

Campbell, J. (with Bill Moyers). (1988). *The power of myth.* New York: Doubleday.

Coles, R. (1996). *The moral intelligence of children.* New York: Random House.

Covey, S., Merrill, A. R., & Merrill, R .R. (1995). *First things first.* New York: Fireside.

Damon, W. (1995). *Greater expectations.* New York: Free Press.

Easwaran, E. (1991). *Meditation.* Tomales, CA: Nilgiri.

Einstein, A. (1954). *Albert Einstein: Ideas and opinions.* New York: Crown.

Emerick, C. D., Tonigan, J. S., Montgomery, H., & Little, L. (1993). Alcoholics Anonymous: What is currently known? In B. S. McCrady, & W. R. Miller (Eds.), *Research on Alcoholics Anonymous: Opportunities and alternatives* (pp. 41–76). New Brunswick, NJ: Rutgers Center of Alcohol Studies.

Engel, G. (1977). The need for a new medical model: A challenge for biomedicine. *Science, 196,* 129–136.

Erikson, E. H., Erikson, J. M., & Kivnick, H.W. (1986). *Vital involvement in old age.* New York: Norton.

Folkman, S. (in press). Positive psychological states and coping with severe stress. *Social Science and Medicine.*

Frank, R. H., & Cook, P. J. (1995). *The winner take all society.* New York: Free.

Friedlander, Y., Kark, J. D.,& Stein, Y. (1986). Religious orthology and myocardial infarction in Jerusalem: A case-central study. *International Journal of Cardiology, 10,* 33–41.

Friedman, H., Rosenman, R., & Carroll, V. (1958). Changes in the serum cholesterol and blood-clotting time in men subjected to variation in occupational stress. *Circulation, 17,* 852–861.

Freidman, M., Thoresen, C. E., Gill, J., Ulmer, D., Powell. L. H., Price, V. A., Brown, R., Thompson, L., Rabin, D., Breall, W. S., Bourg, W., Levy, R., & Dixon, T. (1986). Alternation of Type A behavior and its effects on cardiac recurrences in postmyocardial infarction patients: Summary results of the Recurrent Coronary Prevention Project. *American Heart Journal, 112,* 653–665.

Gallup, G. (1985). *Religion in America, 50 years: 1935–1985.* Princeton, NJ: Princeton Religious Research Center.

Gallup, G. (1995). *The gallup poll: Public opinion 1995.* Wilmington, DE: Scholarly Resources.

Glass, L., & Mackey, M. (1988). *From clocks to chaos: The rhythm of time*. Princeton, NJ: Princeton University.

Goldbourt, U., Yaari, S., & Medalie, J. J. (1993). Factors predicting of long-term coronary heart disease mortality among 10,059 male Israeli civil servants and municipal employees: A 23-year mortality follow-up in the Israeli Ischemic Heart Disease Study. *Cardiology, 82,* 100–121.

Goleman, D. (1995). *Emotional intelligence*. New York: Bantam.

Goleman, D., & Gurin, J. (Eds.). (1993). *Mind body medicine: How to use your mind for better health*. NewYork: Consumers Union.

Hardesty, P. H., & Kirby, K. M. (1995). Relation between family religiousness and drug use within adolescent peer groups. *Journal of Social Behavior and Personality, 10,* 421–430.

Hawks, S. R., Hull, M. L., Thalman, R. L., & Richins, P. M. (1995). Review of spiritual health: Definitions, role, and intervention strategies in health promotion. American *Journal of Health Promotion, 9,* 371–378.

Hill, P. C., & Hood, R. W. (in press). *Measures of religious behavior.* Burmingham, AL: Religious Education.

House, J. S., Landes, K. R., & Umbertson, R. (1988). Social relationships and health. *Science, 240,* 540–545.

James, W. (1902). *Varieties of religious experience*. NewYork: Random House.

Jarvis, G. K., & Northcott, H. C. (1987). Religion and differences in morbidity and mortality. *Social Science and Medicine, 25,* 813–824.

Keen, S. (1994). *Hymns to an unknown God*. New York: Bantam.

Koenig, H . G. (1993). The relationship between Judeo-Christian religion and mental health among middle-aged and older adults. *Advances, 9,* 33–38.

Koenig, H. G., & Futterman, A. (1995, March 15). *Religion and health outcomes: A review and synthesis of the literature.* Presented at the National Institute of Aging Conference on Spiritual and Religious Factors in Health, Durham, NC.

Larson, D., Swyers, J., & McCullough, M. (1997). *Scientific research on spirituality and health: A consensus report.* Rockville, MD: National Institute for Healthcare Research.

Levin, J. (1994). Religion and health: Is there an association, is it valid, and is it causal? *Social Science and Medicine, 38,* 1475–1484.

Lukoff, D., Lu, F., & Turner, R. (1992). Toward a more culturally sensitive *DSM-IV:* Psychoreligious and psychospirited problems. *Journal of Nervous and Mental Disease, 180,* 673–682.

Mandell, A. J. (1980). Towards a psycholobiology of transcendence: God in the brain. In J. Davidson, & R. J. Davidson (Eds.), *The psychobiology of consciousness.* New York: Plenum.

Marwick, C. (1995). Should physicians prescribe prayer for health? Spiritual aspects of well-being considered. *Journal of the American Medical Association, 273,* 1561–1562.

Matthews, D. A., Larson, D. B., & Barry, C. (1993). *The faith factor: An annotated bibliography of clinical research on spiritual subjects.* Rockville, MD: National Institute for Healthcare Research.

McAdams, D. P. (1993). *The stories we live by.* NewYork: Guilford.

McCullough, M. E., Larson, D. B., Hoyt., K., Koenig, H. G., & Thoresen, C. E. (1998). *A meta-analytic review of research on religious involvement and mortality.* Unpublished manuscript.

Miller, W. R., & Bennett, M. E. (1997). Toward better research on spirituality and health: The Templeton Panels. *Spiritual and Religious Issues in Behavior Change, 10,* 3–4. (Official Newsletter of Association for Advancement of Behavior Therapy [AABT], Special Interest Group).

Miller, W. R., & Thoresen, C. E. (in press). Spirituality and health. In W. R. Miller (Ed.), *Integrating spirituality into treatment.* Washington, DC: American Psychological Association.

Moore, T. (1992). *Care of the soul.* NewYork: Harper Collins.

National Institute of Healthcare Research. (1997). *Final report: Scientific progress in spiritual research.* Rockville, MD: Author.

Ornish, D., Brown, S .E., Scherwitz, L. W., Billings, J. H., Armstrong, W. T., & Ports, T. A. (1990). Can coronary artery disease be reversed? *Lancet, 336,* 129–133.

Oxman, T. E., Freeman, D. H., & Manheimer, E. D. (1995). Lack of social participation or religious strength and comfort as risk factors for death after cardiac surgery in the elderly. *Psychosomatic Medicine, 57,* 5–15.

Pargament, K. (1996). Religious methods of coping: Resources for the conservation and transformation of significance. In E. Shafranske (Ed.), *Religion and the clinical practice of psychology* (pp. 102–121). Washington, DC: American Psychological Association.

Peck, M. S. (1978). *The road less traveled.* New York: Bantam.

Polanyi, M. (1958). *Personal knowledge.* Chicago: University of Chicago.

Propst, L. R., Ostrum, R. Watkins, P., Dean, T., & Mashburn, D. (1992). Comparative efficacy of religious and nonreligious cognitive behavioral therapy for the treatment of clinical depression in religious individuals. *Journal of Consulting and Clinical Psychology, 60,* 94–103.

Remen, R. N. (1996). *Kitchen table wisdom: Stories that heal.* Los Angeles: Rinerhead.

Richards, P. S., & Bergin, A. E. (1997). A spiritual strategy for counseling and psychotherapy. Washington, DC: American Psychological Association.

Richards, T. A., & Folkman, S. (in press). Spiritual aspects of loss at the time of a partner's death from AIDS. *Death Studies.*

Roush, W. (1997). Herbert Benson: Mind-body maverick pushes the envelope. *Science, 276,* 357–359.

Schor, J. B. (1991). *The overworked American.* NewYork: Basic.

Schwartz, G. E., & Russek, L. G. (1997). The challenge of one medicine: Theories of health and eight "world hypotheses." *Advances, 13,* 7–23.

Seeman, T. E., Kaplan, G. A. Knudsen, L., Cohen, R., & Guralnik, J. (1987). Social network ties and mortality among the elderly in Alameda County Study. *American Journal of Epidemiology, 126,* 714–723

Seligmann, M. E. P. (1991). *Learned optimism.* NewYork: Knopf.

Smith, H. (1989). *The world's religions.* San Francisco: HarperSanFrancisco.

Spiegel, D., Bloom, J. R., Kraemer, H. C., & Gottheil, E. (1989). Effects of psychosocial treatment on survival of patients with metastatic breast cancer. *Lancet, 14,* 888–891.

Strawbridge, W. J., Cohen, R. D., Shema, S. J., & Kaplan, G.A. (1997). Frequent attendance at religious services and mortality over 28 years. *American Journal of Public Health, 87,* 957–961.

Thomson, K. S. (1996). The revival of experiments on prayer. *American Scientist, 84,* 532–534.

Thoresen, C. E. (1997). *The spiritual side of health.* Unpublished manuscript, Stanford University, Stanford, CA.

Thoresen, C. E., Worthington, E. L., Swyers, J. P., Larson, D. B., McCullough, M. E., & Miller, W. R. (1997). Religious and spiritual interventions. In D. B. Larson, J. P. Swyers, & M. E. McCullough (Eds.), *Scientific research on spirituality and health: A consensus report* (pp. 104–128). Rockville, MD: National Institute for Healthcare Research.

Thoresen, C. E., Luskin, F., & Harris, A. H. S. (in press). Science and forgiveness interventions: Reflections and recommendations. In E. K. Worthington (Ed.), *The foundations of forgiveness.* Radner, PA: Templeton Foundation.

Walsh, R., & Vaughn, F. (1993). *Paths beyond ego: The transpersonal vision.* New York: Putnam.

Worthington, E. L., Kurusu, T. A., McCullough, M. E., & Sandage, S. J. (1996). Empirical research on religion and psychotherapeutic processes and outcomes: A 10-year review and research prospectus. *Psychological Bulletin, 119,* 448–487.

Young, E. (1984). Spiritual health: An essential element in optimum health. *Journal of American College Health, 32,* 273–276.

Zuckerman, D. M., Kasl, S. V., & Ostfeld, A. M. (1984). Psychosocial predictors of mortality among the elderly poor. *American Journal of Epidemiology, 119,* 410–423.

18

Future Directions and Current Debates: Where Do We Go Now That We're Here?

Cheryl Carmin
Sari Roth-Roemer
Sharon E. Robinson Kurpius

As with any other group, psychologists do not view their profession with a single unified vision. Several of the preceding chapters have outlined controversial issues affecting each author's particular medical populations. These concerns are notable for their influence on psychology as a profession and on counseling psychology in particular. Most of all, they lead us to consider how these controversies may be transformed into the new directions our profession will take. Three of the most pressing debates related to counseling health psychology include specialty training, prescription privileges, and managed care.

Specialty Training

There has been considerable discussion within the American Psychological Association (APA) regarding the need for clinical training beyond the doctoral level, with members hotly debating whether the current predoctoral internship requirement should become a postdegree requirement. Regardless of the timing of this internship, students in counseling psychology must first have generalist internship training to provide them with a basic foundation for any specialization training to follow. There is no reason this generalist internship cannot take place at a medical setting. As the debate continues to rage, it should be remembered that one advantage for those who are investigating careers in health care is that the shift of the internship to the postdegree period would put the psychology intern on a similar footing with first-year medical residents.

Moving applied experiences to after the completion of the doctoral degree still does not address what we currently refer to as postdoctoral training or what is perhaps more accurately described as specialty training. One of the questions that arises as a result of this move toward advanced training is whether such specialty skills should be mandated. To clarify the issues involved in this question, an analogy with the medical profession might be helpful. Anyone who has been a hospital patient or whose family member has been hospitalized quickly learns to appreciate the specialized technical skills of the physicians and allied health professionals who are providing treatment. For example, this person would be less than content with a general internist performing cardiac surgery. Similarly, we also would not want a mental health professional who is unfamiliar with the process of congestive heart failure being part of a team assisting the patient and his or her family in disease management, counseling them if invasive procedures are required, and helping them adjust during the posttreatment period. Just like the internist who has completed a fellowship in cardiology in order to provide the requisite high quality of care, mental health professionals are also in need of this kind of expertise. The type of expertise needed can be obtained through specialty training at the postdoctoral level.

Not all postdoctoral positions focus exclusively on clinical training. In many cases, the postdoctoral experience concentrates or at least focuses heavily on research. As is the case in clinical training, postdoctoral fellows need to be attentive to their role on the research team, the team's productivity, and potential for authorship. It is also important to determine how state licensing boards regard clinical versus research fellowships. Many states will not permit research hours to be accumulated for licensure. Likewise, certifying agencies (e.g., National Register of Health Service Providers in Psychology) may not allow such hours to be accrued for their certification.

One final note with regard to postdoctoral training. The predoctoral internship process has become progressively more competitive and this will, no doubt, also be the case for postdoctoral training. As has been stressed in previous chapters, it is essential to secure experiences in medical settings throughout one's training. If all of one's training has been in university counseling centers or settings unrelated to medical centers, students will not effectively compete with clinical and counseling psychology peers who have worked hard to obtain relevant experiences.

Clearly, a strong generalist foundation is necessary but not sufficient when working in a highly specialized area such as health care. For those individuals who are interested in pursuing careers in health-related areas or are interested reshaping their careers with a health focus, specialty training is strongly encouraged.

Prescription Privileges

Another controversial topic is that of prescription privileges. The APA is advocating for the right of psychologists to prescribe psychotropic medications. *The Report of the Ad Hoc Task Force on Psychopharmacology* (APA, 1992) has proposed several stages of training in response to the increased frequency in which psychologists are faced with psychopharmacologic issues today (Lorion, 1996). The three levels of preparation parallel "the degree of involvement with and responsibility for aspects of intervention" desired by psychologists (Lorion, p. 222). These three levels are as follows:

> *Level 1: Basic Psychopharmacology Education:* Competence at Level 1 implies a knowledge of the biological basis of neuropsychopharmacology, including the neurobiology of brain function and the subcellular and cellular mechanisms by which these drugs affect neurotransmitter systems. A second focus of training at this level involves mastery of the psychopharmacology of classes of medications commonly used to treat mental disorders, including both their use in treatment and their abuse. (APA, 1992, p. 57)

> *Level 2: Collaborative Practice:* Level 2 training builds on Level 1 and reflects the necessary knowledge base to participate actively in managing medications prescribed for mental disorders and integrating these medications with psychosocial treatment. . . . Level 2 training includes more in-depth knowledge of the pharmacology of psychoactive medication and drugs of abuse, but it also includes knowledge of psychodiagnosis, physical assessment, physical function tests, drug interactions, and drug side effects. (APA, 1992, p. 58)

Level 3: Prescription Privileges: Level 3 training for psychologists would be similar to training in other professions that have independent prescription privileges limited only by scope of practice and training, e.g., dentists, optometrists, podiatrists, and nurse practitioners. Under these conditions, one can prescribe from a formula that is congruent with the currently accepted scope of practice. The Task Force acknowledges that, in some settings, optimal patient care may require psychologists to have limited prescription privileges. This would allow them to work independently of physicians but would also require a substantial commitment to training, as well as a commitment to developing licensure provisions for this class of practitioner on a state-by-state basis. (APA, 1992, p. 59)

The Task Force proposed that Level 1 training, familiarization of psychologists with frequently prescribed psychopharmacologic medications, be a minimum level of competence for all psychologists providing mental health services. On the other hand, Level 3 training, training for prescription privileges, had no such mandate. The only mandates accompanying Level 3 were educational and licensing requirements. Interestingly, given the settings that most counseling health psychologists work in and the populations they serve, it is likely that many already have the equivalent of Level 1 and possibly even Level 2 knowledge.

The training for psychologists to become prescription providers has already begun with the Department of Defense Psychopharmacology Demonstration Project. Since 1991, the Department of Defense has offered training at the postgraduate level in psychopharmacology to psychologists within the armed forces. They have outlined a comprehensive postgraduate curriculum. Graduates of the program have recommended that any training for psychologists in psychopharmacology be postdoctoral and postlicensure. They further state that "an adequate grounding [and training] in psychodiagnostics and techniques of psychotherapy" are essential before adding psychopharmacology as an additional clinical tool (Sammons, Sexton, & Meredith, 1996, p. 233).

Supporters of prescription privileges assert that it is the natural evolution of our profession to move forward into being responsible for the complete mental health care of our patients (DeLeon & Wiggins, 1996; DeLeon et al., 1996; Sammons & Olmedo, 1997). Furthermore, supporters of prescription privileges argue that since close to 20 percent of all prescribed medications are for psychotropic drugs, psychologists must be trained to recognize the effects of these drugs and their influence on psychological treatment

(Lorion, 1996). Recognizing the importance of this, six states (California, Hawaii, Louisiana, Florida, Tennessee, and Missouri) are already working on legislation related to prescribing privileges for psychologists (Sammons & Olmedo, 1997).

Other arguments in favor of our prescribing involve the usefulness of our diagnostic and assessment skills in preventing the overmedication of individuals who could best benefit from some other form of intervention. With the privilege of prescribing comes the privilege of not prescribing, as well as "unprescribing" (Sammons, 1994). The example of children with attention deficit disorder is often cited in this context; 15 percent of children are diagnosed with ADD and treated with Ritalin compared with the 2–3 percent prevalence figures cited in the *Diagnostic and Statistical Manual of Mental Disorders (fourth edition) (DSM-IV)* (DeLeon, Sammons, & Sexton, 1995).

Despite the APA's advocating for prescription privileges for psychologists, this issue does not have unanimous support. Hayes and Heiby (1996) suggest that the practice community's argument favoring prescription privileges is driven largely by professional pressures, intellectual changes, and market forces. That is, there may be expanded practice opportunities and economic incentives for psychologists since managed care organizations may be more interested in hiring psychologists who are able to prescribe. In support of this argument, Evans (1991) claimed that the issue of prescribing was "introduced solely as a desire to help the professional psychologist gain wealth, prestige, personal power, etc., rather than a desire to help patients" (p. 4). Of course, one must consider that along with increased salaries could come increased malpractice insurance premiums as this is a new skill area for psychology (DeNelsky, 1996). DeLeon, Bennett, and Bricklin (1997) caution psychologists not to use their position of "societal trust" (p. 519) to unfairly advance the profession by attempting to obtain prescription privileges.

DeLeon and colleagues (1996) countered the antiprescription privilege argument with what is, perhaps, the most simplistic argument—that being able to prescribe will "medicalize" psychology. Whether this is the case is difficult to ascertain. Hayes and Heiby (1996) noted that few psychologists have a background in basic science (e.g., courses in biology and organic chemistry). No doubt, these courses can be successfully completed but significantly more hours of didactic instruction accompanied by supervised clinical training would be necessary for Levels 2 and 3 of certification as noted above. This would either add considerable time to one's doctoral program or require additional postdoctoral training and continuing education hours. Currently there is a discrepancy between existing training models and the training that would be necessary to prepare psychologists for prescribing (Riley, Elliott, & Thomas, 1992). In order to obtain the appropriate course-work, more time would need to be spent on physiology, biochemistry, and other such courses, rather than on areas such as learning theory, which could necessitate that graduate programs in psychology move to medical settings, thereby losing their grounding in arts and science (Hayes & Heiby, 1996). Given these requirements, DeNelsky (1996) worries that "psychologists who prescribe will be spending more time studying medicine and less time learning psychology" (p. 209).

While it may not so much be "medicalizing" psychology, those against prescription privileges argue that it is unclear what will differentiate psychologists from psychiatrists should prescription privileges become a reality (DeLeon et al., 1995). Further, given turf issues, prescription privileges have a strong potential for increasing adversarial relationships between psychology and psychiatry.

It should also be noted that there is as yet no vehicle for policing the standards for or the quality of programs that purport to offer training for prescription privileges. There have been mass mailings to licensed professionals and advertisements in the APA *Monitor* for weekend seminars for such privileges even though psychologists are not yet credentialed in this domain.

In addition, the subtleties of working with patients with multiple medical problems, as is the case in counseling health psychology, raises the level of complexity required to prescribe psychotropic medications. When working in medical settings it is rare to see a patient with a straightforward presentation of anxiety or depression. Rather, the patients being treated often have a long list of medical problems and an equally lengthy list of medications prescribed for these disorders. The chances of a medication interaction and the complications of polypharmacy are serious, if not life-threatening. Psychotropic medications have complexities and physiologic side effects (e.g., interactions with heart and liver function) that may compromise a patient's current medical problems.

Clearly there exists a diversity of opinions regarding prescription privileges for psychologists. There are many compelling reasons both for and against psychologists becoming licensed to prescribe psychotropic medication. Perhaps only time will lead to resolution of this debate.

Managed Care

The impact of managed care has reverberated throughout the health care profession. Its effect on psychology has been felt in several areas. As alluded to above, a number of internship sites have closed their doors or eliminated positions due to the fact that unlicensed professionals are not reimbursed by certain third-party payors, such as Medicare or managed care entities in the form of health maintenance organizations (HMOs) and preferred provider organizations (PPOs). Psychology, however, should not feel singled out in this regard; the effect on medical residency training has been similar.

Managed care has also affected the private practitioner. As insurers take greater control of the health care dollar, they are severely limiting the number of outpatient visits. In some cases, this limit is not only per year but also per diagnosis. Thus, if you have been treating someone for depression over the past year within the allowed number of sessions, no new sessions may be authorized for the treatment of that depression during the next benefit period. Further, some managed care groups do not include private practitioners on their provider panels.

The way in which one delivers services has also been touched by managed care. Most groups ask for treatment plans whose outcomes are defined in objective, behavioral terms. Similarly, they tend to authorize treatments that are empirically validated. Thus, the question "What works for whom?" has become a prevailing theme in how treatment is provided or at least which treatments are supported by managed care reimbursement. The treatments that tend to have the greatest empirical support are cognitive-behavioral. Given the focus of cognitive-behavioral therapy on brief, problem-centered interventions and skills training, it is very compatible with the services offered in medical settings. In contrast, interventions focusing on underlying dynamic issues tend to be lengthier and are, therefore, less likely to be covered by a managed care organization.

Ethical dilemmas are also raised in the context of managed care coverage. As stated previously, length of treatment is now often dictated by the insurance company rather than by patient needs. Unfortunately, the responsibility for this inadequacy of treatment length is now falling back onto the practitioner. Legal cases are now beginning to emerge in which the psychologist is being held liable for not fighting with the insurance company to increase length of coverage. In 1986, the court ruled in *Wickline v. State* that a clinician has a responsibility on the patient's behalf to contest an adverse decision by a health maintenance organization regarding treatment. Even though psychologists may have petitioned an insurance company to extend care, if the psychologist did not re-petition upon first denial, he or she has been found negligent. This ruling was challenged in *Wilson v. Blue Cross of Southern California,* 1990, in which the court held that the patient's family had a right to bring a malpractice suit against Blue Cross of Southern California for its denial of needed mental health services which resulted in the suicide of the patient (Appelbaum, 1993).

Another area where managed care has had an impact on health psychology is length of hospital stay. As noted in chapter 4, Working in Medical Settings, the timely response to a consultation request is imperative. If there is a delay, the patient may be discharged from the hospital. All areas of service delivery have been affected by cost-saving measures resulting from reduced lengths of stay. A hospital's contract with a managed care entity may be contingent on its length of stay statistics. The more a hospital stays within the parameters of these statistics, the more likely its contract will be renewed. The renewal of these contracts translates into jobs. A no-win vicious cycle has been created.

An issue that often complicates the mental health provider's role is when the insurer relegates approval of different treatments to different arms of its organization. For example, with some insurers it can be unclear who is responsible for authorizing treatments for a problem such as chronic pain. Is this the domain of the medical arm of managed care or the mental health arm? Is biofeedback a medical treatment (and some companies will only reimburse if a physician administers biofeedback) or a psychological treatment? Unfortunately, these questions are not always considered by the insurer, which leaves the patient squarely in the middle without an answer. Even more frustrating is that coverage varies from company to company and even within a managed care group. Each situation may be handled idiosyncratically.

In light of these problems, we are left to find innovative answers to the dilemmas created by the managed care climate. One answer is capitation. Fundamentally, this means that there is a fixed pool of dollars that an insurer pays out to the provider organization per person per month. The mental health professional is not reimbursed per patient per visit. The dollar incentive is no longer attached to keeping the patient in treatment as long as possible but is attached to keeping the patient healthy. The goal is to keep people well by providing prevention and health promotion or, should disability occur, to treat the problem as efficiently as possible.

Many medical centers are attempting to negotiate directly with insurance companies in order to reclaim the ground they have lost to the middle man of managed care. The advantage of holding a capitated contract is that the expense of having an outside agency authorize and review treatment plans is eliminated, resulting in an immediate cost savings. It also means that the medical center must have an efficient method for assessing quality of care and compliance with the capitated contract. In other words, the enemy becomes us. One's colleagues are responsible for chart review and assuring all parties involved that standards are being met. There may be a team composed of staff members who authorize treatment. As a result, you are not angry at some unknown person who has denied further sessions—it could be your colleague in the office down the hall who has just turned you down.

Within the context of capitation, a growing trend is the integrated delivery network (IDN). Shortell, Gilles, and Anderson (1994) defined this system as "a network of organizations that provides or arranges to provide a coordinated continuum of services to a defined population and is willing to be held clinically and fiscally responsible for the outcomes and the health status of the population served" (p. 47). Included within such networks are primary care and specialty medical service providers, ambulatory care centers, home health care agencies, medical centers, etc. While in the recent past these networks were allied with insurance carriers or HMOs, the movement is now for provider service groups (e.g., hospital systems, physician groups, and home health care agencies) to form such alliances (Newman & Reed, 1996). These authors further note that "the best way to control health care value, that is, cost and service, is to control all of the organization, financing, and delivery of health care as closely as possible, in ways that are responsive to regional demographics and economics. Only integrated delivery systems can offer a seamless, coordinated continuum of health care" (p. 15).

It would seem that we are moving toward an era where the economics of health service delivery are an overriding concern. Since psychological services may be viewed as a luxury item by some, how do we justify our place in this streamlined network? What we must not forget and what we must stress to policymakers is that the provision of mental health services is not a luxury; it results in health care cost reduction and improved quality of life (Cummings, 1996; Cummings & Follette, 1968; Pallak, Cummings, Dorken, & Henke, 1995).

Where Do We Go from Here?

Over recent years, some leaders in our profession have suggested that the death knell of psychology can be heard ringing in the distance. Certainly there has been support for this observation given the reduction in internship positions and the impact of managed care on service delivery. This, however, is the view of the nay-sayers and those individuals who view managed care, or any change, as a threat.

For those of us who take a different view of the future, particularly with regard to health psychology, the future seems considerably rosier. There are several reasons for optimism.

First, we need to expand our self-view. Those who aspire to or who are already working in the health care arena need not view mental health service delivery as our defining characteristic. Instead, we need to view ourselves as health (not simply mental health) care providers and *partners* in the treatment team (Cummings, 1996; DeLeon et al., 1996, Newman & Reed, 1996). We need to remember that the treatments we provide are effective at assisting in the prevention and management of disease and disability. We also need to take a more active role in self-promotion, educating our medical colleagues as well as policymakers as to our value.

In addition, we need to rethink how we are delivering services. While figures vary, one study noted that 60 percent of physician visits were for physical problems resulting from emotional distress (Pallak et al., 1995). Since the majority of such patients are never seen in a mental health professional's office (e.g., Klerman, Weissman, Ouellette, Johnson, & Greenwald, 1991; Pollard, Henderson, Frank, & Margolis, 1989), it would seem incumbent upon counseling health psychologists to go to the patient. The nature of integrated delivery networks is such that providing services within the context of the medical office visit is supported, which further facilitates the collaboration of physicians and mental health practitioners in preventing, diagnosing, and treating problems in an integrated fashion. Disappointingly, only a handful of psychologists have opted to define their role within a multidisciplinary practice.

It will also be important for counseling health psychologists to go beyond some of the territorial issues within psychology. For example, a recent political battle was fought over the clinical service delivery guidelines approved by the APA. Counseling psychologists, understandably, were taken aback by health psychology guidelines being titled "clinical health psychology." The distinctions between counseling and clinical are important only within the profession, not outside of it. Our medical colleagues are more concerned about whether a psychologist can do the job; they have little appreciation for the distinctions between the disciplines. While psychologists preoccupy themselves with such issues, the door is left open for others to take advantages of the schisms created. At the recent meeting of the APA, the President of the Association of Medical School Psychologists observed that if nurses ever could agree on anything, they would be a formidable lobbying force. He noted that the same could be said of psychologists (Wedding, 1997).

Conclusions

In the face of current debates within and surrounding our profession, it appears our task is to learn to appreciate and make good use of our diversity of skills. Hopefully, counseling psychology's emphasis on empirically derived practice will guide us not only in resolving the dilemmas currently before us but will also be our foundation for looking toward the future and finding creative solutions to the changing health care environment. The health care arena needs counseling psychologists and other mental health professionals to become active members of treatment and research teams in order to meet the complex and multidimensional needs of patients. Many of our colleagues have paved the way for our expanded roles in the health care setting. We hope the readers of this book accept the challenges of working within this environmental context and as a result experience the rich and fulfilling rewards possible.

Suggested Resources

There are several excellent sources that address the areas of current debate for counseling psychologists. With respect to prescription privileges, two journals have recently devoted special issues to the topic. In *American Psychologist* (1996, Vol. 51), authors for both sides of the debate make articulate arguments for their position. In addition, *Professional Psychology: Research and Practice* (1997) also published an entire volume (Vol. 28) devoted to the issue of prescription privileges for psychologists. The articles in this edition present the most current debate on the prescription privileges.

The two best resources on the issue of managed care are "The New World of Managed Care: Creating Organized Delivery Systems" (Shortell et al., 1994) and "The New Structure of Health Care and a Role for Psychology" (Cummings, 1996). Each of these articles presents the major issues and dilemmas important for psychologists practicing under the auspices of managed care.

Finally, in order to understand more fully the evolving role of psychologists in our society, the reader is referred to "Expanding Roles in the Twenty-First Century" (DeLeon et al., 1996).

Discussion Questions

1. What are the pros and cons of specialty training at the postdoctoral level?
2. What are the arguments for and against prescription privileges for psychologists?
3. How is managed care influencing the practice of psychology?

References

Applebaum, P. S. (1993). Legal liability and managed care. *American Psychologist, 48,* 251–257.

American Psychological Association. (1992). *Report of the Ad Hoc Task Force on Psychopharmacology.* Washington, DC: Author.

Cummings, N. A. (1996). The new structure of health care and a role for psychology. In R. J. Resnick, & R. H. Rozensky (Eds.), *Health psychology through the life span: Practice and research opportunities* (pp. 27–38). Washington, DC: American Psychological Association.

Cummings, N. A., & Follette, W. T. (1968). Psychiatric services and medical utilization in a prepaid health setting: Part II. *Medical Care, 6,* 31–41.

DeLeon, P. H., Bennett, B. E., & Bricklin, P. M (1997). Ethics and public policy formulation: A case example related to prescription privileges. *Professional Psychology: Research and Practice, 28,* 518–525.

DeLeon, P. H., Howell, W. C., Newman, R., Brown, A. B., Keita, G. P., & Sexton, J. L. (1996). Expanding roles in the twenty-first century. In R. J. Resnick, & R. H. Rozensky (Eds.), *Health psychology through the life span: Practice and research opportunities* (pp. 427–454). Washington, DC: American Psychological Association.

DeLeon, P. H., Sammons, M. T., & Sexton, J. L. (1995). Focusing on society's real needs: Responsibility and prescription privileges? *American Psychologist, 50,* 1022–1032.

DeLeon, P. H., & Wiggins, J. G., Jr. (1996). Prescription privileges for psychologists. *American Psychologist, 51,* 225–229.

DeNelsky, G. Y. (1996). The case against prescription privileges for psychologists. *American Psychologist, 51,* 207–212.

Evans, I. M. (1991, November). *Values in behavior therapy: Implications for training clinical studens from the "me" generation.* Paper presented at the meeting of the Association for the Advancement of Behavior Therapy, New York.

Hayes, S. C., & Heiby, E. (1996). Psychology's drug Problem: Do we need a fix or should we just say no? *American Psychologist, 51,* 198–206.

Klerman, G. L., Weissman, M. M., Ouellette, R., Johnson, J., & Greenwald, S. (1991). Panic attacks in the community: Social morbidity and health care utilization. *Journal of the American Medical Association, 265,* 742–746.

Lorian, R. P. (1996). Applying our medicine to the psychopharmacology debate. *American Psychologist, 51,* 219–224.

Newman, R., & Reed, G. M. (1996). Psychology as a health care profession: Its evolution and future directions. In R. J. Resnick, & R. H. Rozensky (Eds.), *Health psychology through the life span: Practice and research opportunities* (pp. 11–26). Washington, DC: American Psychological Association.

Pallak, M. S., Cummings, N. A., Dorken, H., & Henke, C. J. (1995). Effect of mental health treatment on medical costs. *Mind/Body Medicine, 1,* 7–12.

Pollard, C. A., Henderson, J. G., Frank, M., & Margolis, R. B. (1989). Help-seeking patterns of anxiety disordered individuals in the general population. *Journal of Anxiety Disorders, 3,* 131–138.

Riley, W. T., Elliott, R. L., & Thomas, J. R. (1992). Impact of prescription privileging on psychology training. *The Clinical Psychologist, 45,* 63–70.

Sammons, M. T. (1994). Prescription privileges and psychology: A reply to Adanis and Bieliauskas. *Journal of Clinical Psychology in Medical Settings, 1,* 199–207.

Sammons, M. T., & Olmedo, E. (1997). The prescription privileges agenda in 1997: Forward progress, future goals. *Professional Psychology: Research and Practice, 28,* 507–508

Sammons, M. T., Sexton, J. L., & Meredith, J. M. (1996). Basic science training psychopharmacology: How much is enough. *American Psychologist, 51,* 230–234.

Shortell, S. M., Gilles, R. R., & Anderson, D. A. (1994). The new world of managed care: Creating organized delivery systems. *Health Affairs, 13,* 46–64.

Wedding, D. (1997, August). *The evolving role of counseling psychology in medical settings.* Presentation at the 105th annual meeting of the American Psychological Association, Chicago.

Name Index

445

447

Subject Index

abuse, sexual:
eating disorders and, 270–71
Acceptance of Disability Scale, 213
accountability, 19, 20
Accreditation Council for Graduate Medical Education, 398
acculturation, 90, 359–360, 366, 368–370
acquired immune deficiency syndrome, *see* AIDS
adherence, treatment:
in children/adolescents, 292–94, 298
see also compliance
adjustment (issues):
to cancer and AIDS, model for, 169–178 (figure)
disorders, 169, 198
interventions promoting, 180–83
medical context and, 173–74
in older adults, 312
psychological context and, 175
see also coping
ADL assessment, 317, 326
adolescents, illness and, 286, 292, 298
see also children
adults, older:
African American, biases against, 374–75
ageism, 325
assessment of, 315–19, 325, 326
complex interaction of factors in, 309–310, 314–15, 324
controversies in treating, 324–25
diagnostic/assessment considerations, 315–19, 325, 326
discussion questions, 327
heterogeneity of, 311–12
interventions with, 320–24
mental health problems in, 312–13
normal aging vs. disease, 313–14, 315, 318–19, 326
overview of salient concerns regarding, 309–311
psychological/medical comorbidity in, 314–15
resources, suggested, 326–27
risk factors for, 311, 313, 314
special concerns with, 321–23
spiritual/religious factors and, 417–18
see also assessment, geriatric
African American population:
healing system in, 376

health status of, 372–75
values of, 375–76
Agency for Health Care Policy and Research, 26
aging, *see* adults, older
AIDS:
adjusting to, model for, 169–178 (figure)
coping, domains determining, 166–69
coping, following diagnosis, 163–64
coping, reactions to treatment, 164–66, 169-178 (figure)
discussion questions, 184–85
duty to warn/protect, 68
medical management of, 159
in minority populations, 368, 373
overview of, 158–59
pediatric, 305
"positive illusions," 164, 167, 168, 183
psychosocial treatments for, 178–183
resources, suggested, 184
see also pain
alcoholism:
Alcoholics Anonymous (AA), 382, 417
in Native Americans, 381, 382
spiritual/religious factors and, 417, 418
Alzheimer's disease, 313, 322, 346
American Board of Clinical Neuropsychology (ABCN), 21, 248
American Board of Professional Psychology (ABPP), 21, 45, 48, 248
American Cancer Society (ACS), 2, 337, 338
American College of Psychology, 46, 48
American Heart Association, 2, 95, 96, 99, 102, 123, 127, 152
American Medical Association (AMA) Council on Ethical and Judicial Affairs, 331
American Psychiatric Association, 79, 235, 254, 255, 256, 258, 259, 260, 271, 398
American Psychological Association (APA), 8, 10, 11, 12, 21, 22, 25, 26, 31, 32, 35, 38, 40, 41, 44, 46, 48, 56, 66, 68, 69, 71, 79, 98, 198, 199, 235, 311, 313, 314, 318, 326, 432, 434, 435, 436, 437, 441, 442
Board of Professional Affairs, 66
Committee on Aging, 327
Committee on Women's Health, 351
Council of Representatives, 48

453